RESIDUE REVIEWS

VOLUME 46

RESIDUE REVIEWS

Residues of Pesticides and Other
Contaminants in the Total Environment

Editor
FRANCIS A. GUNTHER

Assistant Editor
JANE DAVIES GUNTHER

Riverside, California

VOLUME 46

Springer Science+Business Media, LLC
1973

Originally published by Springer-Verlag New York Inc. in 1973.
Softcover reprint of the hardcover 1st edition 1973

Library of Congress Catalog Card Number 62-18595.

New York: 175 Fifth Avenue, New York, N. Y. 10010
Heidelberg: 6900 Heidelberg 1, Postfach 1780, West Germany

ISBN 978-3-662-39250-8 ISBN 978-3-662-40267-2 (eBook)
DOI 10.1007/978-3-662-40267-2

Preface

That residues of pesticide and other contaminants in the total environment are of concern to everyone everywhere is attested by the reception accorded previous volumes of "Residue Reviews" and by the gratifying enthusiasm, sincerity, and efforts shown by all the individuals from whom manuscripts have been solicited. Despite much propaganda to the contrary, there can never be any serious question that pest-control chemicals and food-additive chemicals are essential to adequate food production, manufacture, marketing, and storage, yet without continuing surveillance and intelligent control some of those that persist in our foodstuffs could at times conceivably endanger the public health. Ensuring safety-in-use of these many chemicals is a dynamic challenge, for established ones are continually being displaced by newly developed ones more acceptable to food technologists, pharmacologists, toxicologists, and changing pest-control requirements in progressive food-producing economies.

These matters are of genuine concern to increasing numbers of governmental agencies and legislative bodies around the world, for some of these chemicals have resulted in a few mishaps from improper use. Adequate safety-in-use evaluations of any of these chemicals persisting into our foodstuffs are not simple matters, and they incorporate the considered judgments of many individuals highly trained in a variety of complex biological, chemical, food technological, medical, pharmacological, and toxicological disciplines.

It is hoped that "Residue Reviews" will continue to serve as an integrating factor both in focusing attention upon those many residue matters requiring further attention and in collating for variously trained readers present knowledge in specific important areas of residue and related endeavors involved with other chemical contaminants in the total environment. The contents of this and previous volumes of "Residue Reviews" illustrate these objectives. Since manuscripts are published in the order in which they are received in final form, it may seem that some important aspects of residue analytical chemistry, biochemistry, human and animal medicine, legislation, pharmacology, physiology, regulation, and toxicology are being neglected; to the contrary, these apparent omissions are recognized, and some pertinent manuscripts are in preparation. However, the field is so large and the interests in it are so varied that the editors and the Advisory Board earnestly solicit suggestions of topics and authors to help make this international book-series even more useful and informative.

"Residue Reviews" attempts to provide concise, critical reviews of timely advances, philosophy, and significant areas of accomplished or needed endeavor in the total field of residues of these and other foreign chemicals in any segment of the environment. These reviews are either general or specific, but properly they may lie in the domains of analytical chemistry and its methodology, biochemistry, human and animal medicine, legislation, pharmacology, physiology, regulation, and toxicology; certain affairs in the realm of food technology concerned specifically with pesticide and other food-additive problems are also appropriate subject matter. The justification for the preparation of any review for this book-series is that it deals with some aspect of the many real problems arising from the presence of any "foreign" chemicals in our surroundings. Thus, manuscripts may encompass those matters, in any country, which are involved in allowing pesticide and other plant-protecting chemicals to be used safely in producing, storing, and shipping crops. Added plant or animal pest-control chemicals or their metabolites that may persist into meat and other edible animal products (milk and milk products, eggs, etc.) are also residues and are within this scope. The so-called food additives (substances deliberately added to foods for flavor, odor, appearance, etc., as well as those inadvertently added during manufacture, packaging, distribution, storage, etc.) are also considered suitable review material. In addition, contaminant chemicals added in any manner to air, water, soil, or plant or animal life are within this purview and these objectives.

Manuscripts are normally contributed by invitation and should be in English; French or German manuscripts will be considered under exceptional circumstances. Preliminary communication with the editors is necessary before volunteered reviews are submitted in manuscript form.

Department of Entomology
University of California
Riverside, California 92502
January 24, 1973

F.A.G.
J.D.G.

Foreword

The following remarks include, in the general part, considerations of problems which arise from the application of organophosphate esters on edible domestic animals. The special part was thought to be a casuistic collection in order to underset the problems with quantitative data. Since residue numbers of certain residue quantities alone are usually not satisfactory, additional selected data of toxicity and metabolic and excretion processes were included in the text. This was done to round off the picture. It was possible that we did not succeed in surveying and registering all the reports of the world literature, a claim which the authors did not want to intimate; however, they hope to contribute with this survey to the conveyance of knowledge and they have tried to impart an easy understanding, also, for the non-specialist professional worker by including formulas, information of use, etc. This was done at the risk of repeating, inevitably, some facts which had already been dealt with in *Residue Reviews.* * The attempt of the authors to compare generally the different literature reports of some authors in a critical form—for instance in tables—was very quickly given up with the exception of, for example, Coumaphos, since time, dosages, mode of application, and other factors varied too much. The reports of data from the literature were possible only in the continuous text. Here, we tried to follow a certain order, for instance, of the animals: mouse, rat, sheep, cattle, etc.; or to consider the means of application for the respective kinds of animals. The metabolism and residue data from smaller test animals serve the purpose of comparison only.

We are grateful to numerous firms for submitting literature or reports of unpublished data.

The following remains to be said for understanding the next:

1. The designation ® for trade-mark was omitted; however, this does not mean that there is not adequate legal protection.
2. The reports of alternate names do not claim to be complete; they are only a reference to the numerous synonyms in the literature—which generally complicate the survey—as well as in trade and, here again, names differ according to application taking place either in plant protection or in veterinary medicine.

---

* Editor's note: See especially vol. 36 "Chemistry of pesticides."

3. The discussions of specific organophosphate esters follow the alphabet.
4. The denotations are based on the German spelling.
5. Denotations which do not exist in the German language are cited in the original language.
6. Special abbreviations:

a.i.	=	active ingredient
ADI	=	acceptable daily intake
ChE	=	cholinesterase
EC	=	emulsive concentrate
glc	=	gas liguid chromatography
i.m.	=	intramuscular
i.p.	=	intraperitoneal
i.v.	=	intravenous
μg.	=	microgram
ng.	=	nanogram
p.p.m.	=	parts per million
s.c.	=	subcutaneous
TLC	=	thin-layer chromatography
WP	=	wettable powder

Institute for Pharmacology,
Toxicology, and Pharmacy
of the Tierärztliche Hochschule
Hanover, West Germany

K. Kaemmerer
S. Buntenkötter

Table of Contents

The problem of residues in meat of edible domestic animals after application or intake of organophosphate esters

By

K. KAEMMERER * and S. BUNTENKÖTTER *

Contents

---

* Institute for Pharmacology, Toxicology, and Pharmacy of the Tierärztliche Hochschule, Hannover, W. Germany. Translated from German by Annemarie Westlake; translation edited by authors.

I. Introduction and review of residue problems

a) General considerations[1]

Economic agricultural production requires the use of insecticides. The organophosphate esters have their established position within the available

[1] For comparison of conditions in Germany see also general remarks by BRAUN and KLIMMER (1966).

insecticides. Moreover, in practical veterinary medicine, the organophosphate esters found a more manifold field of application than the organochlorine compounds. The organophosphate esters also gained ground in hygiene for the protection of human health, largely because of the occurrence of insecticide resistance towards organochlorine compounds (ANONYMOUS 33).

Aside from the immediate hazards which threaten the user of such substances, the question of residues in meat of edible domestic animals and, through this, the health of the consumer deserves special attention. The magnitude of hazard is often characterized by the acute toxic symptoms in animals which primarily come into contact with these substances. In the majority of cases, a degradation of effective substance in the animal organism can be expected. In a way, the animal acts as a substance filter before the consumer (TIEWS 1966 and 1967, KAEMMERER 1967). Only in a few cases will it lead to poisoning.

The eating habits of the individual nations are remarkably different and, aside from climatic conditions and ritual regulations, they are also largely dependent on social standards. It is therefore difficult to estimate the risk which arises from intake of different quantities of pesticides residues.

b) Problems of pesticides and metabolites

The following factors should be emphasized for the judgment of meat from edible domestic animals: (1) the intact effective substance, (2) the non-poisonous or poisonous metabolites, (3) the total quantity of effective substance and metabolites remaining in the meat, and (4) the life-time of the residues.

Until now little attention has been given to the fact that not only a single effective substance may be present, but a pesticide and/or its metabolites may occur in the presence of other substances in meat (also compare DURHAM 1967). The animal may have been treated simultaneously with any kind of chemical from medication to food additive. A person takes in such residues or residue mixtures not only with the meat, but he himself may have a substance reservoir that also stretches from medication to food additive. According to YEARY (1966), approximately 225 food additives, 50 to 100 substances which have been given to the animal *per os* or by injection, and approximately 1,500 preservatives, emulsifiers, etc. reach a person, aside from the natural food ingredients and those which are added to the soil and thus appear through vegetables in the food.

Only a little is known about the effects of the individual substances and metabolites. There is also little knowledge about the interaction of substances which may accidentally come together. For therapeutic dosages and those which obviously reach the limit of compatibility, it can be proved in acute cases that occasionally an involution of incompatibility will result (KAEMMERER 1963). It was also reported about involution of effects, although the dosages of the experiments involved range much higher than the determined residue quantities (DU BOIS 1958; PALMER and RADELEFF 1963; GAINES 1962; FRAWLEY *et al.* 1952, 1957 a and b; MOELLER and RIDER 1967). However, antagonistic effects have also been observed, for instance between several organophosphate esters and organochlorine insecticides (e. g., KIMMERLE and LORKE 1968, TOMOV *et al.* 1966, FRAWLEY 1965).

c) General criteria for judgment

The difficulty in judging the possible danger quota lies in the uncertain factors under practical conditions. In an acute case of poisoning, specific symptoms of poisoning are observed in connection with the intake by the treated animal, and establishing the connection of cause is easily possible. For edible domestic animals, the following are almost never known: (1) whether and when the animals were treated or might have taken in effective substances, (2) which quantity of a substance and in what formulation it was consumed, and (3) which effective substance was incorporated.

A routine testing of slaughtered animals within the frame of meat control has not been common until now and a search for suspected residues even impossible. There are no specific tissue changes, after intake of organophosphate esters, which could macroscopically be detected; and the least changes would be expected when the intake of effective substance takes place in non-sickening quantities. Although a veterinarian carries a high responsibility in his profession, as well as in the frame of meat and foodstuff control (DURBIN 1963), it cannot be ignored — despite multifarious scientific knowledge about individual compounds — that the "ad hoc" diagnosis of residues (of their presence) of any kind has not been possible until now.

d) About the intake of effective substances by animals

The intake of substances, especially of organophosphate esters, follows from their relatively wide fields of application. If intention or mistake are excluded in this respect, there are:

1. Primary contacts:
   (a) Through cutaneous intake after application as insecticide against ectoparasites.
   (b) Through medical application in the form of injections or *per os,* eventually effective as systemic insecticide; or as a means of nematode control in the organs, and through continuous feeding for "disinfection" against insect larvae in feces.

2. Secondary contacts:
   Through intake of fresh fodder-plants and parts of vegetable food which have been treated with insecticides within the program of plant and storage protection, and that with the intact effective substance or in form of its metabolites. However, sometimes no problems are seen despite high toxicity of the organophosphate esters, since these substances are easily decomposed and are not stored in the body. The special mode of application in veterinary medicine shall be developed more exactly

in the following text, because considerable consequences for a judgment result in dependence from the intake modality, the location of application, and from the high dosages.

(a) Externally against ectoparasites and bot-flies (e. g., ROGOFF *et al.* 1960) as powder; as dust (FIEDLER 1965); as spray, wash, with "jetten" (FLUCKE 1968, ENDREJAT 1967, BEHRENZ 1962), and with back rubber, back oiler, and dust bags (e. g., RAUN and FRENCH 1961, ALLEN 1966); as dip (jump dip, spray dip) (FIEDLER 1958, ENDREJAT 1967); as pour-on (ROGOFF and KOHLER 1960, ROGOFF 1962); and as spot-on formulation.

(b) Internally with probe or as drench (HEBDEN and HALL 1965), as bolus (KNAPP 1960), as tablet (BOLLE and OTTE 1958), and as feed additive for endoparasite and fly larvae control (KNAPP 1965, DRUMMOND and MOORE 1960).

(c) Parenteral application [e. g., at times in Australia with trichlorfon against endoparasites (KEITH 1964, NEEL 1958, LYONS *et al.* 1967, RIECK and KEITH 1958)].

Not only chemical structure and absolute quantity of effective substance, but also number and frequency of applications and intervals between the treatments (HARRIS 1956) as well as the various ways of resorption are of importance for the absolute quantities of substances and their metabolites in the tissues. For external application, a high persistence with considerable adherence capability of the effective substance on skin and hair (e. g., diazinon, lujet, and others) in a suitable formulation may be economically useful for achieving a long residual effect towards ectoparasites (e. g., blowflies). With regard to residues in the meat, this would mean investigation of the question of possible continuous resorption and it would have to be clarified from case to case.

Also, the kind of vehicle for the effective substance may have an important influence on the resorption rate. Emulsifiers, solvents, solvent mediators, or carriers which are used in the formulations cause a higher absorption rate and also a higher toxicity (CESARO *et al.* 1965), of which DMSO (cf. WHETSTONE *et al.* 1966, VILLENEUVE *et al.* 1969) became specially known because of its unbelievably high penetration ability. Furthermore, those formulations deserve attention which prolong effectiveness and which might form "resins" through polymerization processes from utilization of gelatin, glycerin, formalin, and urea (MEDLEY and DRUMMOND 1962).

e) General problems of intake by human beings

MAIER-BODE (1968) shows a scheme of basic pathways of pesticides in the food chain; however, he emphasizes that organophosphate esters can be expected in the beginning of the food chain only (see Fig. 1).

MILLS (1963) found residues of eight different organophosphate pesticides in the total food of a representative diet; these pesticides belong predominantly to the phosphate or thiophosphate type and included demeton,

Trithion, malathion, and parathion. Many authors point out the possibility, although in a very generalized form, of endangering people by intake of organophospate esters, especially in meat (e. g., MAJAT 1964, GREGOIRE *et al.* 1959, DECKER 1959). Without doubt the fact that a human being is not only a meat consumer but also that he consumes only limited quantities reduces the risk factor. Furthermore, it should be kept in mind that the individual person does not take his daily meat from the same animal type or from the same origin. The danger of possible accumulation in the individual case is thus reduced.

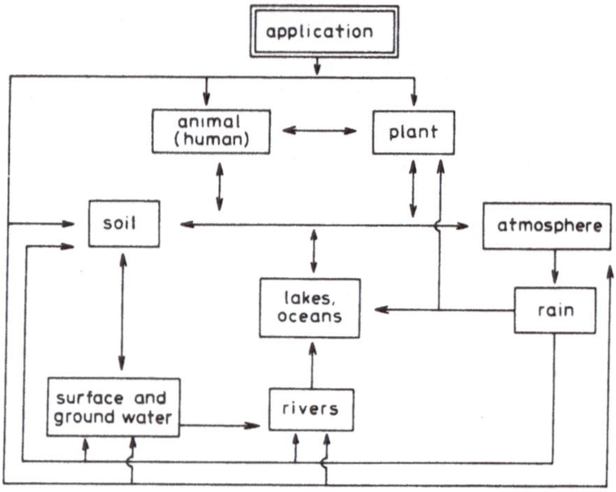

Fig. 1. Basic pathways of pesticides in the food chain (MAIER-BODE 1968).

In the United States the meat consumption per person is estimated to be one-half pound daily (ANONYMOUS 4). The consumption of meat derived from "high consumption" values in the United States is shown in Table I.

Table I. *Summary of daily meat consumption in the United States according to FAO* (ANONYMOUS 20).

Type of meat	High consumption (g./person/day)
Meat and poultry total	500
Meat, total	400
Beef	250
Veal	50
Pork	150
Lamb, mutton	50
Variety meats and game	50
Poultry, total	120
Chicken	110

In the German Federal Republic the yearly meat consumption per person was 68.2 kg. in 1967; this is 0.187 kg./day. This is about 25 percent lower than in the United States (Table II). These key numbers are important as a guideline for the evaluation of the so-called tolerance formula, since the absolute consumption numbers are generally lower for meat than for vegetables, of which the basic value is assumed to be 400 g.

Table II. *Summary of meat production and meat consumption in 1967 in the German Federal Republic* (ANONYMOUS 3).

Type of meat	Production (1,000 tons)	Import (1,000 tons)	Annual consumption (kg./person)
Beef	1,044	135	19.7
Veal	97	24	2.0
Pork	1,932	114	34.2
Poultry	204	210	6.9
Inner organs and other meat	277	49	5.4
Total	3,554	532	68.2

Furthermore, a critical survey of possible residues in meat also requires information about quantities with regard to each type of animal, since the intake of phosphate insecticides is strongly dependent on the feed intake (kind) and the different veterinary indication fields. With mass concentration of animal stock, large parts of the population receive contaminated meat (cf. KINGMA 1967). Lastly, international trade requires consideration of the country of production and its common application and handling methods of insecticides in plant protection and veterinary medicine.

Meat imported into the German Federal Republic comprises about 15 percent of the total consumption. This import comes mostly from countries such as Argentina, where insecticides are used to a considerable extent, especially organophosphate esters directly on the animal against parasites. The world-wide importance of production and trade of residue-free meat may also be seen in the report by TAYLOR (1963): 1,069,338,033 pounds of meat from 28 countries were imported into the United States in 1961/62, in comparison with an export of 699,388,761 pounds.

There are some reports about the magnitude of total pesticide intake. OSER (1966) established that the total intake of residues is far below the quantity which would be expected if all foodstuffs would contain the tolerable residue amount. The approximate residue level lies at a range of 0.003 p.p.m. (ANONYMOUS 21) for all organophosphate esters in well-balanced nutrition. This value agrees with the data of Table III which gives a survey of the presence of organophosphate ester residues in comparison with other pesticides in balanced average human ratios.

The study by DUGGAN and WEATHERWAX (1967) proves the presence of only the smallest quantities of organophosphate esters in foodstuffs, and they occur here predominantly in cereals and grain. "The incidence and intake of the remaining organic phosphates detected are too low to be meaningful." For example, in meat the ingested quantities of the organophosphates diazinon or ronnel are traces ($<$0.001 mg./day). The largest residue factor is malathion with 80 percent. Its intake with food is reported as 0.001 mg./kg. body weight (ANONYMOUS 2) or 0.1 µg./kg., respectively; the overall judgment for an ADI value of 20 µg./kg. is commented upon as "Pesticide residues, no cause for alarm" (ANONYMOUS 24).

Table III. *Summary of the presence of pesticide residues in human food* (ANONYMOUS 23).

Pesticide group in food	Example	WHO/FAO acceptable value (mg./kg. body wt.)	Residue found (p.p.m.)
Organochlorine	DDT	0.0005 –0.01	0.02
	lindane	0.00006–0.0125	—
Organophosphate	malathion	0.009 –0.02	0.003
Carbamate	carbaryl	0.0012 –0.02	0.05
Chlorophenoxy	2,4-D	—	0.003

SEIDEL (1956) gave the survey in Table IV about qualitative findings in the German Democratic Republic in 1955; he did not differentiate organophosphate esters or their metabolites.

Table IV. *Insecticide findings in the German Democratic Republic* (SEIDEL 1956).

Samples	No. examined	No. containing insecticides
Domestic animals	66	22
Wildlife and zoo animals	8	6
Bees	18	5
Inorganic compounds	11	5
Organic compounds (feces, urine, etc.)	3	3

Any discussion about residues in meat must include their presence in the tissues of wildlife. BECK *et al.* (1968) in Austria did not find residues of organophosphate esters in dead animals (hare, deer) except traces of organochlorine derivatives. BUNYAN *et al.* (1969) reported experimental investigations on pheasants; however, the effect after a continuous intake of trace quantities requires further investigation. There are indications that sometimes a certain tolerance is developed against organophosphate esters in the animal body after a chronic treatment with these esters (DU BOIS 1965, JOLLY 1957, KAEMMERER 1963, RADELEFF 1960).

Without doubt, with regard to the toxicology of the effective substance as well as the possible metabolites, there is a dependency on the chemical structure as reported by TOLKMITH (1966). In some respects, the processes for especially the ruminant have to be considered exceptional. The judgment of importance of a *per os* intake as well as secondary contamination through the feed must take into account that, for the ruminant, numerous organophosphate esters can be degraded in the rumen because of enzyme action in the rumen fluid; however, this is also dependent on the ratio [2], and thus a potential danger from decomposing compounds is strongly reduced, also for the meat consumer. Reports in Table V serve as an example: parathion, chlorthion, EPN, malathion, and (with longer duration of reaction) mevinphos are hydrolyzed; diazinon, trichlorfon, dioxathion, and demeton are resistant. The metabolic products of parathion are reduced from *p*-nitrophenol to *p*-aminophenol. In demeton, the thiono-isomer undergoes fast decomposition, while the thiolo-isomer remains active.

Table V. *Effect of rumen fluid on ten organophosphate pesticides* (COOK 1957).

Pesticide	Min. detectability (μg.)	Fresh fluid, % inhibition at				Boiled fluid, % inhibition at		
		0 hr.	1 hr.	3 hr.	25 hr.	0 hr.	3 hr.	25 hr.
Parathion [a]	0.01	57	8	1	5	95	74	68
Parathion [b]	0.01	69	0	5	—	—	—	—
Paraoxon [a]	0.01	65	1	1	0	—	—	—
Paraoxon [b]	0.01	56	0	0	—	—	—	—
Chlorthion [a]	0.50	88	4	1	5	92	91	—
Chlorthion [b]	0.50	80	3	10	—	—	—	84
EPN [a]	0.25	88	27	4	4	95	96	100
EPN [b]	0.25	96	100	100	100	—	—	—
Malathion [a]	0.50	41	43	26	9	53	49	47
Malathion [b]	0.50	51	51	49	43	—	—	—
Mevinphos	0.25	79	81	97	59	82	80	74
Diazinon [a]	0.005	40	45	37	36	—	—	—
Diazinon [b]	0.005	44	44	57	41	—	—	—
Trichlorfon	1.00	100	100	96	100	—	—	—
Dioxathion	0.50	88	83	54	83	—	—	—
Demeton	0.75	59	63	54	57	—	—	—

[a] High-alfalfa ration.
[b] High-grain ration.

There are only very few acute incidents with treated animals during acute treatment with phosphate esters; this contradicts an overestimation of possible hazards after the intake of contaminated meat. STREET (1965) refers to a personal communication from RADELEFF that poisoning of ani-

[2] So-called secondary poisoning is dependent on the quantity of free inhibitor which is not bonded by esterases (residual inhibitor).

mals from pesticides (total) makes up only 0.5 to 1.0 percent of all intoxicants, while a California statistic says, with regard to human beings, that 75 percent of systemic poisonings with agricultural chemicals are brought about by phosphate esters (HOLMES 1965). Accordingly, the primary contact dominates for the humang being. However, during 20 years of phosphate ester application no provable cases have shown where, after intake of contaminated meat, damage to human beings has been reported (cf. DORMAL 1960). Of course, in general, the maximum possible intake of effective substance is the most important factor of judgement. The quantity differs with the kind of consumed tissue. The effective substances have not necessarily an even distribution in the animal body so that different residue quantities have to be expected in, for instance, muscle, liver, and kidney. Also those cases are objectionable in which, after injection treatment with normally slightly soluble substances (for instance, suspensions), a significant substance depot of non-resorbed particles remains at the location of injection after resorption of the solvent and other vehicles; these may be secluded partially in tissue (KAEMMERER 1963). Such spots surely often elude the organoleptic meat inspection.

f) Measures of legislation

Factors of uncertainties cannot be eliminated completely even with the attempt to enforce protection measures by law. In the Federal Republic of Germany the food law of January 17, 1936, in the version from December 21, 1958 [3], makes regimentation possible. It is forbidden:

Section 3, 1 a. To obtain, produce, prepare, pack, store, transport, or treat otherwise any foodstuff for others in such a way that its consumption is able to damage human health.

Section 4 b, 4. To offer, keep on hand, keep for sale, sell, or otherwise bring to the public, food which contains inside or outside plant protection substances and pesticides, preservatives, and substances to prevent sprouting of potatoes, substances to influence fructification or fruit drop or to accelerate fruit ripening, or their metabolites, and which *exceed the allowable tolerances.*

An authorization for a prohibition norm extends the protection measures, which are provided by law:

Section 4 d. Regardless of the regulations of section 4 a, paragraph 1, and section 4 b, No. 3, the Minister of the Interior is authorized, in agreement with the Ministers for Food, Agriculture, and Foresty, and Economy, *to forbid* procedures of treatment of foodstuff by judicial proceeding and with the consent of the Federal Council, if they impart a condition which is critical for human health. The authorization according to sentence 1 refers only to food, which is determined to be brought to the public by trade or for members of associations or similar unions, or to be supplied to establishments for co-operational care.

---

[3] A change or new version is in preparation.

Certain economic, hygienic, etc. requirements could make it necessary to permit justifiable exceptions:

Section 4 a (1). Foreign substances may be added during raising, production, or preparation to food, which is determined to be brought to the public by trade, *only, if it is categorically permitted.* In the sense of this law, the bringing of food to the public by trade stands equal to supplying food for members of associations or similar unions, or establishments for cooperational care.

Paragraph 1 is also valid:

If foreign substances are only added to the surface of foodstuff, which is not meant for consumption.

Finally, section 5 a (1) contains the authorization to enact allowable tolerances; according to number 5, plant protection substances and pesticides are subject to this. Furthermore, accordingly, certain substances can be excluded from use as a plant protection substance or pesticide — as far as this is necessary for the protection of the consumer and to prevent a condition of food which is apt to endanger human health.

The so-called allowable tolerance-decree from November 30, 1966 accommodates these enactments. However, it is only valid for vegetable foods. The number values, which are fixed for them, should also be directive for meat and meat products, although the legislators used the authorization only for the mentioned food groups.

Generally, enactments aim at only one specific effective substance, which is seized and can be excluded from use. The gamut of possible effective substances or their effects, respectively, when several factors come together, is not seized. This fact could be seen in the light of a statement, which TAYLOR (1965) made for the United States: "We can reasonably conclude that every meat animal in this country is produced in a constant environment of agricultural chemicals, and/or is administered one or more drugs during its life time." However, this statement becomes important only with regard to effectively determined residues. The often-used forms of alarm are confronted by the necessity of increased meat production. Increased meat production may be advocated if it is done by means of fattening and with health care, with substances which leave no or only negligible and harmless residues in the tissue. The goal must be to continue to give maximum security to the consumer.

g) Organophosphate esters in meat and criteria for residue questions

The tendency to accumulate organochlorine pesticide derivates, especially in fatty tissue, has often led to the prohibition of such substances for ectoparasite control on domestic animals and to permission to use only such preparations which leave no residues, or the residues of which are so small that they are excreted from the animal body within a short time. Generally, organophosphate esters belong to the latter group (ENDREJAT 1967). Not all of the O-P compounds can be classified as non-persistent; however, the extensive development of such substances encourages the belief that other and "better" ones will follow (RADELEFF 1967).

The total amount, which includes the agricultural and veterinary sector, can be estimated from the following reports. In the United States >60,000 pesticide formulations are based on >900 chemical compounds (ANONYMOUS 5). REID (1966) has reported WALKER who said that in 1965 the total quantity of synthetically produced organic pesticides was 763,000,000 pounds, which was ten percent higher than in previous years. According to SALZER (1968) the annual world consumption of organophosphate esters is 80,000 tons of effective substances; of these, 50,000 tons yearly are of parathion alone (ANONYMOUS 2). In the United States in 1964, 84 percent of the pesticides was used in plant protection, 11 percent for domestic animals, and four percent otherwise (IVERSON 1967). Necessarily, with increasing world population, the need for food and the problem of contamination will also increase.

Organophosphate esters are poisons. SCOTT (1967) classifies poisons in the following groups:

Highly toxic: LD_{50} of less than 50 mg./kg. of substance included in the Agricultural (Poisonous Substances) Regulations
Moderately toxic: LD_{50} between 50 and 500 mg./kg. of chemical included in the Poisons List
Slightly toxic: LD_{50} greater than 500 mg./kg.

Accordingly, a categorization of organophosphate esters is as listed in Table VI.

Table VI. *Classification of organophosphate esters as poisons* (SCOTT 1967).

Highly toxic	Moderately toxic	Slightly toxic
Azinphosmethyl	diazinon	malathion
Chlorfenvinphos	dimethoate	menazon
Demeton-*S*-methyl	formothion	trichlorfon
Dichlorvos	morphothion	
Dimefox		
Disulfoton		
Ethion		
Mevinphos		
Oxydemeton-methyl		
Parathion		
Phenkapton		
Phorate		
Phosphamidon		
Schradan		
Vamidothion		

The residues of such substances which remain in the animal tissue undergo a kind of dilution process, if the common approach of today is followed of a qualitative relation to the animal body weight. The quantity of effective substance which comes to the human being as a consumer of meat from edible domestic animals is always only a fraction of the total dosage which had been applied to the animal, whereby the intake of residues by humans takes place *per os*. The different enteric resorption conditions, which are characteristic for each substance, have to be included in a total evaluation. This also holds for the possibly occuring "poison reactions" during metabolizing.

According to TIEWS (1967) improved agricultural production offers itself as a huge field test in which, for instance, the harmlessness of the feed additives used is proved every day, aside from its economic advantages. Aside from the actual feed additives, drugs and substances for parasite control should, without doubt, be included here. Their harmlessness for the animal has to be proved beforehand, although they are applied in by far higher dosages for this use than they can be passed on in residue form through the meat. Also, those substances which become poisonous during metabolizing should already show effects on the treated animal. For the safety of the consumer, a long-duration animal test is required on two species and is incorporated according to known criteria. Such studies should last at least 90 days (ANONYMOUS 22).

Animal tests allow a statement about the behaviour of a substance in the human being only with a certain probability (HAUSCHILD 1965). Absolute data which are obtained in experiments on test animals are of scientific interest for transformation into practical use insofar as they serve to provide knowledge concerning the behavior of a specific substance.

The German Committee for Substances for Plant Protection, Plant Treatment, and Storage Protection (ANONYMOUS 17) still considers it questionable as to how far the results which are obtained by animal testing can be transferred to the human being. Without doubt this holds especially for the acute toxicity and also for the possible different metabolic processes.

The general claims of DECKER (1959) are still of topical interest:

"1. For every compound there is a level of intake below which there is no discernible effect upon health.
2. Each compound must be considered on the basis of its particular physical, chemical, and toxicological properties.
3. An arbitrarily selected fraction of the "safe dose" should not be used to define the upper limit of a zone of inconsequence for all materials.
4. Chemicals used in food production and processing may occur in foods in amounts so small as to be inconsequential in relation to public health, and in such instances regulatory activity is not required."

There are no binding directions, at least not in Germany, for the judgment of possible endangerment of the consumer by organophosphate esters in meat and meat products. The commonly used formulas for the limitation of tolerable quantities, which have ben recommended by FAO/WHO in the frame of plant protection, remain (in Germany) restricted to vegetable products. In Germany, so far, there are no fixed tolerance values or waiting times before slaughtering, not even for medically aimed application of organophosphate esters to the animal. The substances which have been secondarily taken in without control are inaccessible at any rate. A ChE inhibition, which eventually may have been found, also does not conclude anything about the chemistry of the substance and its metabolism. There are no objections to applying the mentioned formulas for residues in meat, also. This is done in the basic considerations of FAO/WHO (Anonymous 34) for the use of evaluation formulas. Such formulas do not say anything in detail about the substance as such, its excretion, and its metabolism; however, they give information about its compatibility. They do offer a considerable, also not an absolute, measure of safety (Kaemmerer 1967).

With regard to "acceptable daily intake", Van Esch (1966) discusses critically the judgment modalities for pesticide residues. The no-effect level should better give way to the no-toxic-effect level. At first a test, which should be limited to and last 1/10 of the lifetime (of a rat) and which would be considered a semichronical test, may lead to a temporary ADI. With the protection of such knowledge and data, all the remaining toxicity and metabolism data may be worked out in the framework of long duration testing and the carcinogenic effect may be tested. The safety factor of 100, which is used to establish the formula for the ADI, was also criticized, although the strict requirement of a safety factor of 100 is not even fulfilled by many naturally occurring food ingredients (Oettel 1967).

The arbitrarily established factor of 100 (see also Bär 1964 b, Maier-Bode 1965) for the ADI is commented on by WHO/FAO (Anonymous 35): "In the absence of any evidence to the contrary, the Committee believes that this margin of safety is adequate." This factor, which is not scientifically founded, is sufficient for practical use. Some authors have determined the safety factor scientifically. The results show that the factor 100 is rather too high than too low (Van Esch 1966). However, in cases of insufficient toxicological investigation it should be higher (perhaps 500 to 1,000), just as it could be set 20 times lower in other cases (Van Esch 1966). If the no-effect level (= *dosis tolerata*) is based on ChE inhibition measurement, the safety factor in the United States is set lower, according to Möllhoff (1967); in Canada it is 20 for inhibition of the plasma ChE and 40 for inhibition of erythrocyte ChE.

In regard to permissible level, the critic of this formula, which was inaugurated by Van Genderen (1960) (see Wilson and Baier 1963), in part uses the above-mentioned arguments, namely that the animal test must not necessarily give representative values for the human being. However, it is supported by the requirement that two animal species have to be included in the tests. In these formulas no account is taken of the different quantities of intake and the sensitivity of some people such as children, pregnant women, and nursing mothers so that, for instance, factors for child protection (= 2.5) (Hötzel 1965) have been proposed. Van Esch (1966) wants child nutrition to be judged altogether separately. The formulas arbitrarily presuppose an average body weight of 70 kg. and a food intake of 400 g. of foodstuff daily per individual. Obviously, it has also not been taken into account that not all foodstuffs must always contain residues.

The Committee for Plant Protection of the German Research Association explains as follows (ANONYMOUS 16): "So far there is no generally acknowledged basis for the transformation calculation from the acceptable daily dosage to the highest tolerable residue quantities" and "the residue values have to be established in such a way that the acceptable daily dosage of a substance is not exceeded with regard to the expected compositions of the daily food and the totally present residues of a certain effective substance." Futhermore, the climatic conditions vary locally.

In regard to tolerances, the tolerance values serve for the protection of the consumer; they are not irrevocable and have to be reestablished each time it seems necessary (ANONYMOUS 15). Tolerance values differ from country to country; they should not exceed the permissible level values. The discussion about the validity of tolerance values is also not concluded as yet. The terms "no residue" or "zero tolerance" are considered unsustainable, scientifically as well as administratively (ANONYMOUS 5) and should give way in favor of "negligible residue" or "permissible residue", respectively (ANONYMOUS 35). Since the term "tolerance" was interpreted inconsistently, it was proposed to define the word "tolerance" — if it is used alone — as the concentration that is permitted in or on food (ANONYMOUS 20). It follows, hence, that different tolerance types are possible; for example, a temporary one, which is a tolerance which is permitted for a certain time. Table VII gives acceptable daily doses and tolerance values according to FAO/WHO (1966).

Table VII. *Acceptable FAO/WHO daily dosages and tolerance values for some organophosphate esters* (ANONYMOUS 20).

Compound	Acceptable daily dosage (max.) (mg./kg. body wt.)	Recommended tolerance (p.p.m.)
Dichlorvos	0.004	none for 1966
Malathion	0.02	fruits and vegetables 3.0–8.0
Diazinon	0.002	none for 1966
Dimethoate	0.004	none for 1966
Phosphamidon	0.001	none for 1966

The Committee for Plant Protection of the German Research Association proposes permissible quantities of pesticide residues for plant products, which are listed in Table VIII. A permissible quantity regulation in Hungary [4] also includes products of animal origin; the tolerance values for organophosphate esters have been extracted from this regulation and are reported in Table IX.

[4] Kindly communicated by Professor Dr. J. KOVACS, Budapest.

Table VIII. *List of residue values proposed by the Committee for Plant Protection, Plant Treatment, and Storage Protection Substances of the German Research Association from April 5, 1965* (ANONYMOUS 16).

Pesticide	Acceptable daily dose (mg./kg. body wt.)	Permissible level (p.p.m.)	German tolerance (p.p.m.)	U.S. tolerance [a] (p.p.m.)
Azinphosmethyl	0.0025	0.45	0.2	2
Demeton	0.0025	0.45	0.1	0.3–1.25
Methyl demeton	0.0025	0.45	0.1	NR
Diazinon	0.00375	0.66	0.175	0.75
Dimethoate	0.004	0.7	0.2	NR
Dioxathion	0.0022	0.39	0.1	2.1–4.9
Disulfoton	0.0025	0.45	0.1	0.75
Malathion	0.02	3.5	1	8
Parathion	0.005	0.9	0.2	1
Methyl parathion	0.01	1.75	0.5	1
Trichlorfon	0.18	32	0.5	NR

[a] NR = no residue permitted.

Table IX. *Limit values of pesticide residues in animal products* [extracted from Hungarian permissible regulation (ANONYMOUS 31)].

Pesticide	Limit values (p.p.m.) in commodities										
	Fresh meat	Canned meat, meat preparations	Fish	Liver, other inner organs	Fat, fat tissue	Egg	Egg powder	Milk	Milk powder	Butter	Other milk products, cheese, sour cream, etc.
Toxaphene	0.2	0.2	0.1	0.5	0.5	0.1	0.2	0.01	0.03	0.05	0.0
Dichlorvos	0.0	0.0	0.0	0.0	0.0	0.0	0.0	0.0	0.0	0.0	0.0
Trichlorfon	0.0	0.0	0.0	0.0	0.0	0.0	0.0	0.0	0.0	0.0	0.0
Diazinon	0.1	0.1	0.1	0.2	0.1	0.05	0.1	0.01	0.01	0.05	0.2
Malathion	2.0	3.0	2.0	3.0	0.0	0.02	0.05	0.02	0.05	0.05	0.0

With respect to the conditions in the German Federal Republic, a regulation for permissible tolerances was enacted on the grounds of legal authorization on November 30, 1966 and it became effective January 1, 1968. Again, this regulation deals only with plant products so that these data are valid only with reservation and only as a lead for an analogous evaluation of effective substances and their residues in meat (ANONYMOUS 36):

azinphosethyl and -methyl	total 0.4 p.p.m.
bromophos	0.1–0.5 p.p.m.
demeton	0.4 p.p.m.
demeton plus demeton sulfoxide	0.4 p.p.m.
diazinon	0.5 p.p.m.
dimefox	0.1 p.p.m.
dimethoate	0.5 p.p.m.
dioxathion	0.4 p.p.m.
disulfoton	0.2 p.p.m.
fenitrothion	0.4 p.p.m.
formothion	0.1 p.p.m.
malathion	0.5 p.p.m.
mevinphos	0.1 p.p.m.
parathion and methyl parathion	total 0.5 p.p.m.
phosphamidon	0.5 p.p.m.
triamphos (Wepsyn)	0.03 p.p.m.
trichlorfon	0.5 p.p.m.
zinophos (thionazin)	0.1 p.p.m.

In the German Democratic Republic, a tolerance list for several organophosphates is proposed for tolerances on some plant products, but not for meat, fish, animal fat, and eggs (Table X).

Table X. *Proposed tolerance values in the German Democratic Republic* (LAUE 1968).

Pesticide	Tolerance (p.p.m.)	
	Vegetable products	Animal products
Trichlorfon	1	0
Dichlorvos	0–1	0
Methyl parathion	0–0.5–1.0	0
Dimefox	0	0
Methyl demeton	0–0.5	0
Dimethoate	0–0.5	0
Mevinphos	0	0
Malathion	0–3	0

In the German Federal Republic a limit within the range of one p.p.m. has been established for most insecticides. Damage to (human) health is unimaginable in this so-called homoepathic dosage range ("D6") and has never been observed; food from German markets which has been analyzed for residues so far always contained under the permissible tolerances (OETTEL 1967). These findings are supported by KRZEMINSKI and LANDMANN (1963): "The organic phosphates do not give any residues under the present conditions of application. Residues in meat or meat products only occur from those compounds which either are not metabolized or are rapidly excreted."

However, the still present overall uncertainties of residues evaluation — in dependence upon the sensitivity and accuracy of the analytical method and with inclusion of sufficient safety factors — may be seen in the recent efforts of the FDA in the United States. In order to characterize the situation, it is cited literally (ANONYMOUS 19):

"When the data show that finite residues will actually be incurred in milk, eggs, meat and/or poultry, a tolerance will be established on the raw agricultural commodity used as feed, provided that such tolerances can be established at the same time, on the basis of toxicological and other data available, for the finite residues incurred in milk, eggs, meats, and/or poultry. When it is not possible to determine with certainty whether finite residues will be incurred in milk, eggs, meat and/or poultry but there is a reasonable expectation of finite residues in light of data reflecting exaggerated pesticide levels in feeding studies, a tolerance will be established on the raw agricultural commodity, provided appropriate tolerances can be established at the same time, on the basis of toxicological and other data available, for the finite residues likely to be incurred in these foods through the feed use of the raw agricultural commodity or its byproducts."

"When it is not possible to determine with certainty whether finite residues will be incurred in milk, eggs, meats and/or poultry but there is no reasonable expectation of finite residues in light of data such as those reflecting exaggerated pesticide levels in feeding studies and those elucidating the biochemistry of the pesticide chemical in the animal, a tolerance may be established on the raw agricultural commodity without the necessity of a tolerance on food products derived from the animal."

h) Remarks about the analytical methods

A basic statement by COOK (1965) may introduce this section:

"In conclusion, I would like to emphasize that, qualitatively, the phenomenon of residue persistence really exists, but that quantitative relationships of persistence are very difficult to determine except within each experiment. So many important variables are difficult to control that it is hazardous to attempt to relate persistence curves to each other or to assume that one can make an individual analysis and place it on a persistence curve to determine quantitatively what happened before and to predict what will happen."

With regard to and in connection with the Miller Pesticides Amendment in the United States, numerous imponderables have still to be clarified if a just evaluation of organophosphate ester residues shall be made possible. The critical questions, which GUNTHER (1957) states with regard to plants, are also valid for animal tissue in a varied form:

(1) What does the residue consist of?
(2) Where in the animal or in which tissue is the residue localized?
(3) What residue quantity per unit weight (animal or tissue) is present?
(4) What chemical metabolite is present, if the residue is not identical with the (applied) effective substance?
(5) Is the residue or are its metabolites transferred with the animal tissues to the marketed products in significant amounts?

These questions almost initiate a basic analytical program; however, its limits are apparently reached if there is a search for unknown substances and factors. As long as there are no chemically founded criteria and detection methods, auxiliary measures have to be used for the judgment of endangering human beings by residues, provided the primary effective substances are known.

Without doubt the chemist occupies a central position in the team for establishment of criteria of an effective substance and with regard to the identification of the type of residues. It may be important to know both the residue and also the originally applied substance (VORHEES 1956) because changes in molecules can also cause radical changes in the toxicity.

KRZEMINSKI and LANDMANN (1963) discuss the problem of pesticide analyses in meat products in a special survey. The difficulties for the analysis of residues in meat are based on the fact that meat contains substances which are soluble in fat as well as in water. They distinguish three possibilities of analytical procedure: (1) no previous cleanup, (2) potential cleanup, or (3) complete cleanup. The following requirements are made by KRZEMINSKI and LANDMANN (1963) for a screening method which would correspond to a rapid method within the framework of official meat inspections and which is considered necessary by the authors:

(1) The time required for an analysis should be short so that a large number of samples can be processed in one day.
(2) The method should be sensitive enough to respond to the tolerance level of the FDA or to lower concentrations.
(3) It should be possible to neglect obscuring from other components so that difficult separation methods become obsolete.
(4) The method should be simple and not involve longer working procedures.
(5) The necessary equipment should be easy to obtain and simple to use.

A survey of different analytical procedures for the detection of insecticidal phosphate esters and their metabolites in food is reported by MÖLLHOFF (1968). Standard procedures for the determination of appropriate fluorine, *p*-nitrophenol, or alkoxy groups are not specific or not sensitive enough for sufficiently accurate analyses and the absolute quantity of phosphorus, which is offered with the alkylphosphates, is too low in comparison to the phosphorus content of tissues to allow a judgment about residues in tissues by chemical phosphorus-determination (DANGSCHAT 1965). Also, hydrolysis, which is required for some chemical methods and which often leads to characteristic detectable cleavage products, does not predicate anything about the content of "active" substance. Only shortly after intake of an active product is it possible to determine a free effective substance which inhibitis ChE. With respect to the chemical characteristics of alkylphosphate molecules, the nondetectability of an enzyme-inhibiting product is quite often equalized with its being nonpoisonous. With biological testing it is possible to detect the still active enzyme-inhibiting substance residues or their "active" metabolites; these are quite often their oxygen analogs.

The discussions by DANGSCHAT (1965) are to be understood in the sense of the preceding remarks. Furthermore, this author concludes: "With regard to the qualification of meat as food from alkylphosphate-treated animals, biological test procedures allow a quite accurate judgment. There are no basic objections against the use of biological residue determinations." Also, HAZLETON (1955) said: "Under use conditions residue hazard appears to be negligible." For example, either the mosquito test (Aedes) or the fly larvae test may be used for systemically effective organophosphate esters (GUNTHER and BLINN 1955, HEWITT *et al.* 1958, UNTERSTENHÖFER 1960, EDDY 1961, SHERMAN and ROSS 1961, BEHRENZ 1963, and others). Indeed, an identification of metabolites with regard to their chemical configuration is not possible here; however, this way of testing allows a quantitative statement about a still-present insecticidal effect.

The capacity of organophosphate esters to inhibit ChE is used for indirect testing (e. g., the colorimetric determination of ChE inhibition, or ΔpH, or Warburg method). To a certain extent, a quantitative statement about the intact effective substance is possible with this method (NESHEIM and COOK 1959, GUNTHER and BLINN 1955, SANDI 1962). An increase of inhibition is possible for some thionophosphates and thiolophosphates by treatment with bromine water, which transforms them into the actual ChE inhibitor (FALLSCHEER and COOK 1956), and with following determination by paper chromatography on differently prepared papers (MCKINLEY and READ 1962).

FRIEDBERG and SAKAI (1958) and KARLOG and POULSEN (1963) mention the indirect method of detection in animal tissues by reactivation of the blocked enzyme; ACKERMANN (1967) and ACKERMANN *et al.* (1969) developed detection methods with the help of combined TLC and enzyme procedures, especially for biological materials. *

The following basic techniques are often used for complete cleanup and detection: paper chromatography, thin-layer chromatography (TLC), column chromatography, gas chromatography (glc), spectroanalysis in the visible range, spectroanalysis in the IR and UV ranges, mass spectrometry, and NMR.

EGAN *et al.* (1964) described a sensitive detector system for the determination of phosphate esters in the submicrogram range; BRUCE (1967) developed a detector cell which detects less than one ng. of effective substance; and GUNTHER and OTT (1966) reported their fully automatic determination with the AutoAnalyzer. For further general details [5] see ZWEIG (1963 and 1964), EICHLER (1965), MOFFIT (1963), GUNTHER and BLINN (1955), MATOUŠEK and TOMEČEK (1965), DUGGAN *et al.* (1967), RUZICKA

* Editor's note: See MENDOZA, C. E.: Analysis of pesticides by the thin-layer chromatographic-enzyme inhibition technique. Residue Reviews **43**, 105 (1972). This reference was not available to the authors when the present review was prepared.

[5] The cited literature serves only as a reference and does not claim to be complete.

et al. (1967), and SHAFIK and ENOS (1969), as well as COOK and WILLIAMS (1965) (survey and literature), RAGAB (1967) (fluorescence after bromine vapor treatment), EGAN (1967) (multidetector), LOVINS (1969) (determination in mixtures with high resolution mass spectrometry), BECK and SHERMAN (1968), WINTERLIN *et al.* (1968) (TLC), ST. JOHN and LISK (1968 a) (hydrolysis products in urea with glc), PURDUE *et al.* (1969) (double column double electron-capture detector), and many others.

The investigational methods which are specially used for meat differ very much. At present the detection of labelled P^{32} in the molecule is prevalent for directed application (e. g., DEDEK and KÜHNERT 1962). Occasionally the labelling is done at the side chain with C^{14} (CHAMBERLAIN 1965). For these methods, the separation of fractions is necessary for the determination of the various metabolites. Water, chloroform, acetone, acetonitrile, etc. are common as extraction solvents. KADOUM (1968 a) describes a fast micromethod of sample cleanup with benzene-hexane and benzene. Isopropanol combined with either hexane or benzene shows different characteristics. SCHNORBUS and PHILLIPS (1967) describe propylene carbonate as a universal "broad-spectrum" extraction solvent for pesticide residues, which is also suitable for meat extraction. The further separation of chloro- and thiophosphate compounds from propylene carbonate is done with Florisil chromatography. The determination methods for metabolites of organophosphate esters should also be remembered. ST. JOHN and LISK (1968 a) describe a glc method for the determination of dimethylphosphate, thiophosphate, and dithiophospate in bullock's urine as a model.

Since individual methods vary widely and are differently used by various authors, we have to point to the secondary literature for details (e. g., SCHRADER 1963, GUNTHER 1957, and others). However, the question is still open as to the way in which a simple, routine group test can be developed and introduced — for instance, within the frame of veterinary meat inspection — for the purpose of looking for unknown organophosphate esters. Certain analogies are found in the plant protection field, as, for example, the method by BRODERICK *et al.* (1967), who determine surface residues of organophosphate esters on fruit by conversion of the organically bound phosphorus into inorganic phosphate.

A simple separation method (aqueous acetonitrile-hexane) for parathion, methyl parathion, diazinon, malathion, and thimet with following glc determination (0.01 p.p.m.) is described by KADOUM (1968 b and 1969). Automation for pesticide determination should also be considered as has been proposed, for example, by APPLEGATE and CHITTWOOD (1968) for glc; "The goal of pesticide residue research is automation", said SCHECHTER and GETZ (1967). Rapid-test-methods for orientation could be of special interest here; as mentioned above, they would at least allow a group classification. THIER and BERGNER (1966) reported about such a method for vegetables. After acetonitrile extraction and following dilution of the extract with water, it allows organochlorine compounds to be separated by extracting them with ether followed by extraction of the organophosphates with dichloromethane.

In a certain way, the agar-diffusion method (Sandi 1962) represents a rapid method; it is based on enzyme reactions and is applicable on foods for the detection in mg./ml. of the following compounds: parathion 0.003 to 30, methyl parathion 0.03 to 30, chlorthion 0.2 to 100, isochlorthion 0.2 to 100, demeton 0.2 to 20, Metasystox 0.2 to 20, tinox 0.2 to 20, mevinphos 0.1 to 100, phenkapton 0.1 to 100, and malathion 0.1 to 100. The special usefulness of this method for residues in meat would have to be examined.

As a supplement to the previous comments, the reports by Fischer (1968), Fischer and Plunger (1965), and Fischer and Plazer-Altenburg (1969) should be mentioned. They undertook the detection of phosphate inseticides in biological material including meat. The analytical values were obtained after ethanol extraction, saponification with potassium hydroxide, and removal of the resulting fatty acids with magnesium sulfate. The residues were extracted with ether and the solvent was evaporated; in special cases they were cleaned further over polyamide; the final residue contained the basic molecules which are obtained after saponification; they were identified by TLC, based on their characteristic behavior. The $\mathbf{R}_f$ values found by the authors mentioned are summarized and reported in Tables XI, XII, and XIII.

Table XI. R_f *values for TLC of sulfur-containing phosphate esters* (Fischer 1968, Fischer and Plunger 1965).

Pesticide	Developer I [a] (Silica gel G)	Developer II [b] (Silica gel G)	Developer III [c] [Aloxal (Fluka)]
Trichlorfon	36	13	0
Ethyl trichlorfon	57	29	18
Emittol	41	15	5
Phosphamidon	56 and 100	26 and 76	38
Dibrom	40	20	12
Mevinphos	78	40	50
Dichlorvos	50	35	15

[a] Developer I = acetone:*n*-hexane:chloroform (1:1:1).
[b] Developer II = acetone:*n*-hexane (1:2).
[c] Developer III = benzene:ether (2:3).

These tabulated reports have been supplemented recently with values from further organophosphates by Fischer and Plazer-Altenburg (1969) (see Table XIV); here the authors pointed to the significant changing of $\mathbf{R}_f$ values due to different activity of the silica gel. First, the spotting of two thiophosphate esters as reference test substances is therefore necessary and, second, working with both unsaturated and saturated developing chambers is necessary.

Table XII. *Chromatographic values* (Fischer and Plunger 1965).

No. [a]	and substance	Factor [b]	Test tube chromatography [c]				Thin-layer chromatography [c]				Remarks, secondary characteristics
			Developer I		Developer II		Developer I		Developer II		
			After iodacid	Before iodacid	After iodacid	Before iodacid	After iodacid	Before iodacid	After iodacid	Before iodacid	
1	Parathion (E 605)	9.40	40		82		42		84		
1 a	Nitrophenol			50		70		81		90	yellow
2	Diazinon	9.82	50 63		80		44		86		
2 a	Diazine residue			100		82		100		100	Dragendorff +
3	Potasan	10.60	50		84		42 56		88		
3 a	Methylumbelliferone			50		72		80		92	fluorescent
4	Phenkapton	12.18	48 08		82		40 68		98–100		
5	Demeton	8.34	49 58		84		43 58		86		volatile thioether
6	Dioxathion	14.74	50 68		82		42 32 100		94		
7	Ethion	12.40	10 50		34 74		25 38 100		18 78		volatile thioether
8	FAC-20	9.21	50		86		32 98–100		20 80		NH_3 Nessler +
9	Trithion	11.04	50 58		74 86		32 100		76 90		
9 a	Chloro-compound							100		100	Cl-detection

Table XII (continued)

No.[a] and substance	Factor[b]	Test tube chromatography[c]				Thin-layer chromatography[c]				Remarks, secondary characteristics
		Developer I		Developer II		Developer I		Developer II		
		After iodacid	Before iodacid	After iodacid	Before iodacid	After iodacid	Before iodacid	After iodacid	Before iodacid	
10 Azinphosethyl	11.25	50 61		77		42		82		
10 a Benzazimide residue			40		60		24		60	fluorescent Dragendorff +
11 Chlorthion	9.61	42		84		31		82		
11 a Chloronitrophenol			60		76		67		90	yellow
12 Metasystox J	7.44	42 54		84		30 40 48		87		volatile thioether
13 Metasystox R	7.95	42 54		84		30 40		87		less volatile thioether
14 Malathion	10.67	42 22 64		80 90 56 30		32 44 58 66		99–100		
15 Thiometon	7.95	40 60		84		34 28 58		90		volatile thioether
16 Methyl parathion	8.50	41		84		31		82		
16 a Nitrophenol			50		70		81		89	yellow
17 Azinphosmethyl	10.34	43		80		32		70		
17 a Benzazimide residue			40		60		24		60	fluorescent Dragendorff +
18 Lebaycid	8.98	40 60 100		82		30 50		54 80		

19	Endothion	9.05	56 100		74		18 98–100		56 100		
19 a	Pyrone cleavage product							0		22	fluorescent
20	Perfekthion	7.40	10 40 71		60 84		68 92		32 52 90		NH_3 Nessler +
21	Formothion	8.50	11 38		42 67		10 20		15 36		volatile aldehyde Schiff reagent
22	Reduced parathion		49		82		42		84		
22 a	*p*-Aminophenol			78				90			amine reagent +
23	Paraoxon (Mintacol)	8.00	71				0				P-reaction + from 68–74
23 a	*p*-Nitrophenol			50		70		81		90	yellow
24	O,O-Diethyl phosphorothioic acid		49		82		42		86		

[a] No. 1–10 = diethyl esters, no. 10–21 = dimethyl esters, no. 1–22 = phosphorothioic or phosphorodithioic acid esters, no. 23 = phosphoric acid ester, and no. 24 = phosphorothioic acid ester reference.

[b] Factor for the calculation of weight from thiophosphoric ester and phosphoric ester from phosphorus values, which have been obtained by quantitative determination.

[c] R_f values reported × 100; developer I = *n*-butanol:water:acetone:ammonia (10%) in ratios 8:2:2:1, developer II = methanol:water:ammonia (1%) in ratios 19:1:1.

Table XIII. *Organophosphate insecticide determinations in biological materials by detection of spots on chromatograms* (FISCHER 1968).

No.	and substance	Factor [a]	Test tube chromatography [b]				Thin-layer chromatography [b]				Remarks, reactions of cleavage products
			Developer I		Developer II		Developer III		Developer IV		
			After iodacid	Before iodacid	After iodacid	Before iodacid	After iodacid	Before iodacid	After iodacid	Before iodacid	
1	Zinophos	8.01	50		85		43		84		detection of
					75						NH_3
2	Disulfoton	8.83	50		81		41		83		volatile
			94		90		84		96		thioether
3	Azinphosethyl	11.20	51		84		40		91		
					45		72		87		
									42		+ light blue
				39		62+		22		62	fluorescence,
											no Dragendorff
4	Bayer 45515	8.49	42		81		31		86		
							86				
							59				
							20				
4 a	3-Nitrophenol			50		71		97		88	orange
5	Fenitrothion	8.95	42		83		30		85		
	Folithion		35				49				
							22				
5 a	3-Methyl-4-nitrophenol			62		78		85		95	yellow
6	Metasystox S	8.40	41		90		32		85		volatile
			96		80		87		95		thioether
							10				
7	Menazon	9.07	40		81		31		82		detection of
			19		32		58		98		NH_3
							93				

8	Cidial	10.32	40 55 25		84 67		30 22		86 65 22		
								30 25		79 59	$KMnO_4$-reaction + purple, increased with NH_3 vapors
9	Fenchlorfos	10.38	43 35		85 68		31 70 25		80 97		
				81		74		87		93	halogen detection +
10	Bromophos	11.80	43 80		83 95		30 80		82 94 49		
				35		64		83 27		81 69	halogen detection +
11	Supracid	9.75	41 90		85 65		31 88 12		81 97 16		
				80		89		91 59		93	amine reaction positive
12	Vamidothion	9.26	42 29 16		85 71		31 54 72		82 57		volatile thioether
				45		75		95 69 51		79	amine reaction positive

[a] Factor for the calculation.
[b] R_f-values reported × 100; developer I = butanol:water:acetone:ammonia (10%) in ratios 8:2:2:1, developer II = methanol:water:ammonia (1%) in ratios 19:1:1, developer III = methanol:methylene chloride:ammonia (10%) in ratios 20:80:3, developer IV = methanol:methylene chloride:ammonia (10%) in ratios 35:60:5.

Table XIV. *TLC values from further organophosphates regarding significant changes due to different activities of the silica gel* (FISCHER and PLAZER-ALTENBURG 1969).

No. and substance		R_f values								Secondary characteristics to "before iodacid"
		Large plates without chamber saturation				Small plates without chamber saturation				
		Developer I		Developer II		Developer I		Developer II		
		After iodacid	Before iodacid	After iodacid	Before iodacid	After iodacid	Before iodacid	After iodacid	Before iodacid	
					Diethyl-compounds					
1	SRA 7502 (Bayer 77488)	38		73		32		70		HCN-detection after saponification
2	Asuntol	13	13	43	43	10	10	40	40	fluorescence
		38		73		29		70		
			67				60			
			81		95		70		94	
3	Ethyl bromophos	33	84	77		30	75	70		fluorescence with developer I
4	Phosalone [a]	32		8		32		9		volatile thioether
		53		78		50		71		
		100		90		100		86		
					Dimethyl compounds					
5	Metaisosystoxsulfone	27		63		23		58		volatile thioether
		100		100		100		100		
6	Folimat (omethoate)	0–10 [b]		36	15	0–10		32	13	fluorescence and volatile thioether
7	Thiometonsulfoxyde	25		15		22		61		volatile thioether
		100		65		55		100		
				100		100				

					Test substances					
8	Parathion	36	80	73	90	37	76	70	87	yellow
9	Chlorthion	28	69, 75, 81	66	81 (89)	24 25 (85)	54, 62, 73 53	60	79, 88	yellow saturation
10	Potasan [c]	34	48, 71							
11	Azinphosethyl [c]	34 100	23							
12	Disulfoton [c]	38 100								
13	Thiometon [c]	25 100								
14	Metasystox R [c, d]	14 87								
15	Metasystox S [c, d]	14 81								
16	Parathion [c, d]	20 88	51							
17	Chlorthion [c, d]	15	30, 37, 47							

[a] A dithio ester, therefore the low R_f value.
[b] Finger-shaped spot, not found for any other thiophosphoric esters (to No. 6).
[c] Fischer and Plunger (1965), Fischer (1968).
[d] Large plates with chamber saturation.

i) Summarized review

The residue problem is still a genuine problem today which has not been solved (Hauchild 1965), especially because not only dosage problems are involved. The concentration poisons, which are dependent on dosages, are confronted by the summation poisons which are dosage independent. The irreversible tissue damage is followed by new damages in the sense of an effect summation, although the effective substance is no longer present and has been excreted or decomposed. Such damage can be induced by the smallest amounts and nothing is known yet whether and to what extent a summation poisonous effect is developed from insecticides; Hauschild (1965) emphasizes that in these cases, as well as with cumulation tendency, the granting of tolerance values should not be permitted.

In comparison to the duration of organochlorine preparations with their high affinity for fatty tissue, the organophosphate esters — especially the systemically effective ones — represent a danger which is to be estimated as less.

With regard to organophosphate esters, Sinell (1967) states: "The organophosphate and carbamate esters are of little interest here, since they are — despite the high acute toxicity of especially the organophosphate esters — rapidly decomposed and inactivated so that hardly any residues may be expected in food." It remains to be proved whether these general conclusions do justice to the chemically and biologically multifariousness of effective substance from the series of organophosphate esters. This is true, at least, for the dialkyl- and arylthiophosphates, which, *in vivo* and *in vitro*, are subject to hydrolysis to alkyl- and arylphosphates * (Plapp and Casida 1958 b); this means thiophosphate derivatives are hydrolysed rapidly after *per os* application to mammals and are excreted in large amounts with the urine, to a lesser extent with the feces (Robbins *et al.* 1957, Plapp and Casida 1958 a, Krueger *et al.* 1959 a). Also, Unterstenhöfer (1968) considers the overall development as being favorable. The possibility which is given for organophosphate esters "to be able to select compounds, which have a high effect on pests but exclude a danger for mammals or, at least, prevent it by reliably realizable regulations," involves the increasingly more favorable evaluation of organophosphates with regard to their toxicity or hazard, respectively. However, this does not mean that they or their residues are harmless. The magnitude of a "danger" factor is dependent on the time of slaughter after treatment. In an extreme case, for instance, at emergency slaughtering following a treatment with organophosphate esters, the total incorporated pesticide quantity actually may still be present in the animal body. Besides, there is a discrepancy between intended therapeutical effect and pesticide level per time. What is welcome from the standpoint of

* Editors note: See Bull, D. L.: Metabolism of organophosphorus insecticides in animals and plants. Residue Reviews **43**, 1 (1972). This report was not available to the authors when the present review was written.

food hygiene may be unsatisfactory for applied therapy. LINDQUIST (1960) considered systemically effective insecticides to be of little effect for the control of flies, aphids, and ticks because such phosphate esters are excreted from the animal body within one or two days after a single treatment.

Thousands of organophosphate esters have been synthesized during the past two decades. Part of these synthesized products found application in plant protection and within the framework of general pest control. Only a small part of these is used for direct application on domestic animals. However, knowledge about absolute residue quantities in animal tissue is scanty and needs to be completed. Substances which are predominantly applied to plants have often been investigated thoroughly with regard to their metabolism and elimination from their residual quantities in the plants; however, quite often the second necessary step of investigation of these substances, that is in and on the domestic animal which can take in these substances directly or indirectly through the plants is missing. However, it has to be considered that statements about residues are dependent solely on the sensitivity of the analytical methods; in recent years some of these methods have been much refined (ANDERSON 1965). Absolute safety is guaranteed only if total freedom from residues is enforced by imposing a waiting time (minimum interval) until complete excretion of the effective substances. This imposition is unrealistic when unknown substances are taken in without control.

Further means for restricting the hazard of residues is seen in using only such organophosphate esters in the future — at least within the framework of veterinary indications — which have only a short lifetime in the organism. However, this would require application formalities for admission which exist, in Germany, only to a limited degree in so far as the regulations of the pharmaceutical law of 1961 are based on the responsibility of the manufacturer and the registration of specialities (section 20) does not allow an actual regulation. The total unclarified situation and the insecurity of residue evaluation in general have also been reflected in the differences of opinions expressed on the occasion of the FDA veterinary drug symposium in June, 1967 (see also ANONYMOUS 21). As long as absolute reports concerning residue quantities and their excretion or persistence, respectively, are not known, all statements remain suppositions. Some general considerations to this are summarized in the following list:

(1) The absolute magnitude of danger may be — with restriction — estimated from the acute toxicity. Differences in animal species, as well as differences in sensitivity of the sexes and from the dependence on the cycle for female animals, have to be included here (KAEMMERER 1963).

(2) The balance of an effective substance allows a conclusion *(à posteriori)* of the maximum remaining residue risk (brutto intake — brutto excretion = netto residual quantity).

(3) The netto residual quantity does not necessarily need to consist of the pure incorporated substance only. The danger from metabolites is

usually considered to be less; occasionally metabolites are more toxic. The quantity of metabolites is smaller than the totally introduced effective substance.

(4) The tendency for cumulation, poisonous reactions, and the property of acting eventually as a summation poison have to be considered for a judgment.

(5) It has to be proved whether an influence — in the sense of an additive or potentiating effect — by other foreign substances in the food is possible.

(6) At the present time, the extent of animal contamination and the frequency and quantity of intake from meat consumption by human beings has to be denoted as unknown. The residue quantities of organophosphate esters, which are transferred to the consumer through meat, are so small as to be neglected, if the application of pesticides to the animal took place through its food. The residue quantity in the meat of animals which have been treated for veterinary reasons and, therefore, with larger (therapeutical) quantities, is larger, depending on the elapsed time between treatment and slaughtering; however, this is restricted to individual cases and, in addition, the animals are distributed to a larger group of consumers.

(7) For routine investigations of samples taken off-hand, the detection of organophosphate ester residues in meat will, therefore, be poorly efficient, as is also seen for other foodstuffs (Heinemann *et al.* 1965 [6], Duggan *et al.* 1966 [7]) and milk (Durham 1963).

II. Data on the problem of residues

a) General comments

The individual organophosphate esters have been discussed very differently in the literature with regard to reports about residues in animal tissues [8]. In the following subsection c), the discussion of the individual compounds, which with regard to their application form belong properly to two different groups, shall be given together:

(1) The group of organophosphate esters which are applied in veterinary medicine, because the quantity of effective substance which is applied into or onto the animal is generally larger in this application section than for the accidentally collected organophosphate esters.

---

[6] Heinemann *et al.* (1965): "In the organophosphate pesticides the studies detected no residues at the established detection levels."

[7] Duggan *et al.* (1966): "No residues of organophosphorus chemicals ... at or above the quantitative sensitivity limits were found in the samples."

[8] It is known that much more comprehensive data are in the manufacturers' files and also at the registration offices than can be found in technical journals. These reports are mostly "confidential" and therefore are not available. Consequently, in the present report references can be made only to the available literature.

(2) The organophosphates, which are used (in the widest sense) for plant protection and which generally only secondarily get into the animal body.

Since the products of organophosphate esters which are listed in this group come into contact with the domestic animal only secondarily under normal circumstances, it is difficult to give the magnitudes of residues and/or their metabolites, which are approximately estimated correctly, and how much are incorporated with the plants. The absolute incorporated quantity is certainly smaller than the dosages which are applied in most test experiments for residue determinations. The residue quantity which remains in the plants can be used to a certain point for the estimation of quantity intake of the substances of the second group. One should expect that generally the (official) regulations for application have been observed in this case so that permissible tolerances may serve as a guide line. Within these groups, the presupposition for the judgment of possible remaining residue quantities is a critical valuation, and is based on the knowledge of degradation rate and metabolic pathways. For this reason, the bibliographic (available) experimental data regarding this question are also reported in this casuistic survey. However, since residue data in meat or tissue of edible domestic animals, respectively, often do not exist, data from laboratory animals has to be drawn upon for comparison. References to absolute toxicities, predominantly for laboratory animals, serve for further orientation. Details have to be taken from secondary literature.

In order to avoid a too personally emphasized selection of data, they have been taken and printed more in the sense of a casuistic report, partially from original tables from the various authors; this allows an impartial comparison, although with the danger that this casuistry occasionally may become too extensive.

b) Short remarks about the metabolism of organophosphate esters [9]

Alkylphosphates are not stored in the body (Dangschat 1965, Klimmer 1963). However, in a general reference Plapp *et al.* (1960) reported that an insecticide which has been given to test animals can either be stored as such or as its oxidation product, or it can be excreted after its decontamination. It is known that most phosphate insecticides — especially the vinylphosphates and phosdrin (Whetstone *et al.* 1966, Casida *et al.* 1958) — are decomposed and excreted rapidly by mammals. The major paths of excretion for water-soluble excretion products are with the urine and they are predominantly decontaminated degradation products of the insecticides. The pathway of excretion with the feces is of less importance. The same is true for thiophosphate derivatives (Robbins *et al.* 1957, Plapp and Casida 1958 a, Krueger *et al.* 1959 a, Plapp and Casida 1958 b).

For some dimethylphosphate amides, organic thiophosphates, and dithiophosphates, the toxically active ChE inhibitors are formed in the body by

[9] See also a survey by O'Brien (1960); for toxicology see Garner (1968).

oxidation to the O-analog (CASIDA 1956). Part of their toxic condition is dependent on a possible cumulation of these O-analogs in the organism and, also, on the degradation rate of the starting substances (of the O-analogs) in the tissues which are deactivated by hydrolases and by other degradation processes (MURPHY 1966). The liver shows a special degradation activity (DANGSCHAT 1965); it may contain 30 to 50 times more residues than muscle tissue.

MOUNTER (1963) gives a comprehensive survey concerning enzymatic hydrolysis processes of the molecules of organophosphate esters by tissue enzymes and specific (serum-) esterases; in addition, other esterases attack the alkylphosphate and arylphosphate bonds, respectively, for decontamination. Further metabolic processes correspond to the steps which are reported by CASIDA (1956) (see below). The degree of ChE inhibition, however, does not predicate anything about the quantity of substance and/or its metabolites which have remained in the tissue. Some degradation products are formed by hydrolysis, which generally goes very fast; these products no longer exhibit a specific enzyme inhibition. Hydrolysis attacks the bond between the phosphorus atom and the acid or alkyl group. With the cleavage of the alkyl bond, little (or no) toxic hydrogen phosphates are formed and which are excreted by the organism in the urine in a few hours.

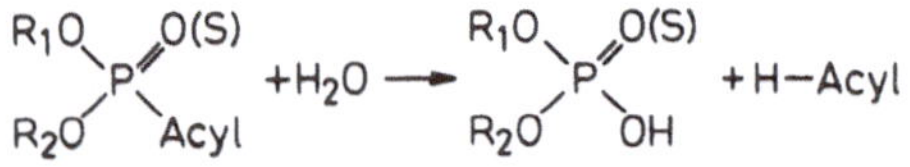

Acid residue   Basic residue

CASIDA (1956) gave the steps of chemical changes in more detail [10]:

(1) Thiophosphate oxidation

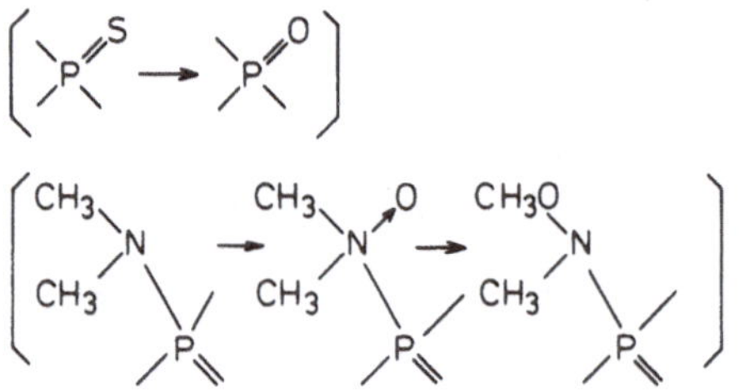

(2) Dimethylphosphoramide oxidation

(3) Thioether oxidation ($-P-OR_1SR_2$ or $-P-SR_1SR_2 \rightarrow$ sulfoxide $\rightarrow$ sulfone)

[10] For correlation between chemical configuration and toxicological effect see KODAMA *et al.* (1955) and MELNIKOV (1971) (Residue Reviews **36**, 1 ff.).

(4) Triphenylphosphate activation (possible introduction of $-OH$ and conjugate formation)
(5) Carboxyl ester hydrolysis
$(-P-OR_1C(O)OR_2 \rightarrow -P-OR_1C(O)OH+R_2OH)$
(6) Phosphoryl phosphatases $(R_1R_2P(O)X \rightarrow R_1R_2P(O)OH+HX)$

Finally, the organism decomposes phosphoric and phosphonic acid esters to dialkylphosphoric acid or to orthophosphate, respectively, which is either excreted or incorporated into the phosphorus metabolism of the body.

Since insecticides as, for instance, Co-Ral or Ruelene are decomposed to phosphoric acid and the phosphorus can be built into natural phosphorus-containing metabolites, DOROUGH and ARTHUR (1961) fed 100 p.p.m. P^{32}-phosphoric acid and O,O-diethyl thiophosphate to hens with their food ration over a period of seven days. Of these 46 or 37 percent, respectively, were excreted within two weeks. These amounts lie between the corresponding values for Co-Ral with 76 percent (DOROUGH *et al.* 1961 a and b) and Ruelene with 30 percent (BUTTRAM and ARTHUR 1961 b). Liver, bones, and kidneys incorporate more P^{32} than the other tissues. After discontinuation of test substance feeding, the concentration in the tissues decreases after one week, with the exception of the concentrations in brain, breast, thighs, and skin. The residue quantities in the tissues correspond to those of Co-Ral or Ruelene, respectively (Table XV).

Table XV. *Phosphoric and phosphorodithioic acid equivalents in tissues of laying hens fed radioactive feed* (DOROUGH and ARTHUR 1961).

Tissue	Equivalents (p.p.m.) after					
	Phosphoric acid			Diethyl phosphorodithioic acid		
	1 day	3 days	7 days	1 day	3 days	7 days
Blood	0.10	0.08	0.33	0.14	0.33	0.19
Bone	0.22	0.80	1.69	0.57	1.28	3.09
Brain	0.01	0.07	0.22	0.48	0.09	0.19
Breast	0.07	0.16	0.49	0.14	0.19	0.38
Drumstick	0.09	0.17	0.40	0.09	0.28	0.43
Fat	0.06	0.05	0.13	0.19	0.19	< 0.01
Feathers	0.02	0.02	0.05	0.66	0.09	< 0.01
Gizzard	0.20	0.44	0.75	0.08	0.41	0.16
Kidney	0.55	0.88	1.42	0.86	1.33	1.05
Liver	1.02	1.26	2.17	1.05	1.76	1.81
Skin	0.04	0.10	0.25	0.09	0.18	0.09

After phosphoric acid treatment only small amounts of radioactive substances are found in the liver (0.12 p.p.m.); they are soluble in acetonitrile. The concentration in feces is very small. After dithiophosphoric acid treatment within the food, the acetonitrile-soluble residues from the liver are also very small, while they are somewhat higher in the feces and amount to approximately one p.p.m. on the third day (Table XVI).

Table XVI. *Acetonitrile-soluble radioactive residues in liver and feces from hens receiving phosphoric acid and diethyl phosphorodithioic acid in the feed* (DOROUGH and ARTHUR 1961).

Days after treatment	Residues (p.p.m.)			
	Phosphoric acid		Diethyl phosphorodithioic acid	
	Liver	Feces	Liver	Feces
0	< 0.01	< 0.01	< 0.01	0.02
1	< 0.01	< 0.01	0.03	0.53
3	0.12	< 0.01	0.04	0.92
7	0.01	0.02	0.03	0.77
14	< 0.01	< 0.01	< 0.01	0.14

With Celite chromatography, 99 percent of the radioactive acetonitrile-soluble substances from the liver could be transferred to the methanol fraction. The methanol fraction was free of phosphoric acid, as were the water-soluble P^{32} residues from the feces. The P^{32} fractions which could not be extracted could be separated as reported in Table XVII. Phospholipids and ribonucleic acid contained the highest P^{32} quantities.

These findings give important references for the further utilization of phosphorus from metabolized insecticides of the organophosphate group.

Table XVII. *Fractionation of unextractable P^{32}-materials from feces and livers from hens receiving P^{32}-phosphoric acid in the diet* [a] (DOROUGH and ARTHUR 1961).

Substrate	Days after treatment	Total residue (p.p.m.) [b] as			
		Acid-soluble compounds	Phospholipids	RNA	DNA
Feces	0	—	—	—	—
	1	1.75	0.38	0.23	0.07
	3	1.79	0.35	0.21	0.07
	7	1.51	0.66	0.36	0.10
	14	0.09	0.02	0.00	0.00
Liver	0	0.57	0.12	0.00	0.00
	1	0.44	0.18	0.06	0.00
	3	0.46	0.26	0.09	0.01
	7	0.65	0.39	0.23	0.02
	14	0.32	0.17	0.10	0.03

[a] Hens fed P^{32}-phosphoric acid in feed at 100 p.p.m. for seven days.
[b] Averaged from four determinations at each time interval after treatment.

c) Residue data from available literature

1. ABATE. — O,O,O′,O′-Tetramethyl O,O-thiodi-*p*-phenylene phosphorothioate

Alternate names: Compound CL 52160, Abate.
Application: For mosquito and gnat control.
Toxicity: Subacute oral dosages of 1 mg./kg. body wt. which are applied over a period of one month have no effect on the ChE of mammals (LAWS *et al.* 1967); for further reports on subacute toxicity for several kinds of animals, see GAINES *et al.* (1967). Table XVIII summarizes these data.

Table XVIII. *Acute oral toxicities of Abate for mouse and rat.*

Animal species	Sex	LD_{50} (mg./kg.)	Remarks	Reference
Mouse	♂	4,700	tech. charge A	GAINES *et al.* (1967)
Mouse	—	4,000	—	LAWS *et al.* (1967)
Rat	—	2,000	pure substance	FREAR (1965)
Rat	—	4,000	—	LAWS *et al.* (1967)
Rat	♂	8,600	tech. charge A	GAINES *et al.* (1967)
Rat	♀	13,000	tech. charge A	GAINES *et al.* (1967)
Rat	♀	4,000	tech. charge B	GAINES *et al.* (1967)
Rat	♀	4,000	tech. charge C	GAINES *et al.* (1967)

Detection: With glc according to DALE and MILES (1969).
Metabolism and residues: BLINN (1969) conducted metabolism studies with H^3-Abate. The known metabolites can be elucidated as in Figure 2.

After oral application of Abate in sesame oil, the level in blood of rats reaches its maximum in five to eight hours. It decreases with a half-life of ten hours. The maximum for guinea-pigs is not as high by far as it is for rats. Two hours after treatment, 24 percent of the chloroform-soluble radio-

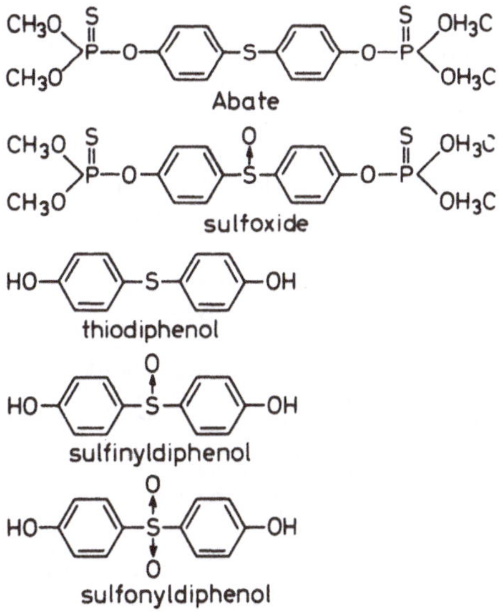

Fig. 2. Metabolites of Abate (BLINN 1969).

active parts of rat blood consists of Abate. Within 48 hours they decrease to seven percent. For guinea-pigs, Abate decreases from 12 percent after four hours to 1.4 percent after 24 hours. The water-soluble thiodiphenol increases from seven percent after two hours to 20 percent after eight hours and remains on this level for 40 hours; the sulfinyldiphenol increases from 20 percent two hours after application to 40 percent after five hours, and again decreases within 48 hours to ten percent (Blinn 1969).

The excretion of Abate takes place mainly with the urine and feces, whereby 95 percent of the radioactive material is recovered. The excretion rate with the feces is higher for guinea-pigs than for rats. Abate, its sulfoxide, and sulfinyldiphenol have beeen identified as metabolites in the feces; in addition, there are mixtures of thiodiphenol and sulfonyldiphenol recognizable on a chromatogram, as well as five not-identified components in smaller amounts (Blinn 1969).

Three major groups can be distinguished in the urine: (1) extractable substances from nonhydrolyzed urine, (2) extractable substances from urine after acid hydrolysis, and (3) nonextractable substances from hydrolyzed urine.

According to Blinn (1969), Abate, 4,4′-thiodiphenol, 4,4′sulfinyldiphenol, and 4,4′-sulfonyldiphenol are present in nonhydrolysed urine as chloroform- and ether-soluble substances. They represent 67 percent of the radioactive substances present in this fraction which, in turn, contains 17 percent of the total radioactivity of the urine. Another 74 percent of urine radioactivity is distributed on two peaks with Silica gel chromatography, after methanol-acetone extraction, while a third peak was not examined.

After acid hydrolysis, approximately 80 percent of the radioactive substances in urine can be extracted with ether and chloroform; 75 percent of these is again 4,4′-thiodiphenol, eight percent is 4,4′-sulfinyldiphenol, two percent is 4,4′-sulfonyldiphenol, and 11 percent is three components not identified. For further reports about identification of sulfuric acid ester conjugates in the urine through enzymatic influence, see Blinn (1969).

The residues in rat tissues are seen in Table XIX.

Table XIX. *Residues in rat tissues after per os application of radioactive Abate in oil* (Blinn 1969).

Tissue	Residues calculated as Abate (p.p.m.)	
	Dosage and time after intake	
	970 µg./rat, 48 hr.	1,357 µg./rat, 72 hr.
Fat	1.25	1.75
Intestines	—	0.51
Kidney	0.07	0.09
Liver	0.17	0.19
Muscle	0.03	0.02
Stomach	0.04	0.24

The residues in fat could be identified as Abate and a smaller amount as its sulfoxide.

No data exist about residues in meat of edible domestic animals.

2. AZINPHOSMETHYL. — Phosphorodithioic acid, O,O-dimethyl ester, *S*-ester with 3-(mercaptomethyl)-1,2,3-benzotriazine-4(3H)-one

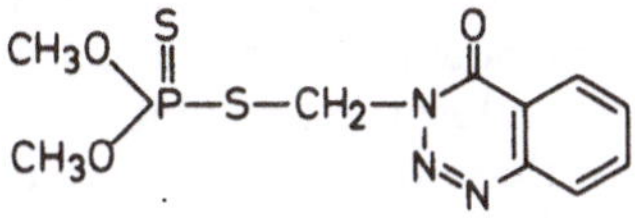

Alternate names: Guthion, Gusathion.
Application: Effective against insects on cotton; mites; long residual effect (MARTIN 1961).
Toxicity: Strong ChE inhibition after activation in the liver; toxicity dependent on the sex (DUBOIS *et al.* 1957). No mortality was caused by one mg./kg. body wt./day in the food within 60 days (MARTIN 1961). One mg./kg. a. i. *i. p.* daily for 60 days showed no special effects on rats (DU BOIS *et al.* 1957); five p.p.m. in the food over a period of 120 days were tolerated by rats without showing any effects; 20 p.p.m. given over 12 weeks did not bring forth toxic symptoms. Dogs also tolerated five p.p.m. over 12 weeks without showing any special effects (ANONYMOUS 12). Table XX summarizes these data.

Table XX. *Acute toxicities of azinphosmethyl for various animals.*

Animal species	Sex and remarks	Mode of application	Toxic dosage (mg./kg.)	LD 50 (mg./kg.)	Reference
Mouse	♂	*i. p.*	—	5,4	DUBOIS *et al.* (1957)
Mouse	♀	*i. p.*	—	3,4	DUBOIS et al. (1957)
Rat	♂	*i. p.*	—	11,6	DUBOIS et al. (1957)
Rat	♀	*i. p.*	—	5,7	DUBOIS et al. (1957)
Rat	♀	*per os*	—	16,4	DUBOIS et al. (1957)
Rat	—	*i. p.*	—	6–12	(ANONYMOUS 12)
Rat	—	*per os*	—	10–18	(ANONYMOUS 12)
Sheep	—	*per os*	max. nontoxic 12.5; min. toxic 25	—	RADELEFF & BUSHLAND (1960)
Calf	1–2 weeks	*per os*	max. nontoxic 0.1; min. toxic 0.5	—	RADELEFF & BUSHLAND (1960)

Tolerances: In the U.S.A., 0.2 to 5 p.p.m. in plants, alfalfa hay, clover hay (FREAR *et al.* 1969).
Detection: Methods are reviewed by MCDOUGALL (1964) and DUGGAN *et al.* (1967). A sensitive fluorometric method involving decomposition to the fluorescent anthranilic acid was proposed by ADAMS and ANDERSON (1966) for the investigation of Guthion residues and its oxygen analog in tissues; it detected 0.02 p.p.m. in tissue, 0.03 p.p.m. in fat. ST. JOHN and LISK (1968 b)

reported a quick sensitive glc detection method after alkaline hydrolysis of Guthion; it cannot be detected simply as such by glc because of its polarity.
Metabolism and residues: Everett *et al.* (1966) treated cows with P^{32}-Guthion *per os* in a single treatment of five mg./kg. body wt.[11], or 2.66 mg./kg. as C^{14}-Guthion[12]. Furthermore, they investigated Guthion in feed which was fed at a low dosage rate .The radioactivity in the blood increased quickly within four to six hours, and decreased markedly in the following 30 hours. However, no chloroform-soluble substance was found. Consequently, it was not Guthion or its oxygen analog in the blood. The P^{32} concentration in urine behaved analogously to that in blood. Of the total P^{32} activity, 40 percent was excreted with the urine, and 17 percent with the feces; milk contained < one percent (C^{14}). The residues were established by Everett *et al.* (1966) five days after treatment as Guthion equivalents — based on the radioactivity — as follows: brain 0.01 p.p.m., meat 0.04 p.p.m., heart 0.12 p.p.m., udder 0.14 p.p.m., kidney 0.57 p.p.m., liver 1.46 p.p.m., renal fat <0.005 p.p.m., omental fat 0.56 p.p.m., and subcutaneous fat 0.08 p.p.m. Only kidney and liver contained conspicuous parts of residues which were soluble in organic solvents; they were 0.06 and 0.1 p.p.m., respectively.

After 17 days feeding of 1.4 p.p.m. Guthion in the food, residues in all tissues were 0.1 p.p.m., determined by fluorimetry. In muscle 0.02 p.p.m. was found, with 0.03 p.p.m. in kidney and fat, and 0.05 p.p.m. in liver.

There is no essentially no hazard for animals from intake of green fodder which is contaminated with two p.p.m. of Guthion and the residues in meat tissues are correspondingly low.

3. AZODRIN. — Phosphoric acid, dimethyl ester, ester with *cis*-3-hydroxy-*N*-methyl crotonamide

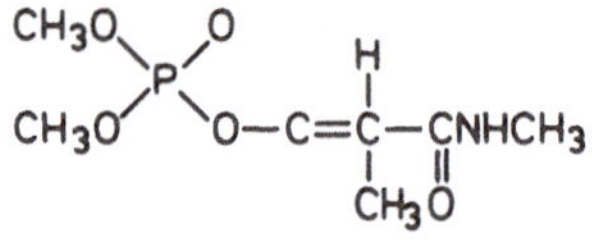

Alternate names: Shell SD 9129, SD 9129.
Application: Insecticide used predominantly in cotton fields; effective both as contact and as systemic poison.
Toxicity: See Table XXI.

Table XXI. *Acute oral toxicity of Azodrin for the rat.*

LD 50 (mg./kg.)	Reference
23	Frear (1965)

[11] Corresponding to 69.5 p.p.m. in the daily ration.
[12] Corresponding to 37 p.p.m. in green fodder.

Metabolism and residues: The decomposition of Azodrin is mainly through hydrolysis at the vinylphosphate and also at the methylphosphate bonds. The metabolism of Azodrin is similar to that of Bidrin (see Bidrin). The metabolic path way of Azodrin with respect to the individual steps for rats, insects, and plants is in Figure 3.

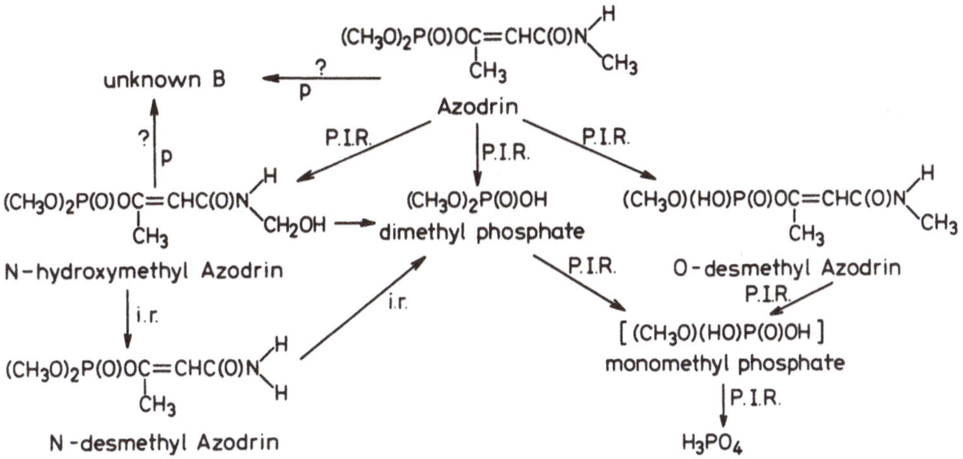

Fig. 3. Proposed composite pathway of Azodrin metabolism: *P* and *p*, in cotton plants; *I* and *i*, in insects; and *R* and *r*, in rats; capital letters indicate major pathways, lowers case letters indicate minor pathways (LINDQUIST and BULL 1967).

After intraperitoneal injection of five mg./kg. body wt. P^{32}-Azodrin, rats excreted 45 percent within six hours. Of these, 46 percent was hydrolysis products and 20 percent methylol derivates. After 24 hours, 58 percent was excreted with the urine and five percent with the feces. Only traces of *N*-desmethyl-Azodrin appeared (BULL and LINDQUIST 1966) (Table XXII).

No special residue data for meat from edible domestic animals are reported in the available literature.

4. BIDRIN. — Phosphoric acid, dimethyl ester, ester with *cis*-3-hydroxy-*N*,*N*-dimethylcrotonamide

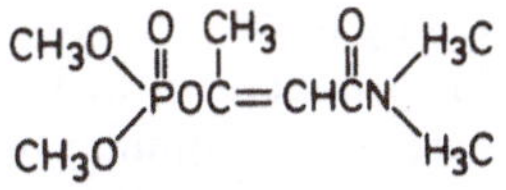

Alternate names: SD 3562, ENT 24/482.
Application: Short-term systemic insecticide against phytopathogenic insects and mites. The technical product consists of 85 percent *cis*- and eight percent *trans*-isomers.
Toxicity: See Table XXIII.

Table XXII. *P^{32} Azodrin and its metabolites in excreta of rats after i. p. injection* [a] (BULL and LINDQUIST 1966).

Hours after treatment	μg. P^{32} Azodrin equivalents of indicated products					
	H_3PO_4	Dimethyl phosphate	O-Desmethyl Azodrin	Hydroxy-methyl Azodrin	Azodrin	Dose excreted (%)
			Urine			
0–2	3.5	89.2	37.7	62.6	152.9	23.1
2–4	2.8	49.4	15.2	38.5	48.8	10.3
4–6	6.0	88.9	14.7	33.9	27.7	11.4
6–8	2.5	39.1	7.1	11.4	11.3	4.8
8–10	1.2	20.6	3.3	5.4	4.8	2.4
10–12	0.7	10.3	1.7	1.9	2.2	1.1
12–24	4.7	46.0	8.7	10.3	9.3	5.3
24–48	7.1	19.5	2.4	3.7	3.8	2.4
			Feces			
0–24	2.6	16.9	15.2	10.1	31.3	5.1
24–48	0.4	6.5	0.9	1.3	1.2	0.7

[a] 5 mg./kg.

Table XXIII. *Acute oral toxicity of Bidrin for rats.*

LD_{50} (mg./kg)	Reference
25	BULL & LINDQUIST (1964)
45	BRADY *et al.* (1960)

Detection: See GIANG and BECKMANN (1969).
Tolerances and restrictions: In the U.S.A. regulated earlier as "Group 4", "zero tolerance", or "no residue" (FREAR *et al.* 1969).
Metabolism and residues: A scheme for the metabolism of Bidrin is in Figure 4. The hydrolysis of the vinyl phosphate bond is the most important degradation step, which leads to dimethyl phosphate.

Rats decontaminated Bidrin very quickly. BULL and LINDQUIST (1964) established 83 percent of the radioactive material in the form of dimethyl phosphate in the urine 20 hours after *s.c.* injections of ten mg./kg. P^{32}-Bidrin. After 24 hours only traces were found in the urine. After two hours there were the rapidly decreasing hydroxymethyl-Bidrin, *N*-methyl Bidrin, Bidrin, and mainly hydrolysis products in the urine. After 24 hours 627 μg. of P^{32}-Bidrin equivalents were water soluble; only 51 μg.-equiv. were excreted with the feces (BULL and LINDQUIST 1964).

MENZER and CASIDA (1965) reported further detailed data for the excretion of Bidrin. The highest excretion rate in urine was reached in six hours for rats; 71 percent excretion in the urine was opposed by six percent in the feces. A survey is given in Table XXIV from which it can be seen that only a very small part of radioactive substances was soluble in chloroform, the largest part of which was Bidrin itself.

Table XXIV. *P^{32}-Bidrin metabolites in urine of various animals 48 hours after treatment* [a] (MENZER and CASIDA 1965).

Animal species	Mode of application	Percent of P^{32}-treatment							
		Total excretion	Products of hydrolysis	*cis*-$(CH_3O)_2P(O)OC(CH_3){=}CHC(O)R$ where R is					
				$N(CH_3)_2$	$N(CH_2OH)CH_3$	$NHCH_3$	$NHCH_2OH$	NH_2	Methanol fraction
Mouse	*i. p.*	71.7	57.0	1.2	0.43	9.9	1.0	0	2.2
Rat ♂	oral	70.1	60.5	2.8	2.8	3.0	0.35	0	0.68
Rat ♀	oral	64.5	53.1	3.2	0.08	5.3	0.09	0	2.7
Rabbit	*i. p.*	72.1	67.7	1.0	0.18	2.8	0.04	0.04	0.36
Dog	oral	97.6	92.2	0.76	0.28	3.3	0.31	0	0.77
Goat [b]	oral	0.05	0.02	0.001	0	0.01	0	0.003	0.01
Goat [c]	oral	10.6	7.8	0.1	0	1.5	0.16	0.53	0.48

[a] One mg./kg.
[b] Zero to one hour.
[c] One to two hours.

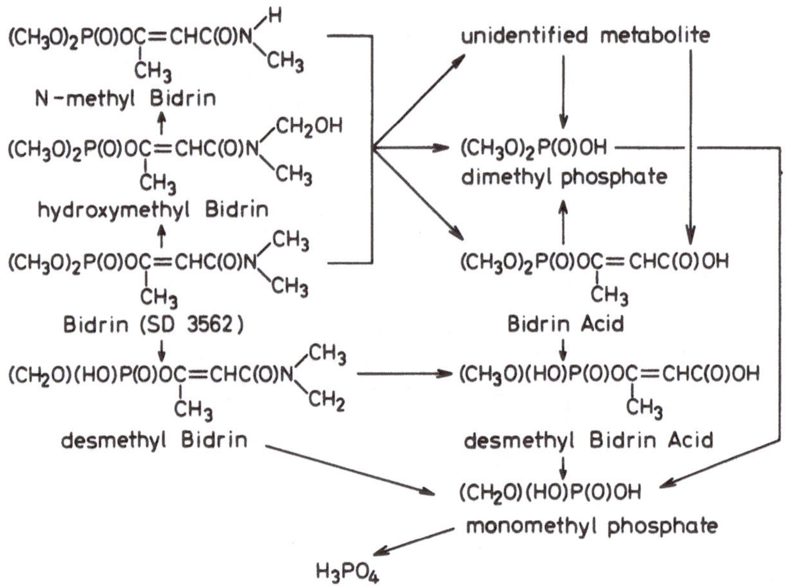

Fig. 4. Tentative pathway for the formation of phosphorus-containing metabolites of Bidrin (Bull and Lindquist 1964).

Forty-eight hours after treatment with one mg./kg. P^{32}-Bidrin, 0.05 p.p.m. Bidrin equivalents were found in blood, 0.29 p.p.m. in the femur, 0.04 p.p.m. in the brain, zero p.p.m. in omental fat, 0.05 p.p.m. in the heart, 0.62 p.p.m. in the liver, 0.34 p.p.m. in the kidney, and 0.01 p.p.m. in the muscle, calculated from the radioactivity present (Menzer and Casida 1965).

After oral Bidrin treatment the excretion rates for goats were as shown in Table XXV.

There are no special reports about detectable residues in edible tissues from mammals; according to the above findings the quantities should be

Table XXV. *Excretion of P^{32}-Bidrin and metabolites for goats after oral application* (Menzer and Casida 1965).

Elapsed time (hours)	Excretion (%)		
	1 mg./kg. dosage	2 mg./kg. dosage	1 mg./kg. dosage P^{32}- and *N*-methyl C^{14}-Bidrin [a]
4	21	4	27
8	55	45	56
16	72	65	78
72	78	82	90

[a] For differences in excretion rates of P^{32} and C^{14}, see original.

immaterial because of the fast metabolism and excretion of the effective substance.

5. BROMOPHOS. — Phosphorothioic acid, O,O-dimethyl O-(4-bromo-2,5-dichlorophenyl) ester

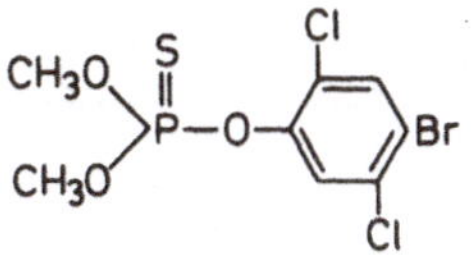

Application: Insecticide against storage and hygiene pests such as beetles, chinch bugs, Diptera, etc, and fly control in stables.

Veterinary application: Dip against *Lucilia sericata* with a dosage-dependent residual effect for nine weeks in the fleece. Applicable against *Chrysomia chlorophyga, Melophagus ovinus, Mallophages,* and *Anoplura (Damalinia).* Inner application with 50 mg./kg. against *Oestrides* (bot larvae); effective against ticks and mites (ANONYMOUS 10).

Application dosage to animal: From 0.01 to 0.5 percent for outside application; 50 mg./kg. *per os* for cattle (bot flies).

Toxicity: The oral compatibility of bromophos is seen from Table XXVI. Bromophos exhibits only a light, indirect ChE inhibition (STIASNI *et al.* 1967).

Residues: The fate of bromophos in test animals was investigated by STIASNI *et al.* (1967) with P^{32}- or H^3-substance; it was given *per os* in ten mg./kg. quantities to rats, whose stomachs had been empty for 24 hours. Bromophos is easily resorbed by the intestine and is eliminated from blood with a half-life value of 14 hours. After 12 hours, P^{32} activities were found in the stomach and small intestine (2.3 percent), large intestine (3.2 percent), liver (2.9 percent), and kidneys (0.9 percent), but the excretion is almost complete after 24 hours without showing a cumulation in the organs. Excretion occured mainly with the urine; after 24 hours 57.6 percent of the P^{32}-material appeared there, and 95.9 percent of the H^3-bromophos. The corresponding values in the feces were 13.7 and 1.0 percent, respectively. Approximately 80 percent of the radioactivity was eliminated through the urine and feces. The remains of the radioactive inorganic phosphorus were transferred to the phosphate pool of the body.

The phenolic moiety of bromophos was also very rapidly and almost quantitatively eliminated with the urine, as shown with H^3-bromophos (STIASNI *et al.* 1967). Bromophos, bromooxon, or monodesmethylbromooxon were not found in the urine. Decontamination took place through hydrolysis of the methylphosphate and/or phenylphosphate bond. After intake of P^{32}-bromophos five metabolites were found, with three after H^3-bromophos intake. The metabolites were more hydrophilic than bromophos; they were phosphate, dimethylthionophosphate, monodesmethyl bromophos, and dichlorobromophenol, while two others were not identified.

Table XXVI. *Acute oral toxicities of 97.0 to 98.5 percent pure bromophos for various animals* (Kinkel *et al.* 1966).

Animal species and sex	Max. dosage without clear clinical symptoms (mg./kg.)	Min. dosage with clinical symptoms (mg./kg.)	Min. dosage with fatalities (mg./kg.)	LD_{50} (mg./kg.)
Rat ♂	1,000	< 2,000	2,000	3,750–4,000
Rat ♀	1,000	< 2,000	4,000	6,100
Mouse ♂	500	~ 1,000	2,000	3,700–5,850
Mouse ♀	—	—	—	2,829
Guinea pig ♂	—	1,000	—	~ 1,500
Rabbit ♂	300	< 600	600	720
Dog ♂ + ♀	175	350	—	—
Cat ♂	1,250	—	—	—
Cat ♀	—	500	750	—
Kitten ♂ + ♀	100	200	—	—
Chicken ♀	250	500	< 8,000	9,700
Pig ♂ + ♀	500	1,000 [a]	—	—
Sheep ♂ + ♀	80	160	1,500 [b]	—
Goat ♀	100	—	—	—
Calf ♂	73–111	—	—	—
Cow ♀	300	400	800 [b]	—
Horse?	400 [b]	800 [b]	(400+400)	—
Honey bee 1 [c]	—	—	—	18.8–19.4
2 [d]	—	—	—	4.7

[a] Sick animal.
[b] One animal.
[c] Effective substance.
[d] 40 percent emulsion (Beran and Stute, private communication).

After *per os* treatment of pregnant rats with 20 mg. of bromophos/kg. body wt., Ackermann and Engst (1970) found 30 minutes after treatment 1,555 ng./g. in the liver tissue, and in the brain, liver, and muscle of the fetus correspondingly 350, 500, and 465 ng./g. of tissue. Only traces of bromooxon were found in the fetal muscles.

Clark *et al.* (1966) did not observe any poisonous effects, aside from a negligible ChE inhibition, in a chronic test: sheep were bathed weekly over a period of nine weeks in a dip of 0.5 percent bromophos (25 percent EC) in xylene-Triton X-100. After cleanup with Celite and chloroform, uptake in petroleum ether, and partitioning into acetonitrile-saturated petroleum ether, averages of 9.8, 2.5, and 3.0 p.p.m. were found after one, eight, and 22 days, respectively, in the omental fat, with glc detection. No special differentiation of bromooxon was undertaken.

6. CARBOPHENOTHION. — Phosphorodithioic acid, *S*-[*p*-chlorophenyl)thiomethyl] O,O-diethyl ester

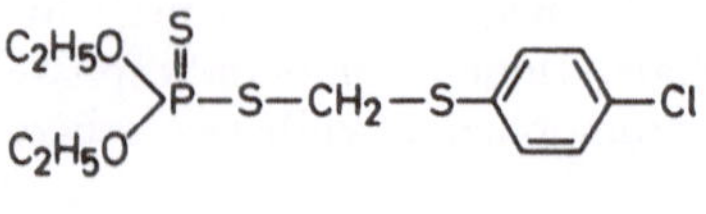

Alternate names: Trithion, Stauffer R 1303.
Application: Insecticide against ectoparasites, acaricide.
Application to the animal: Sheep-dip 0.021 to 0.042 percent against ectoparasites such as blowflies, lice, and keds (TREEBY 1967).
Toxicity: See Table XXVII.

Table XXVII. *Acute toxicities of carbophenothion for various animals.*

Animal species	Mode of application	Toxic dosage	LD_{50} (mg./kg.)	Reference
Rat	*per os*	—	18	BRADY *et al.* (1960)
Sheep	*per os*	— [a]	—	MCCARTHY *et al.* (1967)
Calf	spray	0.05 percent	—	YOUNGER *et al.* (1963)
Cow	spray	1.00 percent [b]	—	YOUNGER *et al.* (1963)

[a] 5 mg./kg. without symptoms.
[b] Suspension.

Detection: For Trithion see MENN *et al.* (1964); for methyl-Trithion see BATCHELDER *et al.* (1964) and DUGGAN *et al.* (1967).
Tolerances: In the U.S.A., 0.2 to 2.0 p.p.m. in plants; 5.0 p.p.m. in fresh alfalfa, alfalfa hay, and clover; zero in milk; and 0.1 p.p.m. in fat and meat of cattle, goats, sheep, and pigs (FREAR and FRIEDMAN 1968).
Metabolism and residues: Depending on the season, external residues remain in the fleece for more than eight to ten weeks; however, no reports about residues in animal tissue are available.

7. CHLORFENVINFOS. — Phosphoric acid, 1-(2,4-dichlorophenyl-2-chlorovinyl O,O-diethyl ester

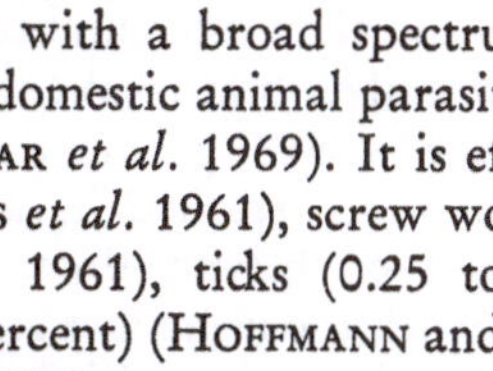

Alternate names: GC-4072, ENT 24969.
Application: Insecticide with a broad spectrum and long residual effect (GRAHAM 1961) against domestic animal parasites; also applicable in stables and chicken houses (FREAR *et al.* 1969). It is effective against bot-flies (0.1 to 0.5 percent) (ROBERTS *et al.* 1961), screw worms *(Callitroga hom.)* (0.25 percent) (WRICH *et al.* 1961), ticks (0.25 to 0.5 percent) (DRUMMOND 1961 b), and lice (0.25 percent) (HOFFMANN and DRUMMOND 1961).
Toxicity: See Table XXVIII.
Detection: With glc after acid hydrolysis of chlorfenvinfos into trichloroacetophenone (five p.p.b.) (CLABORN and IVEY 1965).

Restrictions and tolerances: In the U.S.A., "zero tolerance" or "no residue" regulated as "Group 4" (FREAR *et al.* 1969).
Metabolism and residues: C^{14}-chlorfenvinfos was quantitatively excreted by rats within four days, with 87.2 percent in urine, 11.2 percent in feces, and 1.4 percent in breath. The excretion was 67.5 percent after the first day of treatment (HUTSON *et al.* 1967). Ninety-four percent of C^{14}-labelled material was excreted by the dog in urine and feces within four days; 86 percent was in urine within 24 hours. The metabolism for dogs and rats was so complete that no intact chlorfenvinfos was excreted in urine. The different metabolites in urine are in Table XXIX.

Table XXVIII. *Acute toxicities of chlorfenvinfos for various animals and different applications.*

Animal species	Mode of application	Toxic dosage (mg./kg.)	LD_{50} (mg./kg.)	Reference
Rat	*per os*	—	10	HUTSON *et al.* (1967)
Rat	*per os*	—	13	FREAR (1965)
Guinea pig	*per os*	100	—	DRUMMOND (1960)
	s. c.	50	—	DRUMMOND (1960)
Cattle	*per os*	max. 10 tolerable	—	RADELEFF *et al.* (1961)

Table XXIX. *Metabolites of chlorfenvinfos in the urine of dogs and rats* (HUTSON *et al.* 1967).

Compound	Percent of chlorfenvinfos dosage in	
	Rat	Dog
2-Chloro-1-(2′,4′-dichlorophenyl)vinylethyl hydrogenphosphate	32.3	69.6
[1-(2′,4′-Dichlorophenyl)ethyl-β-D-glucopyranoside] uronic acid	41	3.6
1-(2,4-Dichlorophenyl)-1-hydroxyacetic acid	7	13.4
2,4-Dichlorophenylethandiol glucuronide	2.6	2.7
1-(2,4-Dichlorobenzoylamino)acetic acid	4.3	—

The metabolism of chlorfenvinfos in dogs and rats is in Figure 5.

The resorption pathway causes differences in quantities. IVEY *et al.* (1966) referred to unpublished data from CHAMBERLAIN and HOPKINS, in which two to five times more chlorfenvinfos and its metabolites were found in the blood and urine of cattle after oral intake than after dermal application. CHAMBERLAIN and HOPKINS (1962) proved the very fast dermal resorption with P^{32}-chlorfenvinfos, which reached its maximum after only two hours. The amount of radioactive substance decreased rapidly in the blood. Excretion took place mainly with the urine and reached 25 to 32 percent of the applied dosage after seven days, of which more than half was found after 24 hours. The excretion with the feces was 1.6 to 2.0 percent, which is obviously smaller than with urine. However, most of the nine to ten radio-

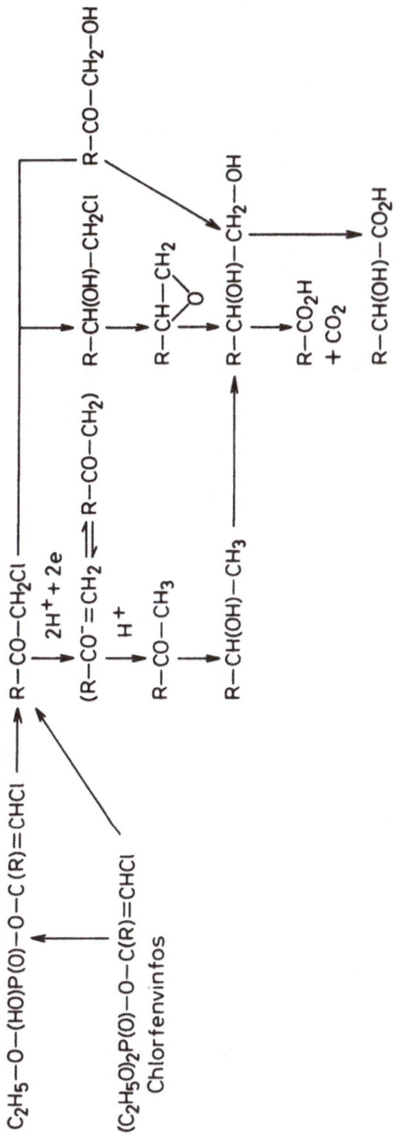

Fig. 5. Chlorfenvinfos metabolism in dogs and rats (Hutson *et al.* 1967); R equals

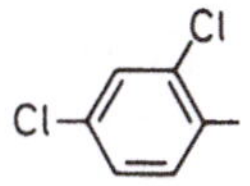

active metabolites which were found in the urine after dermal application remain unidentified; on a chromatogram two to 14 percent corresponded to dimethyl phosphoric acid, 0.4 to 7.0 percent to diethyl-1-methyl-2-chlorovinyl phosphate; two further fractions which made up 49 and 44 percent, respectively, remain unknown.

IVEY *et al.* (1966) found practically no residues (<0.004 p.p.m.) after seven days in muscle, heart, kidney, and liver of cattle which had been sprayed with P^{32}-labelled substance in a 0.25 percent emulsion. After a spray with a 0.5 percent emulsion, the residue concentrations in muscle, heart, and kidney were 0.008, 0.015, and 0.008 p.p.m., respectively. The maximum residue value in fat was not yet reached after one day. The threshold value was on the third day, and afterwards the concentrations rapidly decreased until seven days after treatment. After 15 days, no residue could be established any more. The survey in Table XXX is an attempt to bring together the results of the different test series of IVEY *et al.* (1966) for omental fat. Also, with repeated sprays, the residues in fat remained small. They reached their maximum (0.161 p.p.m.) after the eighth of weekly treatments (0.1 percent). After a corresponding treatment with two-week intervals, the maximum residue value in fat was reached after the fifth spray with 0.247 p.p.m. [13]

Table XXX. *Survey of chlorfenvinfos in omental fat of cattle after spray application* (IVEY *et al.* 1966).

Spray concentration (%)	Residue (p.p.m.) after					
	1 day	3 days	7 days	15 days	16 days	28 days
0.05	—	0.060	0.001	0	—	—
0.25	0.355	—	0.036	—	—	—
0.25	—	—	0.085	—	0.006	< 0.005
0.25	—	0.675	0.055	0	—	—
0.50	—	—	0.223	—	—	—

Apparently detectable residues which are present only in fat were eliminated after 28 days. 2,2,4′-Trichloroacetophenone was not established in fat as a metabolic product.

The following data are important for comparison. Five hours after a spray with five g. of effective substance in 400 or 60 ml., respectively, the largest quantities which were found in milk are those fractions which were soluble in organic solvents. The residues disappeared after ten to 12 days (ROBERTS *et al.* 1961); the values for practical dosages remained small indeed (CLABORN *et al.* 1965).

ROBINSON *et al.* (1966) investigated the behaviour of chlorfenvinfos residues in sheep after a dip or a "tipspray", respectively. The sensitivity of the method was 0.003 p.p.m. No trichloroacetophenone was discovered in fat after a 0.05 percent w/v chlorfenvinfos treatment; after a dip with 0.1 percent w/v concentration no residue of chlorfenvinfos was found in organ tissues after seven days, and also the level of trichloroacetophenone was below the limit of detectability. The highest residue amounts did not exceed

[13] The author points to factors such as fleece, licking, etc. to explain the different residue quantities (intake, excretion).

0.1 p.p.m. in the fat; all residues in the organs were <0.003 p.p.m. Average residue values are reproduced in Table XXXI.
Supplementary remark: Thirty-seven to 53 percent (mashed potatoes), and 56 to 80 percent (mashed cabbage), respectively, of chlorfenvinfos were hydrolyzed during cooking of vegetables for 30 minutes (ASKEW *et al.* 1968).

Table XXXI. *Average residues in body fat of sheep after chlorfenvinfos treatment* (ROBINSON *et al.* 1966).

Treatment	Residues (p.p.m.) after			
	3 days	7 days	14 days	21 days
0.05% Dip	0.011	0.015	0.004	0.009
0.1% Dip	—	0.016	0.004	0.003
0.2% Tip-spray	—	< 0.003	0.003	0.004
Control	< 0.003	—	—	0.003

8. CIODRIN. — Crotonic acid, 3-hydroxy-α-methylbenzyl ester dimethyl phosphate

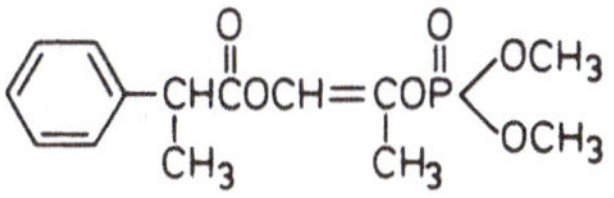

Alternate names: Ciodrin, SD 4294, ENT 24717.
Application: Against insects on domestic animals as face-flies spray, larvae control in feces.
Toxicity: See Table XXXII.

Table XXXII. *Acute oral toxicities of ciodrin for rat and rabbit.*

Animal species	LD_{50} (mg./kg.)	Reference
Rat	125	EICHLER (1965)
Rabbit	384	FREAR (1965)

Detection: See WESTLAKE *et al.* (1969 a and b).
Metabolism and residues: After *per os* treatment with radioactive Ciodrin (579.4 mg./28.4 kg. of a 66 percent product with α- and β-isomers), the maximum level in blood of sheep was established after six hours, based on total radioactivity. However, the largest quantity of chloroform-extractable substances was found after one hour (27 percent) (CHAMBERLAIN 1964 a). After six hours the chloroform extract contained 87 percent dimethylphosphoric acid. Two further unknown components appeared with 11.4 percent of the total activity, while <0.5 percent appeared as SD 4294. The rapid excretion and more rapid decomposition at the P=O−C bond corre-

sponded to the rapid resorption. Likewise, in the urine the maximum total radioactivity was reached after six hours and approximately 79 percent of total substance was excreted within 48 hours. Another approximately 7.3 percent appeared in the feces after 48 hours. Of the radioactive material in the urine, 61 to 90 percent was dimethylphosphoric acid. Further products such as crotonic acid and its derivatives were small. Ciodrin itself appeared only in very small quantities in the urine. Chamberlain (1964 a) reported, with reference to Claborn, the concentration in tissues from sheep as 0.4 p.p.m. for liver and kidney and 0.03 p.p.m. each for fat, muscle, and heart.

The following values were measured after dermal application (spray with an emulsion of 99.2 percent α-substance, 106.8 mg./animal) by Chamberlain (1964 b) in goats. After two hours radioactivity was established in the blood which reached a maximum after four hours and then decreased. The total radioactivity in blood reached only 0.5 percent. Approximately 11 percent of the applied quantity after *per os* treatment of sheep was excreted with the urine, whence it follows that only part of the substance penetrated through the skin into the body. The prevailing metabolite in the urine was, as for sheep, dimethylphosphoric acid with 80 to 91 percent of the radioactive material; however, after dermal application some metabolites which were found in sheep urine were missing in goat urine (compare purities of test substance). Only 0.12 percent of the applied spray appeared in the feces.

9. COLEP. — O-phenyl-O′-(4-nitrophenyl) methylphosphonothionate

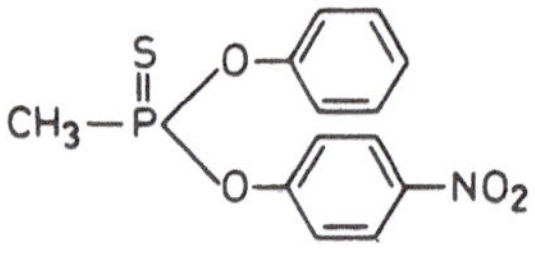

Trade product: Colep.
Application: No longer in use.
Toxicity: See Table XXXIII.

Table XXXIII. *Acute oral toxicity of colep for the rat.*

Sex	LD_{50} (mg./kg.)	Reference
♀	3.0 (2.5–3.5)	Marco & Janowski (1964)
	8.0 (5.25–12.5)	Kelly, cited from Marco & Janowski (1964)
♂		

Metabolism and residues: Marco and Janowski (1964) investigated the metabolism in rats with C^{14}-Colep after *per os* treatment. Rats which received 0.45 and 1.19 mg./kg., respectively, excreted 79 and 68 percent, respectively, of radioactive substances with the urine after 24 hours. The decontamination and excretion process in the tissue ran down within 24 hours. The liver as a decontamination organ and the kidney as an excretion organ contained only small quantities of radioactivity. After 24 hours, liver contained 1.4 to 3.3 percent of radioactive material in the aqueous extraction phase, and 0.1 to 0.3 percent in the chloroform; in the kidney it corresponded to 0.2 to 0.6 percent and zero percent, respectively, and abdominal fat zero percent; 0.7 to 2.0 percent and 0.6 to 0.7 percent, respectively, were found in the feces. The excretion products were identified after TLC and separation with ion-exchange resins as being polar molecules, which give phenol after acid hydrolysis.

10. COROXON. — Phosphoric acid, O-(3-chloro-4-methyl-cumarinyl-7) O,O-diethyl ester

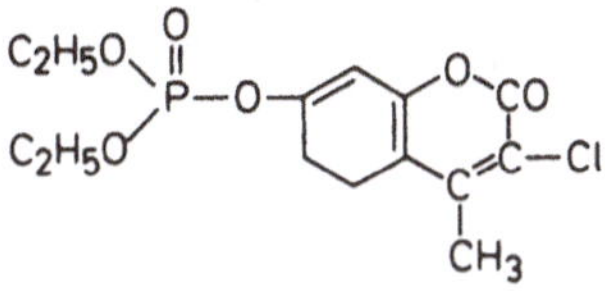

Toxicity: See Table XXXIV.

Table XXXIV. *Acute oral toxicity of coroxon for the rat.*

Toxic dosage (mg./kg.)	LD_{50} (mg./kg.)	Reference
—	10	SCHRADER (1963)
Min. lethal dosage 20 [a]	—	MALONE (1962)
—	30 [b]	MALONE (1962)

[a] 20 percent WP.
[b] Two percent solution in polyethyleneglycol.

Metabolism and residues: Coroxon was resorbed through the skin, which can be demonstrated from the behaviour of ChE activity (MALONE 1962). P^{32}-Coroxon (six mg./kg.), given *per os* in mixture with phenothiazine, was 90 percent excreted with the urine and feces within four to six days; 64 percent and 72 percent left in six and eight days, respectively, with the urine, and 28 percent and 20 percent, respectively, with the feces. However, the major excretion ratio lay in the first 48 hours after treatment.

Ninety-seven percent of the urine radioactivity came from the water-soluble metabolites of Coroxon (PLAPP and CASIDA 1958 c); in particular it was 90 percent diethylphosphoric acid. In the feces 20 to 25 percent of the radioactive materials were water soluble, of which approximately half behaved as Coroxon itself, meaning only two to three percent unchanged Coroxon was present in the feces. Coroxon residues were found by MALONE (1962) in the tissues of sheep after application of six mg. of Coroxon/kg. of body wt.; they were <0.5 p.p.m., calculated as Coroxon from the radioactivity. After six and eight days, respectively, 0.9 and 3.6 p.p.m. were found in the spleen; 1.9 and 1.5 p.p.m., respectively, in the kidney; and 4.0 and 5.0 p.p.m., respectively, in the liver. Five percent of the radioactive material present corresponded to Coroxon and was found in the liver, meaning there was not more than 0.25 p.p.m.; the remainder were metabolites.

11. COUMAPHOS. — Coumarin, 3-chloro-7-hydroxy-4-methyl-, O-ester with O,O-diethyl phosphorothioate

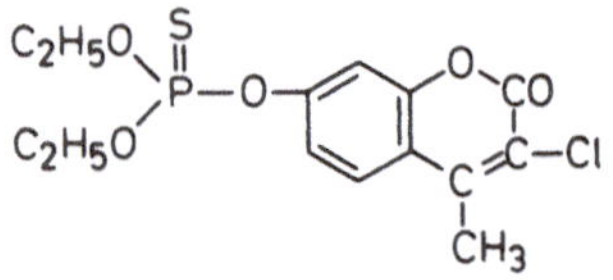

Alternate names: Resitox, Muscatox, Bayer 21/199, Co-Ral.
Application: Insecticide, good effect against flies.
Veterinary application: Outside application against ectoparasites of domestic animals as dip (BEHRENZ *et al.* 1959), spray or pour-on (ADKINS *et al.* 1963, DRUMMOND and GRAHAM 1962) especially against bot-fly attack (SMITH and RICHARDS 1954), back rubber application (ALLEN 1966), dust bath for poultry, and inner application against worms, for instance, in the stomach and intestines of ruminants (HERLICH and PORTER 1958, LEVINE *et al.* 1956, GALVIN *et al.* 1959). In South Africa, the mixture with trichlorphon as anthelminticum was also common. The dosage range for inner application was approximately 25 mg./kg. body wt. for cattle and sheep. For outer application insecticide concentrations of 0.01 to 0.05 percent were used. After outside application there was a considerable residual effect in the fleece of sheep over a period of 14 weeks (BEHRENZ *et al.* 1959). Application of 0.25 percent coumaphos on the skin was protective for three weeks against the turkey mite, *Neoschongastia americana* (DISCHBURGER *et al.* 1969).
Toxicity: See Table XXXV. Coumaphos was resorbed by the animal body not only with *per os* application. BEHRENZ *et al.* (1959) proved the penetration through the cutis with ChE inhibition. After oral intake, coumaphos was not systemically effective (ADKINS *et al.* 1963, KAPLANIS *et al.* 1959 a). During dusting hens proved to be less sensitive toward one percent dust than chickens toward 0.25 percent dust (KRAEMER 1959).
Detection: McDOUGALL (1964); colorimetrically, see CLABORN *et al.* (1960 b). ANDERSON *et al.* (1959) described a procedure — aside from detection with P^{32}-labelled substance — for residues in animal tissue which made use of photofluorimetry and reached a sensitivity for coumaphos and

Table XXXV. *Acute toxicities of coumaphos for various animals.*

Animal species	Mode of application	Toxic dosage (mg./kg.)	LD_{50} (mg./kg.)	Remarks	Reference
Rat	*per os*	—	56–230	tech. product	ANONYMOUS 7
Rat	*per os*	—	20	1:1 in corn oil:acetone	VICKERY & ARTHUR (1960)
Rat	*per os*	—	90–110	as Resitox	KLOTZSCHE (1955)
Rat	*s.c.*	—	285	1:1 in corn oil:acetone	VICKERY & ARTHUR (1960)
Guinea-pig	*per os*	max. sublethal 25	—	—	ROBBINS *et al.* (1959 b)
Cattle	*per os*	max. nontox. 25 min. tox. 50	—	—	RADELEFF & BUSHLAND (1960)
Sheep	*per os*	max. nontox. 15 min. tox. 25	—	—	RADELEFF & BUSHLAND (1960)
Rat [a]	*per os*	—	11	1:1 in corn oil:acetone	VICKERY & ARTHUR (1960)

[a] Treated with coroxon (q. v.) for comparison.

coroxon down to 0.02 p.p.m.; for detection of the related Potasan [14], see GUNTHER and BLINN (1955), BERG *et al.* (1956), RAHN (1962), and BOWMAN *et al.* (1968).

O'BRIEN (1960) pointed out explicitly with regard to methodology that according to KRUEGER *et al.* (1959 a) the chloroform extraction of coumaphos from tissues was difficult and led to losses; he referred to a personal communication from McDOUGALL which says that with the use of acetone and benzene more than 90 percent can be regained. DOROUGH *et al.* (1961 a) then recommended subsequent extraction with *n*-hexane and acetonitrile. CLABORN and RADELEFF (1960) mentioned that the values obtained in the organs (e. g., liver and kidney) by radioactivity measurements were higher than those which were chemically determined. This indicates that with the first method phosphorus-containing degradation products are also detected.

Tolerances and restrictions: Treated animals should not be slaughtered until 60 days after the spray (ANONYMOUS 11); ADKINS *et al.* (1963) considered a "safe" slaughtering 45 days after treatment. Furthermore, in the U.S.A. there is a tolerance of one p.p.m. for meat, meat products, and fat from cattle, sheep, goats, pigs, horses, and poultry (FREAR *et al.* 1969). BÄR (1964 a) required a waiting time of 45 days after bathing or spraying with coumaphos.

Metabolism and residues:

α) General. Coumaphos was rapidly degraded in the organism into several metabolic products which were predominantly excreted as water-soluble metabolites with the urine or feces. The liver was highly responsible for the decomposition (O'BRIEN and WOLFE 1959). Types and amounts of metabolites were strongly dependent on the mode of application. A survey of those metabolites which were found in the mammal is in Figure 6.

The cleavage of the P – O-ethyl group seemed to be important for coumaphos, and an opening of the lactone ring was assumed to occur in dependence on pH in the alkaline range (pH 8.0 to 8.5 in the urine of ruminants); however, VICKERY and ARTHUR (1960) did not find any indication for an alkaline decomposition in biological systems. DOROUGH *et al.* (1961 b) established no opening of the lactone ring for poultry and, moreover, they could not isolate a "desethyl-Co-Ral". Furthermore, hydrolysis also occured in the P – O-phenyl group (PLAPP *et al.* 1960 b). The degradation extended to phosphoric acid. ROBBINS *et al.* (1959 a) assume, especially for degradation after dermal application, that an enzymatic hydrolysis to more polar compounds took place, namely to diethylthiophosphoric acid and diethylphosphoric acid. The latter could be formed by enzymatic

[14] Potasan:

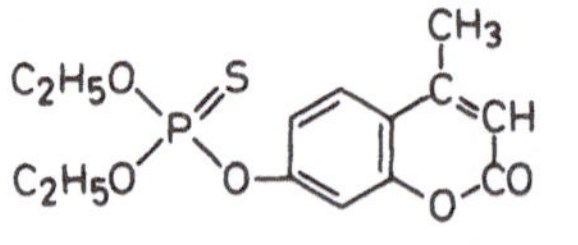

Rat *per os:* LD_{50} 15 mg./kg. (PERKOW 1956) or 20 mg./kg. (1:1 in corn oil:acetone) (VICKERY and ARTHUR 1960).

oxidation, either before or after hydrolysis. One part of the insecticide was completely decomposed to organic phosphorus, which then entered the general metabolic pool and was used for the synthesis of normal phosphorus-containing compounds. Aside from residues of unchanged coumaphos, the only other toxically effective metabolite in animal tissues was coroxon (KRUEGER, cited by ANDERSON *et al.* 1959). 3-Chloro-4-methyl-7-hydroxy-coumarin was formed by hydrolysis. Essential to the accuracy and the limit of detection was the extraction system. LINDQUIST *et al.* (1958) reported, for instance, that in rat tissues after 24 hours 1.3 to 2.3 percent of a coumaphos activity were detectable in the liver, 0.2 percent in the kidney, 0.1 percent in the urine, and only traces in the feces. Thus, the rat organism rapidly excreted coumaphos or decomposed it to nontoxic cleavage products.

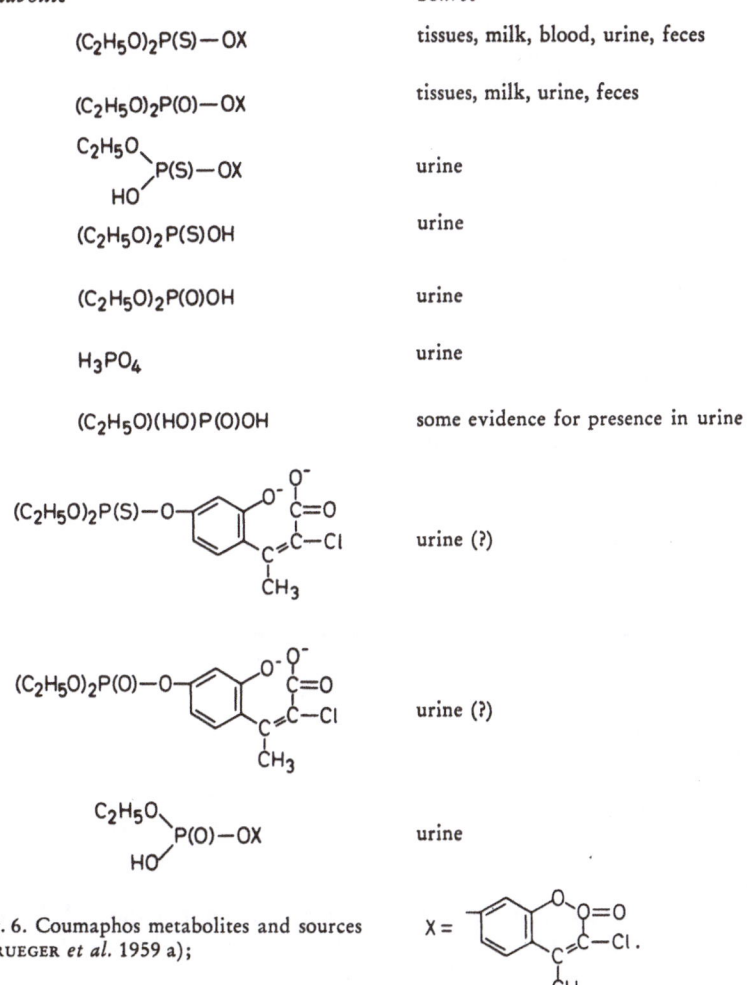

Metabolite	*Source*
$(C_2H_5O)_2P(S){-}OX$	tissues, milk, blood, urine, feces
$(C_2H_5O)_2P(O){-}OX$	tissues, milk, urine, feces
$(C_2H_5O)(HO)P(S){-}OX$	urine
$(C_2H_5O)_2P(S)OH$	urine
$(C_2H_5O)_2P(O)OH$	urine
H_3PO_4	urine
$(C_2H_5O)(HO)P(O)OH$	some evidence for presence in urine
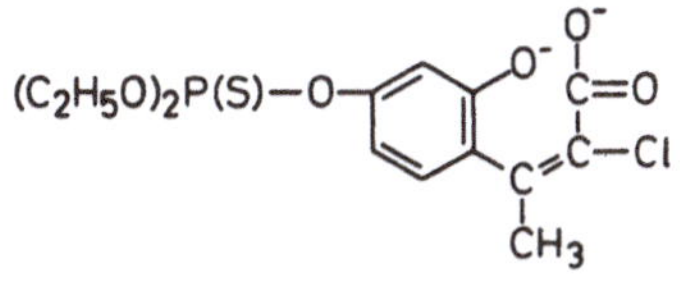	urine (?)
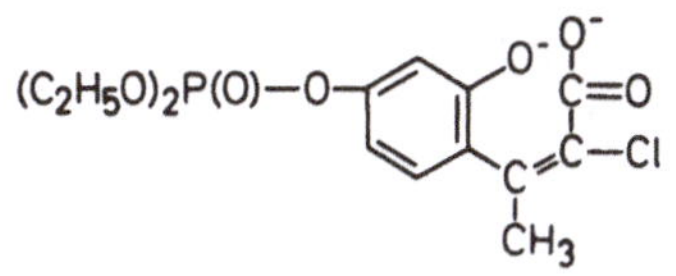	urine (?)
$(C_2H_5O)(HO)P(O){-}OX$	urine

Fig. 6. Coumaphos metabolites and sources (KRUEGER *et al.* 1959 a);

X = 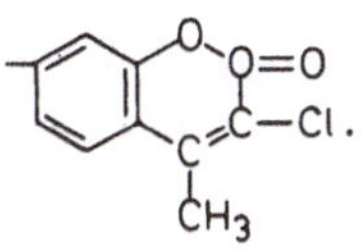

The decontamination processes should not be generalized and transferred from one animal species to another. The liver, which generally is a decontamination organ, is an activation system; indeed, in mice it made coumaphos more poisonous, while in rats and cattle it was mainly decomposed. An activating mechanism, which originates in the liver microsomes, competed with a degrading mechanism in cattle, whereby the latter was more effective. It follows from this that these animals were more resistent to coumaphos (O'Brien and Wolfe 1959). Indeed, there were specific metabolic pathways for coumaphos for each species which are important for the judgment of residues, exactly as the coming together with other substances which may cause changes that, at first, they may become apparent by a higher toxic ratio. The synergistic effect of piperonyl butoxide should be mentioned in this connection, as described by Robbins *et al.* (1959 b). The latter inhibited the enzymatic hydrolysis of coumaphos to more polar degradation products. The substances finally excreted were mostly hydrolysis products, aside from residual coumaphos, coroxon, and a methanol fraction. The concentrations of metabolites were dependent on the mode of application; for instance, the amount of coroxon in the urine of rats was larger after *per os* treatment than after dermal application (Vickery and Arthur 1960). The hydrolysis products after *per os* treatment were identified by these authors as: O-ethylphosphoric acid, O,O-diethylphosphoric acid, and O,O-diethylthiophosphoric acid. These three hydrolysis products appeared at about the same ratio in the urine after dermal application, while after *per os* treatment the diethylthiophosphoric acid prevailed in the urine. With regard to the excretion of coumaphos, O'Brien (1960) collated a table from reports of Krueger *et al.* (1959 a), presented here in a slightly altered form as Table XXXVI.

Table XXXVI. *Excretion of coumaphos by rats* (O'Brien 1960).

Description	Percent excreted			
	Days after treatment	Application (mg./kg. body wt.)		
		per os 50	*s.c.* 40	*dermal* 45
Excretion in urine and feces	4	45	28	10
Excretion in urine and feces	14	52	45	20
Portion of the O,O-diethylphosphorothioate in the urine excretion products	—	65	75	33
of diethylphosphate	—	10	20	33
of phosphoric acid	—	10	0	33
of desethyl-coumaphos	—	15	5	0
Total excretion in the feces	14	33	20	20
Portion of coumaphos or coroxon	—	55	17	55

β) Remarks concerning dermal resorption: Coumaphos showed, for external application, a remarkable residual effect against insects (Graham

1961). This effect was tantamount to the presence of outside-applied effective substances so that a longer lasting source of contamination existed for the animals. This fact caused a factor of uncertainty for the judgment of absolute quantities. The time factor with regard to contamination and possible (uncontrolled) intake did not allow a clear judgment. The lipid solubility of coumaphos allowed a limited passage through the skin. For the same reason, a certain affinity for body fat was to be expected (CLABORN *et al.* 1960 a); however, the quantities which were resorbed by the cutis were small (KAPLANIS *et al.* 1959 a). Also, for chicken a cutaneous resorption of very slight extent was described. The degradation of resorbed substance was fast (DOROUGH *et al.* 1961 a). The degradation after dermal application and resorption corresponded to that after oral treatment (DOROUGH *et al.* 1961 b). The time factor for resorption was conspicuous, for it pointed to the importance of a possible later resportion. VICKERY and ARTHUR (1960), for instance, found a time factor with a maximum of P^{32}-activity in rabbit blood after 24 hours for dermally applied coumaphos; for *per os* treatment, the maximum was reached shortly after application. None of the substances which appeared in the blood could be extracted with chloroform, which pointed to the fast decomposition of coumaphos.

VICKERY and ARTHUR (1960) estimated the rate of coumaphos resorption for rats as $<$ ten percent. After dosages of 100 mg./kg. body wt. only 3.74 percent was excreted with the urine and 1.85 percent with the feces; indeed, after dermal application of coumaphos only fractions of the applied dosage appeared in the urine (PLAPP *et al.* 1960 b). Also, the blood level remained low, but there was only light resorption through the skin. PLAPP *et al.* (1960 b) reported blood level values for cattle after dermal application of 37-to-52 and 40 mg./kg. body wt. which became <0.035 and 0.015 p.p.m., respectively, after 120 hours. The maximum value for dermal application was, with reference to other authors, reported as 0.27 p.p.m. for cattle. According to further reports by KRUEGER *et al.* (1959 a), the blood level of cattle reached its maximum for coumaphos with 0.2 p.p.m. on the sixth day after treatment, and for coroxon with 0.015 p.p.m. on the fifth day, after dermal application of 40 mg./kg. body wt. For goats the dermal application of 30 mg./kg. body wt. showed two maxima after six hours and five days, respectively; however, the blood level was less than 0.004 p.p.m.

γ) Excretion and residues in rat: Rats excreted more metabolic products with the urine than with the feces (VICKERY and ARTHUR 1960). After *per os* treatment, coumaphos was quickly changed into water-soluble compounds and excreted. The excretion speed and ratio gave an indication for the residue quantities possibly remaining in the different tissues. After a *per os* treatment of white rats with 20 mg./kg. of P^{32}-coumaphos (LINDQUIST *et al.* 1958), 78 percent showed within 24 hours as water-soluble metabolites in the urine, and 2.5 percent in the bile; 7.6 to 16 percent were found in the feces. VICKERY and ARTHUR (1960) established for rats, after a ten mg./kg. *per os* treatment, an excretion rate of 54.7 percent in the urine and 14.5 percent in the feces within seven days. VICKERY and ARTHUR (1960) reported about the different tissue residues in rats and, for comparison, in rabbits, after different modes of application (these data are found in Table XLII, No. 1 and 3).

According to Krueger *et al.* (1959 a), rats excreted, especially after dermal application with 45 mg./kg. body wt., four percent with the feces and urine after one day, 11 percent after four days, 16 percent after seven days, 22 percent after 14 days, and 25 percent after 28 days, of the total applied quantity. After *s.c.* treatment with 40 mg./kg. or oral treatment with 50 mg./kg., two-thirds of the applied dosage was eliminated with the urine within 18 or 14 days, respectively. The metabolites in the totally present radioactivity of the urine were distributed according to the individual modes of application (Table XXXVII).

Table XXXVII. *Distribution of coumaphos metabolites in the urine of rats after different modes of application* (Krueger *et al.* 1959 a).

Compound [a]	Distribution (%)			
	Coumaphos		Coroxon	
	50 mg./kg. *per os*	40 mg./kg. *s.c.*	45 mg./kg. *dermal*	20 mg./kg. *per os*
Diethylthiophosphoric acid	50–80	~50–80	+	—
Phosphoric acid	10–20	none	+	50
Diethylphosphoric acid	10–20	~20–40	+	10
Desethylated coumaphos and/or coroxon	5–30	10	none	40

[a] Coumaphos metabolites after 96 hours, coroxon metabolites after 24 hours.

After *s.c.* application the feces contained 17 percent, and after oral and dermal application 50 to 60 percent of radioactive substances read as coumaphos or coroxon. The quantitative residue data in bodies of rats, which were found by Krueger *et al.* (1959 a) after dermal application of coumaphos, are reported in Table XLII, No. 2. The concentrations reached two maxima, namely four to six hours after application, and four to seven days later.

δ) Excretion and residues for domestic animals:

αα) Per os treatment. Numerous investigations have been conducted for cattle. All of these closely considered practical application. Residue data were extensive and were reported in separate tables. The blood level for cattle after oral treatment with 20 mg. of coumaphos/kg. body wt. was 0.02 p.p.m. after 12 hours (Plapp *et al.* 1960 b; cf. Krueger *et al.* 1959 a and Robbins *et al.* 1959 a). The corresponding values after *per os* treatment with ten and 20 mg./kg. body wt. P^{32}-substance reached their maximum in blood of cattle after ten hours with 0.44 and 0.88 microequiv./ml., respectively. In the latter case, the activity was still 0.14 after five days and 0.08 after seven days, while after treatment with ten mg./kg. body wt. it reached zero after 84 hours (KAPLANIS *et al.* 1959 a). KAPLANIS *et al.* (1959 a) also followed up the excretion for cattle after P^{32}-coumaphos treatment. The maxima in the urine were reached after 30 hours with 16.48 percent after ten mg./kg. *per os*, and with 18.97 percent after 20 mg./kg. After 96 hours 32.29 and 36.36 percent, respectively, and after seven days 34.92 and 37.54 percent, respectively, were excreted. Of the excretion products in urine 25 to 26 percent were unknown; about 20 percent was diethylphosphoric acid, and 53 percent was diethylthiophosphoric acid.

The excretion with the feces began four hours after *per os* intake and reached its highest rate after 36 hours with about 17 percent. Of the substances which were excreted with the feces, 56 percent consisted of coumaphos, 32 percent coroxon, and 12 percent polar degradation products. The total excretion after calculation of values was about 26 percent after one day and about 71 percent after four days.

According to PLAPP *et al.* (1960 b), cattle excreted in urine and feces the same quantities of substance after oral intake of P^{32}-coumaphos (approx. 34 percent). The quantities in question were largely unchanged substance in the feces, which pointed to a relatively little resorption through the intestinal wall.

Milk cows, which received oral coumaphos for fly larvae control in the feces, excreted coumaphos and small amounts of Potasan [14], but not coroxon (BOWMAN et *al.* 1968). Because of relatively fast excretion, 2.6 percent of effective substance was found the day after intake in muscles and fatty tissues (ANONYMOUS 7). Only a small amount of effective substance was found in the liquid parts such as blood, lymph, and bile.

Special residue data which were obtained after oral application of coumaphos are summarized in Table XLII.

ββ) Dermal application. For understandable reasons of application mode, the analytical data concerning the behaviour of coumaphos after outside application dominate. Although considerable quantities of unchanged substance remained on the body cover, according to ROBBINS *et al.* (1959 a), after spray treatment of bulls with 1.5 percent EC or WP formulation, respectively, with P^{32}-coumaphos, only small quantities were resorbed. The blood level remained low; however, it was approximately four times higher with a maximum of 0.27 p.p.m. after six days, after application of the EC, than for WP treatment. The isopropyl ether extractives did not behave like the original substances.

The excretion took place through the urine (ROBBINS *et al.* 1959 a), which also has low values in correspondence to the low resorption rate. In 14 days 2.4 percent of the applied dosage after WP treatment, and 6.3 percent after EC treatment, were excreted. The maximum of excretion was on the seventh (WP) or sixth day (EC), respectively. After chromatography only traces of the radioactive material from the urine behaved like unchanged substance; 42 percent corresponded to the $\mathbf{R}_f$-value for diethylthiophosphoric acid, and 18 percent to the one for diethylphosphoric acid; the remainder consisted of more polar degradation products. The P^{32}-level in the feces was low. The highest radioactivity of tissues was found in liver and kidney. After WP treatment, more than half of it fell on the phosphoprotein fraction, and 20 and 24 percent, respectively, on the water-soluble phosphates. Only liver and kidney contained distinct radioactivity, which was soluble in organic solvents (see Table XLII, No. 5).

There were mostly hydrolysis products in liver and kidney and only traces (<0.02 microeq./g.) behaved like unchanged coumaphos, of which the highest content was about 0.1 microeq./g. in *s.c.* fatty tissue after spray with suspension. The enzymatic hydrolysis also led, aside from the mentioned products — for instance, after oxidation to coroxon — to the release of inorganic phosphorus, which again was built into other phosphorus-containing compounds in the bodies of cattle.

Table XXXVIII. *Fractionation of radioactive phosphorus in the liver and kidney of suspension-treated animals* (ROBBINS *et al.* 1959 a).

Fraction	Total P^{32} (%) in	
	Liver	Kidney
Acid-soluble phosphate	20.2	23.9
Phospholipid	11.8	18.7
Nucleic acid	1.5	5.2
Phosphoprotein	66.5	52.2

Also, KRUEGER *et al.* (1959 a) reported about investigations on cattle and goats after spray treatment. After dermal application, the excreted substances in the urine of cows were predominantly hydrolysis products. After one week 99.9 percent of the radioactive material was found in the urine. The maximum excretion for goats was reached after three days. The distribution is seen in Table XXXIX.

Table XXXIX. *Distribution of metabolites of P^{32}-coumaphos in urine and feces after dermal application* (KRUEGER *et al.* 1959 a).

Substrate	Cow (40 mg./kg.)		Goat (30 mg./kg.)	
	%	Remarks	%	Remarks
Urine				
Phosphoric acid	36	0.25–7 days	25	3—4 days
Diethylphosphoric acid	17	—	18	—
Diethylthiophosphoric acid	29	—	37	—
(with desethylated product)	(18)	—	(20)	—
Coumaphos	2.1	up to 6 hr. (Coumaphos and Coroxon)	1.2	3rd day
Coroxon	0.9		1.8	—
Feces				
Coumaphos	32	6 days	31	6 days
Coroxon	6	—	1.6	—

Reports by KRUEGER *et al.* (1959 a) concerning the residues of metabolites after dermal application to cows and goats are summarized in Table XLII. Here, the values in bones are striking. ALLEN (1966) found no residues in tissues seven days after a 0.5 percent spray. PLAPP *et al.* (1960 b) established the largest quantity of insecticide with 0.11 p.p.m. in the subcutaneous fatty tissue two weeks after a spray treatment with 52 mg./kg.; six weeks after dermal application of 40 p.p.m., the residues in all tissues were <0.06 p.p.m. CLABORN and RADELEFF (1960) reported the following colorimetrically determined residues in tissues for cattle, sheep, and goats:

After seven days of 0.5 percent spraying: 0.25 and 0.4 p.p.m. in omental fat
Two days after six weeks of 0.25 percent spraying: 0.07 p.p.m. in omental fat
After two weeks of 0.5 percent spraying: no residues in fat
Four weeks after three twice-weekly 0.5 percent spraying: no residues in fat, liver, kidney, and muscle

After pour-on application in white oil (paraffin oil), coumaphos residues were fluorophotometrically determined by ADKINS *et al.* (1963); the highest of the generally low residue values were found in the back fat seven days after treatment with 0.07 p.p.m. (Table XLII, No. 7).

The back-rubber application of one percent coumaphos in diesel oil for 28 days did not lead to any residue formation in tissues during this time (ALLEN 1966).

ε) Metabolism and residues for poultry: After oral application of 100 p.p.m. of coumaphos in the feed over seven days, laying hens excreted after one day 35 percent, after two days 66 percent, and after seven days 75 percent of the applied quantity (cumulative). After discontinuation of application, the radioactive substances in the feces decreased rapidly and 28 days after the start of treatment 79 percent had been excreted. The excretion products of the first seven days consisted of 85 to 91 percent of hydrolysis products, while four days after discontinuation of treatment the entire radioactive material in the feces came from hydrolysis products (DOROUGH *et al.* 1961 b). The excretion ratio corresponded to the reported amount of 76 percent within two weeks for excretion by hens (DOROUGH and ARTHUR 1961).

If the radioactive substances in the feces of laying hens one to seven days after treatment were fractionated, the water-soluble portions varied from 31 to 34 percent and the chloroform-soluble portion varied from seven to 22 percent. In the latter the major part was coumaphos, while coroxon only reached < one percent. The water-soluble portion contained mono- and diethylphosphoric acid, as well as diethylthiophosphoric acid (DOROUGH *et al.* 1961 b).

During oral application of P^{32}-phosphoric or diethylthiophosphoric acid the residue concentrations increased in proportion to the duration of application. The highest concentrations were found in liver, kidney, and bones. One week after discontinuation of application the residue quantities decreased, except for brain, breast muscle, thigh, and skin. However, the residue concentrations were of approximately the same order as after application of P^{32}-phosphoric acid or its diethyl ester derivatives, respectively (Dorough and Arthur 1961).

The quantitative residue data established for individual tissues after oral treatment are found in Table XLII, No. 13. Liver and kidney contained the highest concentrations, which decreased very rapidly after discontinuation of insecticide application, however. The residues in fat and skin were small. After changing to insecticide-free feed, no toxic residues could be established in the tissues (Dorough *et al.* 1961 b). Fractionation gave the results in Table XL.

Table XL. *Acetonitrile-soluble radioactive materials in tissues of laying hens fed radioactive coumaphos mixed in the feed at 100 p.p.m.* [a] (Dorough *et al.* 1961 b).

Tissue [b]	Radioactive materials (p.p.m.) [c]				
	Days on radioactive feed			Days on normal feed	
	1	3	7	3	7
Blood	< 0.02 [d]	0.03	0.03	< 0.02	< 0.02
Breast	0.02	0.03	0.02	< 0.02	< 0.02
Drumstick	< 0.02	0.03	< 0.02	< 0.02	< 0.02
Fat	< 0.02	0.03	0.02	< 0.02	< 0.02
Gizzard	0.05	0.03	0.05	0.04	< 0.02
Kidney	0.14	0.15	0.12	0.07	< 0.02
Liver	0.05	0.09	0.10	0.04	< 0.02
Skin	0.03	< 0.02	< 0.02	< 0.02	< 0.02

[a] Compare also total contents in Table XLII, No. 13.

[b] The brain and feathers contained no acetonitrile-soluble radioactive materials during the experiment; no tissue contained acetonitrile-soluble radioactive materials after the hens were returned to normal feed for 14 to 21 days.

[c] Averaged from three hens sacrified at each time-interval with duplicate analyses/tissue.

[d] 0.020 p.p.m. = sensitivity of analytical method.

After dusting with 50 mg./kg. coumaphos, hens excreted with the feces approximately 11 percent after a single treatment and 27 percent after two treatments with a weekly interval, within 28 days after the first or second treatment, respectively. More than half of it appeared within the first 24 hours. Fractionation resulted in coumaphos, coroxon, diethylphosphoric, and diethylthiophosphoric acid. Coroxon reached < one percent of the total radioactive material. Most of the non-extractable P^{32}-substances were present in the acid-soluble or phospholipid fraction, respectively (Table XLI).

Knapp (1962) found no residues in inner organs after daily dusting with 0.02 g. a.i./hen with a 0.5 percent powder. Zero to 0.04 p.p.m. residues were found in meat five days after the last treatment. With six hens, the residue quantity after 12 days was 0.08 p.p.m. in the meat. The corresponding control samples showed blank values of up to 0.02 p.p.m. DOROUGH *et al.* (1961 a) found after one or two times dusting a rapid decrease in P^{32}-concentration on skin and feathers. The highest radioactivities were recorded in liver and kidney. Breast- and thigh muscles reached negligible values three days after a single and seven days after a two-time treatment. The relatively high P^{32}-content of bones was due to the incorporation of

Table XLI. *Acetonitrile-soluble radioactive materials in tissues of laying hens dusted with P^{32}-coumaphos* [a] (DOROUGH *et al.* 1961 a).

Days after treatment	Radioactive materials (p.p.m.) [b] in				
	Feathers	Gizzard	Kidney	Liver	Skin
One application					
1	603	0.04	0.04	0.05	1.53
3	252	0.02	0.03	0.02	0.93
7	89	< 0.02	< 0.02	< 0.02	0.36
10	88	< 0.02	< 0.02	< 0.02	0.37
14	24	< 0.02	< 0.02	< 0.02	0.09
21	26	< 0.02	< 0.02	< 0.02	0.15
28	2.7	< 0.02	< 0.02	< 0.02	0.09
Two applications					
7	87	0.03	0.04	0.03	0.84
14	55	< 0.02	< 0.02	0.03	0.83
21	36	< 0.02	< 0.02	< 0.02	0.20
28	6	< 0.02	< 0.02	< 0.02	0.18

[a] One percent Co-Ral dust applied May 15 and May 22, 1959 at approx. 50 mg./kg.

[b] Blood, brain, breast, drumstick, and fat contained less than 0.02 p.p.m. except the drumstick (0.03 p.p.m.) and fat (0.04 p.p.m.) on the first day after one dust application and the breast (0.03 p.p.m.) at seven days following the second application.

coumaphos which had been degraded to inorganic phosphorus (see Table XLII, No. 12).

Acetonitrile-soluble radioactive substances from the inner organs were negligible three days after treatment (DOROUGH *et al.* 1961 a). These acetonitrile-soluble residues were only a very small part of the total P^{32}-residues. The non-extractable P^{32}-substances which remained in the tissues were acid-soluble components, phospholipids, ribonucleic acid, and desoxyribonucleic acid.

Remarks for evaluation: No apparent deviation from taste was recognized by ADKINS *et al.* (1963) in the muscles of cattle after *per os* treatment; also, BROGDON *et al.* (1962), after 0.5 percent coumaphos treatment of cattle, did not observe any deviation from taste on "rib cuts", "round steak", and kidneys, but there was a significant, although light, coloring of the liver.

Table XLII a. *Summary of literature for residue studies after application of coumaphos* (see also Table XLII b).

No.	Animal species	Mode of application	Dosage	Detection method	Reference
1 a	rat	oral	10 mg./kg.	P^{32}, incl. metabolites	VICKERY & ARTHUR (1960)
1 b		dermal	100 mg./kg.		
2	rat	dermal	45 mg./kg.	P^{32}	KRUEGER *et al.* (1959 a)
3 a	rabbit	oral	10 mg./kg.	P^{32}, incl. metabolites	VICKERY & ARTHUR (1960)
3 b		dermal	100 mg./kg.		
4 a	cattle	spray	58 mg./kg.	P^{32}	CLABORN & RADELEFF (1960)
4 b		spray	25 mg./kg.		
4 c		oral	20 mg./kg.		
4 d		oral	10 mg./kg.		
5 a	cattle	dermal emul.	51.9 mg./kg.	P^{32}	ROBBINS *et al.* (1959 a)
5 b		dermal susp.	37.1 mg./kg.		
6	cattle	dermal emul.	0.75%	P^{32}	KRUEGER *et al.* (1959 a)
7 a	cattle	pour-on	7.5 g. a.i. in 375 ml.	photofluorimetry	ADKINS *et al.* (1963)
7 b		pour-on	5.0 g. a.i. in 250 ml.		
8 a	calf	spray (0.5%)	25 mg./kg.	photofluorimetry	CLABORN *et al.* (1960)
8 b		spray (0.5%)	58 mg./kg.		
9	goat	dermal	30 mg./kg.	P^{32}	KRUEGER *et al.* (1959 a)
10 a	goat	spray	not reported	P^{32}-ext. 95% EtOH + Skellysolve B	ANDERSON *et al.* (1959)
10 b	goat	spray	not reported	P^{32}-ext. 95% EtOH + benzene	
10 c		spray	not reported	$CHCl_3$ + benzene	
10 d		spray	not reported	acetone + benzene	

11 a	laying hens	oral [a]	0.5 mg./kg. daily for 10 days	photofluorimetry	Shaw *et al.* (1964)
11 b		oral [a]	1.0 mg./kg.		
11 c		oral [a]	2.5 mg./kg.		
11 d		oral [a]	5.0 mg./kg.		
11 e		oral [a]	25.0 mg./kg.		
11 f		oral [a]	1.0 mg./kg. daily for 7 days	photofluorimetry	
11 g		oral [a]	5.0 mg./kg.		
11 h		oral [a]	1.0 mg./kg.		
11 i		oral [a]	5.0 mg./kg.		
11 k		oral [a]	1.0 mg./kg.		
11 l		oral [a]	5.0 mg./kg.		
11 m	laying hens	dust in straw	5%	photofluorimetry	Shaw *et al.* (1964)
11 n		spray on straw	25% WP		
12	laying hens	dusting	50 mg./kg. 1 appl.	P^{32}	Dorough *et al.* (1961 a)
13	laying hens	with feed for 7 days	100 p.p.m. (approx. 1.5–2.5 mg./kg. body wt.)	P^{32}	Dorough *et al.* (1961 b)

[a] 50 percent French powder in capsules.

Table XLII b. *Summary of literature on residue values after application of coumaphos* (see also Table XLII a).

No.	Residue (p.p.m.) in										Remarks
	Liver	Kidney	Brain	Heart	Muscle (Flank and leg)	Skin, etc.	Fat				
							Flank	Back	Renal	Omental	
1 a	3.25	1.53	0.14	0.46	0.32	0.27	—	0.20	—	—	after 3 days
	0.86	0.52	0.17	0.25	0.13	0.53	—	0.05	—	—	after 7 days
1 b	2.80	1.85	0.28	0.44	0.56	2.65	—	0.89	—	—	after 3 days
	4.63	1.62	0.25	0.58	0.37	0.99	—	1.10	—	—	after 7 days
2	0.2 *a*	—	—	—	—	186 *a*	—	2.8 *a*	—	—	after 1/2 day
	0.4 *b*	1.2	0.2	0.2	—	16 *b*	—	0.4 *b*	—	—	
	2.7 *c*	—	—	—	—	457 *c*	—	1.6 *c*	—	—	
	0.4 *a*	—	—	—	—	222 *a*	—	2.4 *a*	—	—	after 1 day
	0.7 *b*	2.9	0.3	0.6	—	11 *b*	—	0.4 *b*	—	—	
	4.2 *c*	—	—	—	—	473 *c*	—	— *c*	—	—	
	0.5 *a*	—	—	—	—	154 *a*	—	2.0 *a*	—	—	after 2 days
	1.8 *b*	3.8	0.6	0.9	—	12 *b*	—	0.3 *b*	—	—	
	7.2 *c*	—	—	—	—	408 *c*	—	1.7 *c*	—	—	
	0.2 *a*	—	—	—	—	94 *a*	—	1.4 *a*	—	—	after 4 days
	1.0 *b*	3.9	0.7	1.6	—	8.8 *b*	—	0.2 *b*	—	—	
	7.4 *c*	—	—	—	—	189 *c*	—	1.4 *c*	—	—	
	0.4 *a*	—	—	—	—	34 *a*	—	— *a*	—	—	after 7 days
	1.7 *b*	1.7	0.8	1.5	—	1.7 *b*	—	2.0 *b*	—	—	
	8.4 *c*	—	—	—	—	64 *c*	—	— *c*	—	—	
	< 0.04 *a*	—	—	—	—	5.7 *a*	—	— *a*	—	—	after 14 days
	0.8 *b*	1.2	0.7	0.6	—	0.5 *b*	—	1.0 *b*	—	—	
	3.7 *c*	—	—	—	—	16 *c*	—	— *c*	—	—	
3 a	1.77	0.41	0.06	0.07	0	0.05	—	0	—	—	after 3 days
	2.26	0.61	0.07	0.08	0.02	0.14	—	0	—	—	after 7 days
3 b	1.15	1.26	0.18	0.20	0.04	—	—	0.11	—	—	after 3 days
	1.89	1.92	0.15	0.39	0.17	—	—	0.27	—	—	after 7 days

4 a	0.48	0.21	—	—	0.01	—	—	—	0.03	0.04	after 14 days
4 b	0.35	—	—	—	0.00	—	—	—	0.10	0.13	after 7 days
4 c	0.40	0.40	—	—	0.02	—	—	—	trace	0.01	after 14 days
4 d	1.35	1.96	—	—	0.04	—	—	—	trace	0.08	after 7 days
5 a	10.8	23.4	0.41	—	0.31	—	—	—	—	—	after 2 weeks [d]
	0.13	0.43	—	—	—	—	s.c. 0	—	0	0	
	12.0	4.5	—	—	—	—	—	—	—	—	
5 b	4.12	3.26	0.19	—	0.08	—	—	—	—	—	after 2 weeks [d]
	0.03	0.09	—	—	—	—	0.14	—	0	0	
	12.1	8.1	—	—	—	—	78.6	—	—	—	
6	1.22	0.96	0.2–0.5	0.2–0.5	0.2–0.5	— [e]	< 2	—	—	—	after 8 weeks
	0.23	0.42	0.13	0.11	0.05 [f]	—	0.16 [i]	—	0.16	0.16	— [j]
	0.02	0.04	0.01	0.02	0.04 [g]	—	0.06 [i]	—	0.05	0.05	
	0.67	0.34	0.1	0.22	0.18 [h]	—	0.03 [i]	—	0.06	0.01	non-extract. CH_3CN
7 a	0.01	0.01	0.04	0.01	0.03	—	0.05	0.07	0.04	0.06	after 7 days
	< 0.01	< 0.01	< 0.01	< 0.01	0.02	—	< 0.02	< 0.02	< 0.02	< 0.02	after 14 days
	< 0.01	< 0.01	< 0.01	< 0.01	< 0.01	—	0.05	< 0.02	< 0.02	< 0.02	after 28 days
	< 0.01	< 0.01	< 0.01	< 0.01	0.01	—	< 0.02	< 0.02	< 0.02	< 0.02	after 42 days
7 b	< 0.01	0.01	< 0.01	< 0.01	0.01	—	0.02	0.02	< 0.02	0.04	after 7 days
	< 0.01	< 0.01	< 0.01	< 0.01	0.03	—	0.03	0.05	< 0.02	0.03	after 14 days
	< 0.01	< 0.01	< 0.01	< 0.01	0.01	—	< 0.02	< 0.02	< 0.02	< 0.02	after 28 days
	< 0.01	< 0.01	0.02	< 0.01	0.01	—	< 0.02	< 0.02	< 0.02	< 0.02	after 42 days
8 a	— [a,b,k]	— [b,k]	—	—	—	—	—	— [l]	—	—	after 7 days
8 b	—	—	—	—	—	—	—	— [m]	—	—	after 14 days
9	3.74	0.9	< 0.2	< 0.2	< 0.2 Back/Loin	0.1–0.5 [n]	—	— [o]	—	—	after 6 days
	< 0.04	0.64	0.01	trace	— [p] trace — [p]	—	< 0.03	0.03	0.03	0.03	— [j]
	0.13	0.24	0.01	0.02	— [q] 0.01 — [q]	—	0.14	0.12	0.16	0.18	
	1.94	0.20	0.01	0.06	— [r] 0.03 — [r]	—	trace	0.03	0.01	0.02	non-extract. CH_3CN
10 a	60 [s]	—	—	—	—	—	—	—	—	—	after 6 days
10 b	70 [s]	—	—	—	—	—	—	—	—	—	
10 c	100 [s]	—	—	—	—	—	—	—	—	—	in acetonitrile
10 d	230 [s]	—	—	—	—	—	—	—	—	—	

Table XLII b (continued)

No.	Residue (p.p.m.) in										Remarks
	Liver	Kidney	Brain	Heart	Muscle (Flank and leg)	Skin, etc.	Fat				
							Flank	Back	Renal	Omental	
11 a	—	—	—	—	—	—	—	< 0.02 [u]	—	—	after 2 days [t]
11 b	< 0.02	—	—	—	—	—	—	< 0.02 [u]	—	—	
11 c	< 0.02	—	—	—	—	—	—	0.05 [u]	—	—	
11 d	< 0.02	—	—	—	—	—	—	0.07 [u]	—	—	
11 e	0.52	—	—	—	0.1	—	—	—	—	—	died
11 f	< 0.02	—	—	—	—	—	—	0.03 [u]	—	—	after 1 day [t]
11 g	0.06	—	—	—	< 0.02	—	—	0.25 [u]	—	—	
11 h	—	—	—	—	—	—	—	< 0.02 [u]	—	—	after 8 days [t]
11 i	< 0.02	—	—	—	—	—	—	0.05 [u]	—	—	
11 k	—	—	—	—	—	—	—	< 0.02 [u]	—	—	after 16 days [t]
11 l	< 0.02	—	—	—	—	—	—	< 0.02 [u]	—	—	
11 m	0.03	—	—	—	—	—	—	0.08 [u]	—	—	after 2 days
	< 0.02	—	—	—	—	—	—	0.04 [u]	—	—	after 7 days
	< 0.02	—	—	—	—	—	—	0.04 [u]	—	—	after 14 days
11 n	0.06	—	—	—	—	—	—	0.14 [u]	—	—	after 2 days
	< 0.02	—	—	—	—	—	—	0.05 [u]	—	—	after 7 days
	< 0.02	—	—	—	—	—	—	0.04 [u]	—	—	after 14 days
12 [v, w]	0.75	0.80	0.05	—	0.04	0.10–2.00 [y]	—	0.09	—	—	after 1 day
	0.84	0.64	0.03	—	0.03	0.11–1.36 [y]	—	< 0.02	—	—	after 3 days
	0.51	0.57	< 0.02	—	< 0.02	0.21–0.60 [y]	—	< 0.02	—	—	after 7 days
	0.42	0.33	< 0.02	—	< 0.02	0.17–0.23 [y]	—	< 0.02	—	—	after 14 days
	0.17	0.15	< 0.02	—	< 0.02	0.06–0.16 [y]	—	< 0.02	—	—	after 28 days
	0.48	0.58	< 0.02	—	0.03	0.33–1.03 [y]	—	0.03	—	—	after 7 days
	0.63	0.42	< 0.02	—	0.03	0.30–0.35 [y]	—	< 0.02	—	—	after 14 days
	0.41	0.25	< 0.02	—	< 0.02	0.22–0.24 [y]	—	< 0.02	—	—	after 21 days
	0.29	0.13	< 0.02	—	< 0.02	0.22–0.29 [y]	—	< 0.02	—	—	after 28 days

Total P^{32}-equivalents (12 v, w: after 1 day – after 28 days)

13 x, z	2.60	2.01	0.03	—	0.04	0.08–0.13 y	—	0.03	—	—	1 day aa
	1.97	1.90	< 0.02	—	0.04	0.02–0.14 y	—	0.04	—	—	3 days aa
	4.05	3.16	0.12	—	0.17	0.17–0.32 y	—	0.05	—	—	7 days aa
	1.07	1.12	0.08	—	0.25	0.02–0.69 y	—	0.04	—	—	3 days bb
	0.59	0.67	0.09	—	0.13	0.04–0.55 y	—	< 0.02	—	—	7 days bb
	0.20	0.32	0.09	—	0.12	0.03–0.55 y	—	< 0.02	—	—	14 days bb
	< 0.02	0.09	< 0.02	—	0.10	0.03–0.65 y	—	< 0.02	—	—	21 days bb

a Extractable with chloroform.
b Water-soluble.
c Non-extractable.
d % extracted with acetonitrile from isopropyl ether extract.
e 0.2—0.5 tongue, 9.6 rib, 0.52 udder.
f 0.45 back, 0.051 loin.
g 0.025 back, 0.044 loin.
h 0.18 back, 0.22 loin.
i Interstitial tissue.
j Acetone-benzene extractives soluble in Skellysolve B.
k Presumably metabolites.
l Abdominal fat 0.12–0.4.
m Abdominal fat 0.04.
n Tongue.
o Abdominal fat 0.2–0.5.
p 0.004 back and loin.
q 0.008 back, 0.009 loin.
r 0.011 back, 0.024 loin.
s Radioactive impulses/minute, in CH_3CN.
t After last intake.
u Back plus renal.
v 0.02–0.045 breast.
w Total P^{32}-equivalents.
x 0.02–0.08 breast.
y Larger values in bone tissues.
z p.p.m. equivalents.
aa Days of feeding.
bb Days after discontinuation of feeding.

12. DDVP. — Phosphoric acid, 2,2-dichlorovinyl-, dimethyl ester

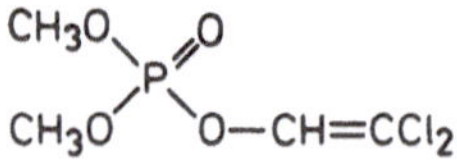

Alternate names: Dichlorvos, Vapona (93%), dichlorphos.
Application: Insecticide against houseflies; also present as "contamination" in trichlorphon (MATTSON *et al.* 1955); application on cattle, goats, sheep, pigs, and poultry; treatment against worms in pigs (BATTE *et al.* 1965), especially against *Oesophagostomum* and *Hyostrongylus rubidus* (JACOBS 1968).
Toxicity: See Table XLIII. FISKEN (1965) reported surprisingly different results; he found for fasting rats the following *per os* LD_{50} values: ♂ 679 mg./kg. and ♀ 382 mg./kg. In a semichronic application, rats tolerated daily about ten mg./kg. over a period of six weeks (KLOTZSCHE 1956). Cattle tolerated 200 p.p.m. DDVP in the feed over 32 days without inhibition of ChE (TRACY *et al.* 1960). The fast resorption through the portal vein after *per os* treatment, which was experimentally established for rats, provided an explanation for the rapid decontamination (LAWS 1966).

Table XLIII. *Acute toxicity of DDVP for the rat after oral and i.p. application.*

Mode of application	LD_{50} (mg./kg.)	Reference
per os	56–80	DEDEK & SCHWARZ (1966 b)
per os	50–80	COCHRANE (1963)
per os [a]	80	DURHAM *et al.* (1957)
per os [a]	73	KLOTZSCHE (1956)
per os [b]	56	DURHAM *et al.* (1957)
i.p.	6	ARTHUR & CASIDA (1957)

[a] Male
[b] Female

Tolerances: In the U.S.A., for tomatoes 0.5 p.p.m. [as naled (Dibrom)] (FREAR *et al.* 1969).
Detection: See GALLEY (1967) and PORTER (1964) for multidetector glc; for naled, see PACK (1964).
Metabolism and residues: DDVP is an easily hydrolysed substance with a high vapor pressure. It underwent a rapid degradation in the body (COCHRANE 1963), meaning it was quickly and completely decontaminated (TRACY *et al.* 1960). According to HODGSON and CASIDA (1962), homogenates of liver, kidney, and spleen of rats and rabbits, cleaved DDVP at the P – O-vinyl group and the P – O-methyl ester bond. Fifty to 85 percent dimethylphosphate and dichlorovinylphosphate were formed. Furthermore, hydrolysis led to monomethylphosphate and inorganic phosphate. The dichlorovinyl part reacted to form mainly dichloroethanol, with dichloro-

acetaldehyde as an intermediate, and traces of dichloroacetic acid were formed.

The DDVP metabolic pathways model for rat tissue *in vitro* are shown in Figure 7 (cf. MILLAR and AITKEN 1965).

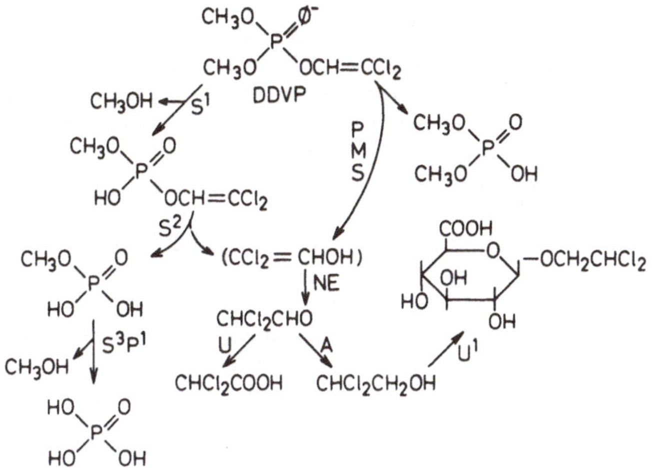

Fig. 7. Metabolic pathways of DDVP in the rat based on *in vitro* studies (HODGSON and CASIDA 1962):

P = plasma enzyme hydrolyzing DDVP to dimethyl phosphate, activators not studied.

P[1] = plasma enzyme hydrolyzing monomethyl phosphate to inorganic phosphate, activators not studied.

S = soluble liver enzyme hydrolyzing DDVP to dimethyl phosphate, activated by Mn^{++}.

S[1] = soluble liver enzyme hydrolyzing DDVP to desmethyl DDVP, activators not studied.

S[2] = soluble liver enzyme hydrolyzing desmethyl DDVP to monomethyl phosphate activated by 1×10^{-4} M Co^{++}.

S[3] = soluble liver enzyme hydrolyzing monomethyl phosphate to inorganic phosphate, no known activators, inhibited by —SH inhibitors, pH optimum 6.8 to 7.2.

M = liver mitochondrial enzyme hydrolyzing DDVP to dimethyl phosphate, activated by Ca^{++}.

A = reduction of dichloroacetaldehyde to dichloroethanol by alcohol dehydrogenase, requires DPNH.

NE = nonenzymatic.

U and *U*[1] = pathway probably present, nature of enzymes not studied.

DDVP metabolism should also be seen in connection with that of trichlorphon (q.v.), since that is cleaved to DDVP. However, the hydrolytic cleavage took place ten times faster in blood than it did in an aqueous system of the same pH *in vitro*. It follows that in addition certain enzyme systems took part in the degradation (KÜHNERT *et al.* 1963).

TRACY *et al.* (1960) established after oral treatment of rats the following in the tissues of the animals: the stomach was highly toxic to flies; brain tissue was toxic to flies one to 16 hours after treatment, but not after 23 hours. Liver, fatty tissue, muscle, blood, and small intestine did not affect flies. It is striking that these types of tissue, in contrast to liver tissue, cannot decontaminate DDVP as such. This statement is also true for the decontamination capacity of liver from cattle, pigs, chickens, and cats.

In the muscles of rats SCHENK (1967) found residues in the range of 0.1 to 1.0 p.p.m., after DDVP treatment with a three-fold LD_{50} quantity, as determined with an indirect ChE inhibition method for the intact insecticide; the rats died four minutes after treatment.

The half-life of DDVP in the blood of cattle was 1.2 hours, according to KÜHNERT *et al.* (1963).

According to EICHLER (1965), no insecticidally effective DDVP could be detected with fly larvae either in the urine or in the feces of cows. General statements say that the DDVP taken in by the mammal organism was about 50 percent excreted after six to 12 hours and that after 24 hours no more DDVP was found in the organism (EICHLER 1965).

After dusting meat products with 0.08 and 0.025 µg./l. FISKEN (1965) recovered 0.5 p.p.m. after three days and 0.2 p.p.m. after seven days, respectively, on the meat. In insecticide-free air, these values dropped 20 to 50 percent within seven days. The above-mentioned values were supported by MILLAR and AITKEN (1965), who did not observe any penetration of DDVP into the meat. The decomposition took place through hydrolysis and enzyme processes. Furthermore, DDVP was completely destroyed by the cooking process: SCHENK (1967) estimated the decontamination time as 1.5 hours of cooking. Frying and cooking decomposed DDVP to dimethylphosphoric acid, monomethylphosphoric acid, and desmethyl-DDVP, aside from some unidentified components.

13. DEMETON GROUP. — See Table XLIV for structures and names and special section on Thimet.

Alternate name: Systox group.

Application: The derivatives of the demeton group (Systox group) are used only in plant protection. Although there is no special application in veterinary medicine, there was an effect against ticks on cattle and blowflies for sheep (MCCARTHY *et al.* 1967).

Toxicity: Systox and IsoSystox belong to a strongly cholinergic-effective group, the effect of which with regard to blood pressure, breathing, intestine, and pupil is similar to that of parathion; however, it exhibited a lower muscarine-like and stronger nicotine-like effect (PERKOW 1956). The toxicities of the trade products were dependent on the ratio of the isomers. Most of the products were highly volatile and penetrated easily through the intact skin. The sulfone of MetaSystox in undiluted form seemed to penetrate only slowly through the skin (DU BOIS and PLZAK 1962). The trade product of MetaSystox consists of an isomer mixture of 70:30 of P – S and P – O MetaSystox, while MetaSystox (1, Table XLIV a) stands for a further development of the sulfoxide of P – O-MetaSystox (NIESSEN *et al.* 1963). DAHM and JACOBSON (1956) gave Systox or demeton to milk cows as such or in contaminated lucerne hay and observed, after treatment of 0.1 mg./kg. body wt., clear poison symptoms and ChE inhibition.

Table XLIV a. *Survey of the demeton group: Structures and names.*

No.	Chemical structure	Chemical names/alternate names
1	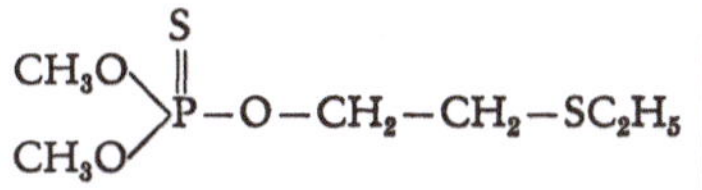	O,O-dimethyl-O-2-(ethylmercapto)-ethyl thionophosphate methyldemeton, P—S-MetaSystox (thiono-form)
2	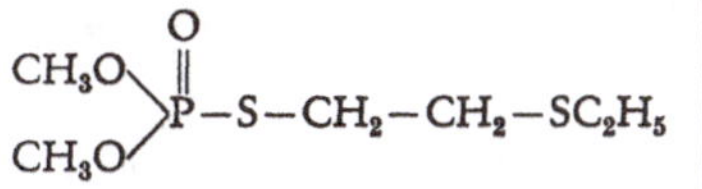	O,O-dimethyl-*S*-2-(ethylmercapto)-ethyl thiolphosphate isomethyldemeton, P—O-MetaSystox (thiolo-form)
3	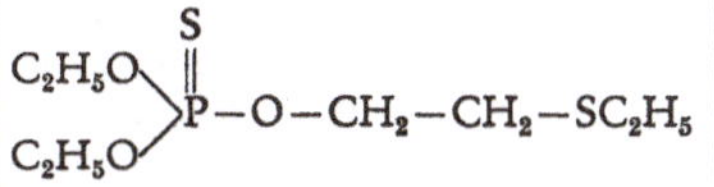	O,O-diethyl-O-2(ethylmercapto)-ethyl thionophosphate demeton, P—S-Systox (thiono-form)
4	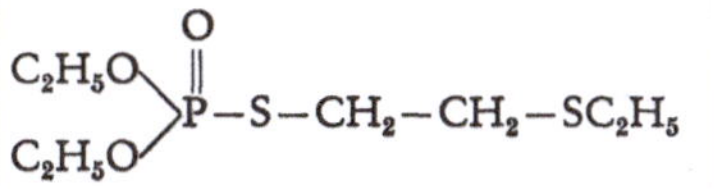	O,O-diethyl-*S*-2-(ethylmercapto)-ethyl thiolphosphate isodemeton, P—O-Systox (thiolo-form)
5	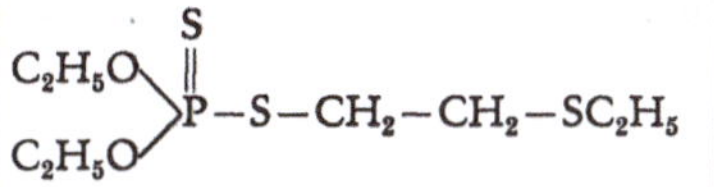	O,O-diethyl-*S*-2-(ethylmercapto)-ethyl dithiophosphate disulfoton, thiodemeton, Di-Syston
6	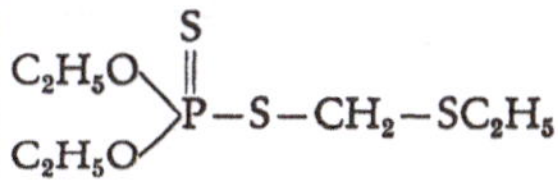	O,O-diethyl-*S*-(ethylmercaptomethyl) dithiophosphate Phorate, Thimet [a]

[a] See special section.

Restrictions and tolerances in the United States:
Demeton in plants 0.2 to 1.25 p.p.m.; in green lucerne, barley, oats, wheat, and green clover five p.p.m.; in lucerne and clover hay 12 p.p.m. (FREAR *et al.* 1959).
Di-Syston (disulfoton) in plants 0.3 to two p.p.m.; in fresh lucerne, green barley, and wheat as green fodder five p.p.m.; in lucerne and clover hay 12 p.p.m.
Detection: The detection of derivatives of the Systox group is difficult for the toxicologist; FISCHER and SPECHT 1957 give a critical survey. For further reports see DUGGAN *et al.* (1967), GELDMACHER *et al.* (1963), NAEVE (1954 a), and BETKER *et al.* 1966); detection of the sulfonium ion III, NIESSEN *et al.* (1963); detection after steam distillation, ether extraction, and oxidation of phosphorus and sulfur, MACHATA (1956); rapid determination in 15 minutes through combination of NMR and glc, BABAD and TAYLOR (1968); detection of Di-Syston, MetaSystox, and Systox, McDOUGALL (1964) and STENERSEN (1967).

Table XLIV b. *Survey of the demeton group: Toxicological properties.*

No.	Indication	Oral toxicity (LD_{50}) against rats and reference (mg./kg.)	Remarks
1	Contact insecticide with systemic effect	250 HOLMSTEDT (1959) 180 MARTIN (1961) 64 KLOTZSCHE (1955) 180 Compound A, FREAR (1965) [a]	—
2	—	60 HOLMSTEDT (1959) 40 MARTIN (1961) 40 FREAR (1965) [b]	—
3	Contact insecticide with systemic effect	30 HOLMSTEDT (1959), WIRTH (1954) 7.5 PERKOW (1956) 7.7 SCHRADER (1963)	Sheep *per os* 2.0 mg./kg. without reaction, 2.5 mg./kg. evoke symptoms (MCCARTHY *et al.* 1967); one p.p.m. in feed inhibits plasma ChE for dog; two p.p.m. inhibit erythrocyte-ChE (FRAWLEY and FUYAT 1957)
4	Contact insecticide with systemic effect	1.5 HOLMSTEDT (1959) 1.7 DU BOIS *et al.* (1956)	—
5	Systemic insecticide	5 HOLMSTEDT (1959) 12.5 [c] BOMBINSKI & DU BOIS (1958) 2.6 [d] BOMBINSKI & DU BOIS (1958)	Rat tolerates 0.5 mg./kg. daily
6	Contact insecticide with systemic effect	2.1 HOLMSTEDT (1959) 3.7 MARTIN (1961)	*In vitro* light ChE-inhibition

[a] "Compound A."
[b] "Compound B."
[c] Male rats.
[d] Female rats.

Metabolism and residues: In this group, the thiol compounds were more toxic than the thiono derivates (WIRTH 1960). Aqueous solutions of P–S-Systox may convert to the toxic thiol form with time. Oxidation processes at the thioether sulfur led to the formation of sulfoxides and sulfones in plants (METCALF *et al.* 1954 and 1955). WIRTH (1960) considered this as being possible also in the animal body. The oxidation products exhibited a slighter ChE inhibition effect for the demeton- and the methyldemeton group than the thiolo- or thiono-form, respectively (WIRTH 1960) (Table XLV). For Di-Syston, a conversion to demeton-S seemed to exist, with the exception of the male rat (BOMBINSKI and DU BOIS 1958, DU BOIS *et al.* 1956). WIRTH (1960) concluded from the strongly increasing ChE inhibition effect *in vitro* that an oxidation took place not only at the sulfur, but that during oxidation highly active thiol compounds were formed. For comparison, plants also formed metabolites which have a stronger ChE inhibition than the starting product (DAHM and JACOBSON 1956). Demeton

Table XLV. *Toxicities of the sulfoxides and sulfones of the demeton group.*

Structure of R	Rat oral LD_{50} (mg./kg.)					
	Methyldemeton $(CH_3O)_2P(=S)OCH_2-R$	Isomethyldemeton $(CH_3O)_2P(=O)S-CH_2-R$	Demeton $(C_2H_5O)_2P(=S)OCH_2-R$	Isodemeton $(C_2H_5O)_2P(=O)S-CH_2-R$	Di-Syston $(C_2H_5O)_2P(=S)S-CH_2-R$	Phorate $(C_2H_5O)_2P(=S)S-R$
$CH_2S(=O)C_2H_5$ (sulfoxide)	600 [a]	♂65 [b] ♀75 [b]	100 [a]	2.0 [a] 2.3 [c]	6.5 [a]	2.1 [a]
$CH_2S(=O)_2C_2H_5$ (sulfone)	500 [a]	40 [a] 80 [b]	90 [a]	2.0 [a] 1.9 [c]	7.5 [a]	1.7 [a]

[a] Holmstedt (1959).
[b] Du Bois and Plzak (1962).
[c] Du Bois *et al.* (1956).

and Di-Syston were only lightly attacked by rumen fluid (AHMED *et al.* 1958).

The demeton compounds (WIRTH 1960) as well as Di-Syston (BOMBINSKI and DU BOIS 1958) were easily resorbed by the digestive tract with 95 percent absorbed by rats within two hours; the residues of P^{32}-labelled substance were excreted within two days. The excretion was very rapid, and no toxic substances were detected in the urine or feces. In rabbits, the pathway of excretion was 90 percent through the kidneys within 48 hours (WIRTH 1954). These excretion products in feces and urine were nontoxic (WIRTH 1954). Traces of P^{32} were still excreted after two to three weeks.

After *i.p.* injection of two mg. of P^{32}-Di-Syston in ethanol, it was slowly excreted by rats with the urine and feces in the form of hydrolysis products (BULL 1965); 14.1 percent after 24 hours and 28.6 percent after 48 hours of the injected radioactivity appeared in the urine. The prevailing hydrolysis products were diethylthiophosphate and diethylphosphate. The fraction as phosphoric acid was 4.1 percent between ten and 12 hours after treatment, diethylthiophosphate was 24.8 percent, diethylphosphate was 61.2 percent, and two unknown metabolites were 2.2 and 7.79 percent. There were only traces of diethyldithiophosphate in the urine. In the liver from 30 to 120 minutes after injection, several also-more-toxic metabolic products were found:

Di-Syston sulfoxide: 11.3 percent (30 minutes) and 12.9 percent (120 minutes)

Di-Syston sulfone: 2.4 percent

Di-Syston-P – O-sulfoxide: 26.7 percent (30 minutes) and 27.2 percent (120 minutes)

Di-Syston-P – O-sulfone: 59.6 percent (30 minutes) and 59.9 percent (120 minutes)

Further residue data exist for methyldemeton only for special kind of animals. BUNYAN *et al.* (1969) established residue values for pheasants and pigeons, after feeding with 100 p.p.m. of methyldemeton for 14, 28, and 42 days (Table XLVI).

Table XLVI. *Residues of methyldemeton in pheasants and pigeons* (BUNYAN *et al.* 1969).

Feeding time (days)	Residue (p.p.m.)			
	Pheasant		Pigeon	
	Fat	Liver	Fat	Liver
14	260	180	3.8	25
14	436	138	< 0.1	28
28	2.7	48	< 0.1	22
28	< 0.1	< 0.1	< 0.1	45
42	5	2	< 0.1	13
42	0.3	2	0.7	5

14. DFP. — O,O-diisopropyl-fluorophosphate

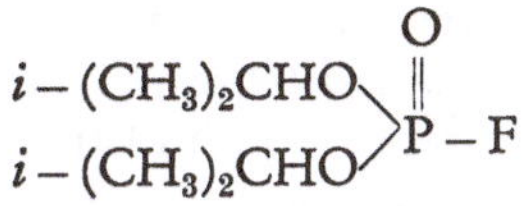

Trade product: No application as insecticide; mioticum in optometry.
Toxicity: See Table XLVII. DFP was a strong ChE inhibitor (MICHEL and KROP 1951). It caused paralysis in hens because of demyelinization (BARNES and DENZ 1953.

Table XLVII. *Acute toxicities of DFP for mouse and rat.*

Animal species	Mode of application	LD_{50} (mg./kg.)	Reference
Mouse	*i.p.*	6.9	RAMACHANDRAN (1966 b)
Mouse	*i.p.*	4.0	HOLMSTEDT (1959)
Mouse	*s.c.*	3.9	RAMACHANDRAN (1966 b)
Mouse	*s.c.*	3.8	RAMACHANDRAN (1966 a)
Rat [a]	*per os*	7.7	FRAWLEY *et al.* (1952)
Rat [b]	*per os*	13.5	FRAWLEY *et al.* (1952)

[a] Female.
[b] Male.

Metabolism and residues: DFP as a prototype of an alkylphosphate has been thoroughly investigated. For DFP hydrolytic cleavage took place at the P – F bond:

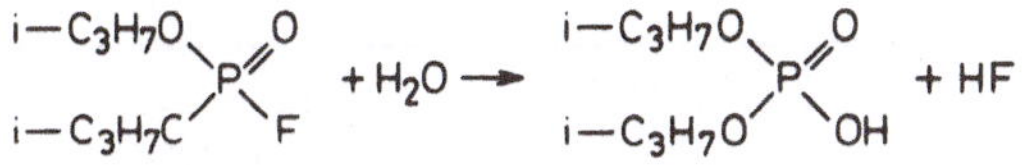

Cleavage resulted in diisopropylphosphate and hydrogen fluoride (MAZUR 1946, SAUNDERS and STACEY 1948, COHEN and WARRINGA 1954); the diisopropyl ester was not cleaved (DANGSCHAT 1965).
According to COHEN and WARRINGA (1954), metabolism of DFP took the following paths:

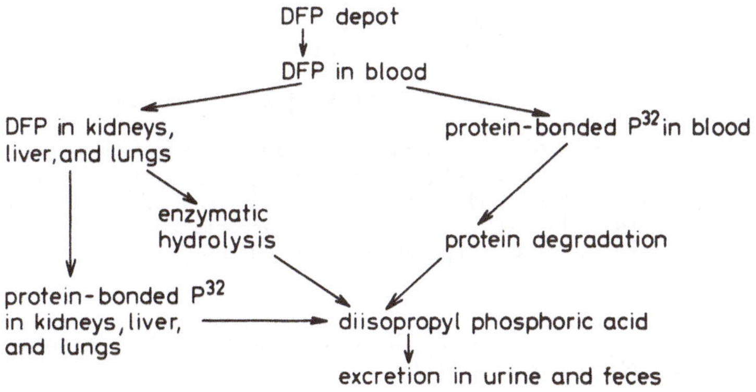

Excretion was mainly through the urine. The ratio of the only hydrolysis product, diisopropylphosphate, was one-third of the applied dosage for the human being within 24 hours, and 60 to 70 percent in ten days. Less than five percent appeared in the feces. A part of the P^{32}-labelled DFP remained as DFP-protein complex in the tissue.

Hydrolytic cleavage in the tissue — for instance, for rabbits and human beings — was carried out by enzymes, predominantly in the liver, kidney, and serum (MAZUR 1946). These ferments, which are also called "MAZUR's-enzymes" by JANDORF and MCNAMARA (1950), belong to the A-esterases (MOUNTER and WHITTAKER 1953). MOUNTER *et al.* (1955 a and b) called them "DFP-ases" and COHEN and WARRINGA (1954) referred to "fluorophosphatases" [15]. MOUNTER *et al.* (1955 a) found this enzyme in various tissues of human beings, rats, cats, guinea pigs, and pigeons, but there was no correlation between hydrolysis of DFP and its analogs by tissue enzymes and the normal metabolic activity. However, RAMACHANDRAN and ÅGREN (1964) and RAMACHANDRAN (1966 a) explained the following: although "DFP-ase" hydrolyses DFP, it is present only in small amounts in rat and rabbit tissues and plays a subordinate roll for decontamination. This can also be seen from the behaviour of excretion of radioactivity in the liver, where it was said: "There is no increased excretion of radioactivity, when DFP^{32} is injected intraperitonally," although DFP would first have to be exposed to the liver enzymes (for comparative values, see Table XLVIII).

Table XLVIII. *Incorporation or excretion of DFP^{32} in rat tissues* (RAMACHANDRAN and ÅGREN 1964).

Tissue	Interval between injection and sacrifice (hours)	Radioactivity [a] when injected		
		s.c.	*i.p.*	*s.c./i.p.*
Liver	1	277	371	0.75
	24	188	303	0.62
Kidney	1	162	81	2.00
	24	58	41	1.41
Lung	1	27	28	0.96
	24	17	18	0.94
Brain	1	4.1	2.3	1.78
	24	2.3	1.1	2.09
Excreta [b]	24	2,190	2,212	0.99

[a] The values are expressed in counts/minute$\times 10^{-3}$. Each figure represents the average of two rats weighing from 290 to 310 g. The rats were injected with 1 ml. each of a DFP^{32} solution (0.8 mg. of DFP/kg.) which contained 3.53×10^6 counts/minute of radioactivity. The animals used in the excretion studies were allowed free access to food and water. The 24-hour values for the organs pertained to these animals.
[b] Urine and feces.

[15] It is noteworthy that bacterial "DFP-ases" in the rumen fluid of ruminants also decompose DFP (MOUNTER *et al.* 1955 b).

Table XLIX. *Radioactivity in the organs and tissues of guinea pigs at intervals after i.v. injection of H^3DFP* (HANSEN *et al.* 1968 a).

Organ or tissue	Radioactivity (nCi or µCi/g. fresh wt.) [a] after							
	1 mg./kg.				3 mg./kg.		6 mg./kg.	
	5 min. (nCi./g.)	30 min. (nCi/g.)	60 min. (nCi/g.)	360 min. (nCi/g.)	5 min. (µCi/g.)	60 min. (µCi/g.)	5 min. (µCi/g.)	30 min. (µCi/g.)
Lung	595±36	423±78	531±30	258±22	16±3	5±1	18±4	11±1
Auricle	128±76	96±27	70±11	75±16	7±1	4±0.2	8±2	5±0.6
Apex of heart	68±9	63±12	40±3	38±8	8±2	5±0.1	11±4	5±0.6
Fat	Ø	Ø	Ø	Ø	7±2	3±0.2	13±2	8±2
Skeleton muscles	Ø	Ø	Ø	Ø	8±2	5±0.1	7±1	4±0.4
Suprarenal gland	37±6	42±6	29±4	30±9	12±2	7±0.2	13±0.5	7±1
Cerebrum	Ø	Ø	Ø	Ø	3±0.1	2±0.1	6±1	3±0.4
Cerebellum	Ø	Ø	Ø	Ø	4±0.2	3±0.2	7±2	4.±0.4
Medulla	Ø	Ø	Ø	Ø	5±0.3	2±0.2	7±2	3±0.4
Nerve ischiadic	Ø	Ø	Ø	Ø	9±3	5±0.1	8±1	5±0.7
Liver	41±7	49±12	34±8	33±10	24±5	15±2	34±5	21±2
Gall	22±7	22±7	18±4	12±2	46±10	8±0.2	27±8	48±7
Kidney	128±29	98±23	61±20	80±20	46±13	13±2	57±9	61±6
Urine	43±15	181±38	402±51	162±12	58±14	192±21	45±16	71±18

[a] The symbol Ø means the amount of radioactivity was under the detection limit.

After application of labelled DFP, radioactivity in blood and plasma decreased very rapidly; in the erythrocytes the elimination was parallel with the regeneration of ChE activity, *i.e.*, it was an expression of cell regeneration; the event took place in 25 days (Cohen and Warringa 1954, Jandorf and McNamara 1950).

Metabolic processes and residues concentrations have been investigated for many test animals. In the serum of guinea pigs, the level of substance decreased in dependence on the dosage within five to 30 minutes to a level which then was maintained over a long period (Hansen *et al.* 1968 a). With a dosage of 0.1 mg./kg. body wt. as *i.v.* application, the concentrations in the organs were usually below the serum level, but after 30 minutes the organ concentration also decreased. The excretion for guinea pigs occurred mainly with the urine, and for higher dosages (six mg./kg.) also with the bile (Table XLIX).

After injection of three mg. of DFP/kg., separation by TLC five and 60 minutes afterwards resulted in about ten percent DFP and predominantly diisopropylphosphate in serum, urine, and bile. Because of the instability of DFP, Hansen *et al.* (1968 a) were not able to analyse the other organs. High concentrations were found mainly in liver, kidney, and lung (Jandorf and McNamara 1950). The serum values were very much dependent on time.

The following concentrations of protein-bonded phosphorus, four hours after subcutaneous injection, in the tissues of mice, depending on the dosage have been found.

Table L. *DFP^{32} derived phosphoprotein phosphorus in mouse organs* (Ramachandran 1967).

Dose of DFP^{32} +DFP (mg./kg.)	Phosphoprotein P (ng./g. wet tissue)				
	Liver	Kidney	Lung	Brain: As protein ^{32}P	Brain: As ^{32}P-ser.-P
3.4–3.8 [a]	921	266	170	27	6.3
4	871	236	136	30	6.8
8	891	236	144	47	7.4
16	831	251	119	54	9.5
32	868	234	208	66	10.8
64	769	280	207	80	—
128	809	212	135	90	—

[a] Control without antidotes. Organs from six to ten animals were pooled and worked up. The results of a single representative series were given in the case of liver, kidney, and lung. Sacrifice was at four hours after DFP^{32}.

See Table LI for the dependence of concentration in tissue on the time after application.

Table LI. *DFP^{32}-derived phosphoprotein phosphorus content of mouse organs at various times after DFP^{32} administration* [a] (RAMACHANDRAN 1967).

DFP^{32}+DFP Time beetwen injection and sacrifice (hours)	Phosphoprotein P (ng./g. wet tissue)			
	Liver	Kidney	Lung	Brain
0.5	1,071	346	216	56
3	1,044	377	259	61
6	890	330	209	62
18	853	266	184	56
24	846	265	141	50
48	565	189	173	56

[a] DFP^{32}+DFP was administered *s.c.* at 32 mg./kg. to mice protected with atropine and Toxogonin. The results were from one representative series, each value being that of pooled organs from six to ten animals.

After *i.p.* injection of DFP, RAMACHANDRAN (1966 a) found more P^{32} in the liver of mice than after *s.c.* or *i.v.* injection; these extensive data should be read in the original paper.

Further distribution studies in organs were conducted by RAMACHANDRAN (1966 b) with high DFP^{32} dosages on mice with antidote protection. There was no influence on the quantity of tissue-bonded DFP. However, the fraction of acid-soluble DFP increased approximately in proportion to the logarithm of the applied dosage.

After ten and 15 mg. of DFP/kg. body wt., DANGSCHAT (1965) found with colorimetric ChE determination in rats up to 1,000 p.p.m. in immediately-killed animals, up to 100 p.p.m. after 15 minutes, and one p.p.m. effective substance one hour after contamination. After two hours, free alkylphosphate was no longer present. With regard to the ability of protein bonding, the fraction in muscle was 0.5 p.p.m. at the most.

JANDORF and MCNAMARA (1950) treated rabbits with 200 to 500 µg. of DFP^{32}/kg. body wt. and with diisopropylphosphate for comparison. The high level of radioactivity in blood plasma in the beginning decreased within a few hours. The P^{32} content of the erythrocytes reached a maximum about one hour after injection, which remained for nine hours. Approximately 50 percent of the total phosphorus which originated from DFP was bound to protein within the first ten minutes in liver, kidney, and lung tissue. After four hours it was approximately 100 percent. The distribution in tissues is reported in Table LII.

In the cat as a model animal, HANSEN *et al.* (1968 b) found, 30 minutes after *i.v.* injection of H^3-DFP, higher DFP values in the arterial serum than in the venous serum. The half-life of DFP in the arterial serum was established in two exponential phases as seven and 200 minutes, respectively. Also for the cat, DFP was rapidly decomposed to diisopropylphosphate and was mainly excreted through the kidneys.

Table LII. *Distribution of P^{32} in rabbit tissues after i.v. injection of labelled diisopropyl fluorophosphate or sodium diisopropylphosphate* (JANDORF and McNAMARA 1950).

Dose (μg./kg.)	Survival (hours)	P^{32} distribution (μg. P/g. dry tissue) in							
		Kidney	Liver	Lung	Brain	Heart	Skeletal muscle	Plasma	RBC
			Diisopropyl fluorophosphate						
2,000	1/4	17.3	7.7	4.7	0.24	1.30	1.01	11.8	0.29
500	5	0.31	0.74	0.39	0.04	0.10	0.04	—	—
500	19	1.12	0.32	—	0.06	0.12	0.03	0.10	0.04
			Sodium diisopropylphosphate						
1,100	18	0.06	0.02	0.03	0.00	0.03	0.01	0.00	0.01
1,100	18	0.04	0.03	0.01	0.00	0.03	0.01	0.01	0.01

There are no residue data for meat and tissues of edible domestic animals so that the above-mentioned data have to be used for analogous conclusions with regard to rapid decomposition and excretion.

15. DIAZINON. — Phosphorothioic acid, O,O-diethyl O-(2-isopropyl-6-methyl-4-pyrimidinyl) ester

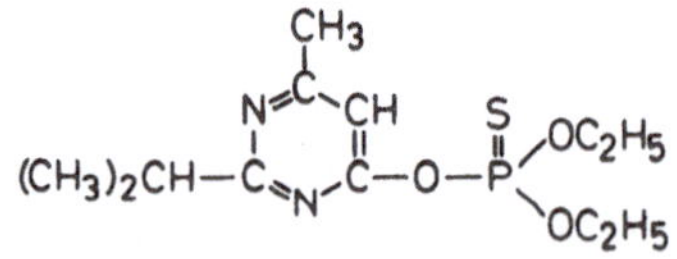

Alternate names: Basudin, Exodin.
Application: Insecticide with a wide spectrum for insect control in agriculture.
Veterinary application: Insecticide for ectoparasite control on domestic animals (except poultry), especially for sheep with a considerable residual effect in the fleece. Effective against *Dermatobia, Lucilia,* lice, ticks, mites, and others (GATTERDAM *et al.* 1962).
Application dosage for animals: 0.06 percent as spray for cattle, 0.02 percent for sheep; 0.03 percent as a bath for cattle, 0.01 percent for sheep; 2.0 percent as a powder.
Toxicity: See Table LIII. Diazinon was resorbed by the skin, the respiration tract, and from the intestines. Rats tolerated 1,000 p.p.m. in the food during a two-year chronic test. There was no tendency of cumulation (ANONYMOUS 25); dogs tolerated 5.3 mg./kg. body wt. daily over 271 days.
Tolerances and restrictions: In the U.S.A., 0.75 p.p.m. in and on fat, meat products from sheep (FREAR *et al.* 1969, ANONYMOUS 30). The label directions specify not to slaughter within two weeks after application [compare U.S.A. imposed tolerances for plants, hay, etc.: 0.75 to 60 p.p.m. (FREAR and FRIEDMANN 1968)].
Detection: see GUNTHER and BLINN (1955), MARGOT *et al.* (1964), DUGGAN *et al.* (1967).

Table LIII. *Acute toxicities of diazinon for various animals.*

Animal species	Mode of application	Toxic dosage (mg./kg.)	LD_{50} (mg./kg.)	Remarks	Reference
Mouse	*i.p.*	—	65	—	HOLMSTEDT (1959)
Mouse	*per os*	—	85–135	tech. in gum arabic	ANONYMOUS 25
Mouse	*per os*	—	80	in corn oil	ANONYMOUS 25
Mouse	*per os*	—	100	—	PERKOW (1956)
Rat [a]	*per os*	—	76	—	ANONYMOUS 25
Rat [b]	*per os*	—	108	—	ANONYMOUS 25
Rat	*per os*	—	150–220	tech. in gum arabic	ANONYMOUS 25
Rat [b]	*per os*	—	100–150	in corn oil	ANONYMOUS 25
Rat	*per os*	—	240	—	PERKOW (1956)
Rat	*per os*	—	~250	—	MÜCKE *et al.* (1970)
Rat	*per os*	—	220–225	90%	KLOTZSCHE (1955)
Chicken	*per os*	—	8.4	—	SHERMANN & ROSS (1959)
Calf	*per os*	max. nontox. 0.5 min. tox. 1.0		1–2 weeks	RADELEFF & BUSHLAND (1960)
Cattle	*per os*	max. nontox. 10 min. tox. 25		—	RADELEFF & BUSHLAND (1960)
Sheep	*per os*	max. nontox. 20 min. tox. 30		—	RADELEFF & BUSHLAND (1960)
Sheep	*per os*	0.25% nontox. 0.06% tox. 0.12% tox.		1-month old 1-week old 3-days old	MATTHYSSEN *et al.* (1968)

[a] Female.
[b] Male.

Metabolism [16] *and residues:* Test animals excreted within a few hours almost the total applied quantity in the form of degradation products (DANGSCHAT 1965). MÜCKE *et al.* (1970) (Table LIV) investigated the metabolic pathway of diazinon in rats with diazinon double-labelled with C^{14} in the pyrimidine ring and in the ethoxy group; it was applied orally in the form of an 8:2 V/V water-ethanol solution. The excretion of diazinon and its metabolites reached 50 percent of the starting quantity within 12 hours. The major excretion pathway was through the kidneys with 69 to 80 percent; 18 to 25 percent appeared in the feces. The limit of detection was reached after five days. No cumulation of diazinon and its metabolites took place in the

[16] The liver microsomes were of vital importance during the degradation of diazinon (cf. NAKATSUGAWA *et al.* 1969).

Table LIV. *Distribution and dissipation of radioactivity in organs and tissues of the rat after subchronic feeding* [a] *of 2-C^{14}-diazinon* (Mücke *et al.* 1970).

Organ or tissue	Radioactive content (%) [b] after				
	0.25 day	1 day	2 days	5 days	8 days
Esophagus and stomach	0.25	0.02	< 0.01	< 0.01	< 0.01
Small intestine	0.65	< 0.05	< 0.05	< 0.05	< 0.05
Cecum and colon	0.76	< 0.05	< 0.05	< 0.05	< 0.05
Liver	0.16	< 0.05	< 0.05	< 0.05	< 0.05
Spleen	0.01	< 0.01	< 0.01	< 0.01	< 0.01
Pancreas	0.01	< 0.01	< 0.01	< 0.01	< 0.01
Kidney	0.04	< 0.01	< 0.01	< 0.01	< 0.01
Lung	0.02	< 0.01	< 0.01	< 0.01	< 0.01
Testis	0.02	< 0.01	< 0.01	< 0.01	< 0.01
Muscle	0.77	< 0.30	< 0.30	< 0.30	< 0.30
Fat	0.23	0.18	< 0.10	< 0.10	< 0.10
Sum	2.92	0.70	—	—	—

[a] 0.1 mg./rat daily during ten subsequent days.
[b] Percent of dose totally applied.

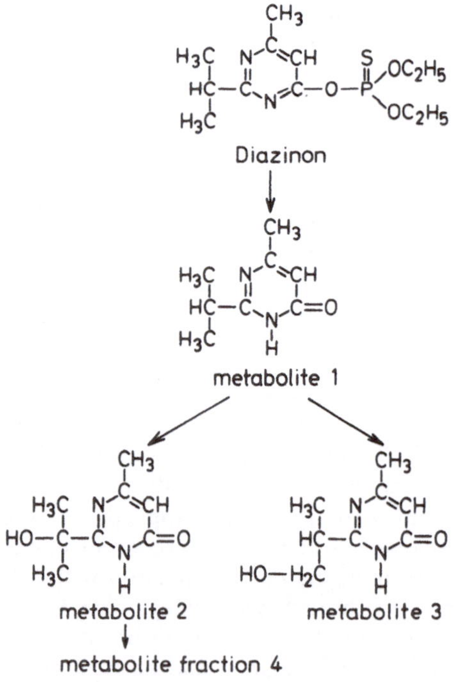

Fig. 8. Metabolic pathway of the pyrimidine moiety of diazinon in the rat (Mücke *et al.* 1970).

tissues, not even with ten days continuous treatment. No radioactivity could be measured any more two days after discontinuation of treatment.

The pyrimidine ring was not broken during metabolism as derived from the lack of radioactive CO_2 after application of ring-labelled diazinon; however, a limited oxidation to $C^{14}O_2$ was observed when the side chain was labelled. Three of four metabolites which were found in the urine and feces — aside from traces of unchanged diazinon — represented about 70 percent of the total radioactivity; the fourth fraction contained a number of polar substances.

Metabolites 1 and 2 (Fig. 8) almost completely lost their ability to inhibit ChE and their oral toxicity was low, with about 2.700 and >5,000 mg./kg., respectively. Degradation occurred mainly through hydrolysis of the ester bond to form 2-isopropyl-4-methyl-6-hydroxypyrimidine, and oxidation on the primary and tertiary C-atoms of the isopropyl side chain.

Millar (1963) established for the dog, after oral dosages of 225 mg./kg. body wt., the residues in tissues ten hours after treatment, radiochemically as well as with enzyme inhibition. The radioactivity in the stomach and urine was attributed to diethylphosphoric acid, which is a degradation product. Unchanged diazinon was essentially missing. The real depots were

Table LV. *Diazinon concentrations in dog organs and tissues* (Millar 1963).

Organ or tissue	Diazinon (p.p.m. wet-wt.) [a]	
	Radiochemical method [b]	Enzyme inhibition method
Hind leg muscle		
Sample 1	20.6 ± 0.6	18.5
Sample 2	20.7 ± 0.7	NE
Hind leg fat	13.6 ± 0.6	12.1
Perirenal fat	81.0 ± 1.3	78.4
Omental fat	17.2 ± 0.6	16.8
Pericardal fat	39.0 ± 0.9	37.0
Temporal muscle	2.6 ± 0.9	NE
Brain	3.3 ± 0.3	NE
Adrenals	31.2 ± 1.4	15.0
Tongue	18.6 ± 0.7	NE
Lung	3.4 ± 0.4	NE
Heart	11.9 ± 0.5	NE
Spleen	17.5 ± 0.7	12.3
Kidney	3.2 ± 0.3	nil
Liver	16.4 ± 0.6	nil
Blood	86.6 ± 2.0	NE
Urine	691.0 ± 1.2	nil
Stomach contents	838.0 ± 4.1	nil

[a] NE = not examined.

[b] Standard error of the mean of three counts.

found in the fat samples, especially in the perirenal fat, pericardal fat, and omental fat (Table LV).

Diazinon as spray residue on consumed fodder plants did not show measurable residues in meat, fat, and organs (Anonymous 25 and 26). Diazinon was resorbed through the skin, as mentioned before. After a single dermal application on cattle the insecticide concentration in the body was below one p.p.m.; this residue was excreted within a few days (Anonymous 25).

After 16 sprays (0.05 and 1.0 percent suspensions), which were applied at weekly intervals, Claborn *et al.* (1963) (Table LVI) found in biopsy samples that small quantities of diazinon were detected in the fat of cattle one to seven days after the last spray, according to the analytical procedure of Geigy [17].

Table LVI. *Diazinon residues in fat samples after spray treatment of cattle* (Claborn *et al.* 1963).

Spray conc. (%)	Residue (p.p.m.)							
	Consecutive spray no.							
	1 (6 days)	2 (6 days)	6 (6 days)	10 (6 days)	11 (1 day)	16		
						1 day	1 day	1 day
					1	1	7	14
0.05	< 0.05–0.06	< 0.05–0.09	0.28	0.20	0.69	0.78	0.29	< 0.05–0.08
0.1	0.57	0.53	0.67	0.78	—	2.3	0.72	< 0.05

The residue quantity was dependent on the concentration of diazinon and the frequency of application. Only with the high concentration was there a considerable residue after the 16th treatment. Degradation (excretion) is fast so that two weeks after the last treatment the lower detection limit was reached.

Twenty mg. of P^{32}-labelled diazinon/kg led to a limited increase of radioactivity in the blood of a milk cow with a maximum after 12 hours; no more radioactivity was detected after 96 hours (Robbins *et al.* 1957). However, only a 18 percent of radioactive material that was soluble in organic solvents behaved like diazinon. The R_f-values of radioactive substances from the aqueous phase corresponded to diethylphosphoric and diethylthiophosphoric acid.

The metabolic processes of diazinon showed some similarities to trichlorfon, but also several differences. Thirty percent of *per os*-applied diazinon was excreted within 12 hours with the urine, and 74 percent within 36 hours. There were mainly polar degradation products, and only 0.24 percent

[17] Geigy Chemical Co. sulfide procedure for the determination of diazinon residues. Geigy Agricultural Chemicals, Ardsley, N. Y. (cited by Claborn *et al.* 1963).

behaved like unchanged diazinon. The metabolic products were diethylthiophosphoric acid (50.5 percent) and diethylphosphoric acid (44.8 percent) (ROBBINS *et al.* 1957). After oral application relatively little radioactive material was eliminated with the feces during a short time period; after 96 hours only traces were detected and after 120 hours no more activity was found. The excretion products were toxic only between the sixth and 48th hour as established in a biological test with fly larvae. The cumulative excretion rate was about 6.5 percent of the applied total activity in 36 hours (ROBBINS *et al.* 1957).

Only personal communications from the manufacturer could be obtained about residues in the tissues (ANONYMOUS 27). Bulls were treated daily for two weeks with diazinon in capsules containing quantities of 1.06 mg./kg. and 5.3 mg./kg. body wt.; after slaughtering, the tissues were investigated for residues with the use of several methods (sulfide method, ChE method, and unspecific biological test with flies). It was found that with a five-fold increase of the dosage the residue increased only two-fold. With the exception of fat, no significant residues were in the tissues one and seven days, respectively, after slaughtering. No residues were in the heart, and in the brain only with the sulfide method in a sample taken the day after treatment with the smaller dosage, at 0.02 p.p.m. One day after treatment with the smaller dosage, the liver contained 0.01 p.p.m. as established with the ChE method. After application of 5.3 mg./kg. body wt., the quantity of residue was dependent on the method and was 0.07 and 0.04 p.p.m., respectively, on the day after treatment, and zero and 0.02 p.p.m., respectively, after seven days (ChE method). The concentrations in muscle tissue and fat are reported in Table LVII.

Table LVII. *Diazinon residues in bull tissues by two analytical methods* (ANONYMOUS 27).

Dosage (mg./kg./day)	Day of slaughtering	Residue (p.p.m.) in			
		Muscle		Fat	
		Sulfide method	ChE method	Sulfide method	ChE method
1.06	1	0.02	0.02	0	0.09
	7	0	0	0	0.09
	1	0.02	0	0.23	0.22
5.30	7	0.09	0.02	0.10	0.16

MILLAR *et al.* (1963) referred to their unpublished results in which, two days after oral application to sheep, diazinon was present in all the body fat samples at approximately the same concentration. After dip or spray of sheep with diazinon, MATTHYSSE *et al.* (1968) established diazinon residues in the tissues only a short time after treatment with the sulfide method. After 15 (dip) or 26 (spray) days most tissues were free of detectable diazinon. The highest quantities were always found in the fat tissue; values were lower after spray treatment than after a dip (Table LVIII).

VIGNE *et al.* (1957) investigated the metabolism of P^{32}-diazinon in goats. The oral dosage was 235.8 mg./36.5 kg. body wt.; this quantity corresponded to a radioactivity of 19.106 c/m. The maximum excretion — mainly in the urine and also in the feces — was reached after one to two days and the concentration then droped very sharply until the fourth day after application. Diazinon was rapidly metabolized, indeed; no ChE inhibiting activity could be found any more in the feces and plasma, and it was only very slightly present in the urine.

BUNYAN *et al.* (1969) established residue values in pheasants and pigeons, after a feeding of 100 p.p.m. diazinon for different lengths of time, which show no relation to the duration of feeding (Table LIX).

Table LVIII. *Diazinon residues in sheep tissues at intervals after treatment* (MATTHYSSE *et al.* 1968).

Treatment	Interval (days)	Residue (p.p.m.) in						
		Fat	Blood	Muscle	Heart	Liver	Kidney	Brain
0.06% dip, not shorn	1	1.45	0.05	0.01	0.16	0.02	0.04	0.01
	15	0.52	0.10	0.08	0.05	0.08	0.02	0.01
	26	0.31	0.35	0.01	0.02	0.03	0.06	0.01
0.06% dip, shorn	1	2.30	0.48	0.02	0.06	0.13	0.13	0.01
	15	0.23	0.04	0.02	0.01	0.08	0.01	0.02
	26	0.04	0.17	0.08	0.01	0.08	0.05	0.02
1% sprinkle, not shorn	26	0.22	0.03	0.06	0.04	0.06	0.03	0.03
1% sprinkle, shorn	26	0.22	0.07	0.01	0.02	0.01	0.01	0.05
0.06% sprinkle, not shorn	1	0.14	0.04	0.01	0.04	0.06	0.03	0.01
	15	0.11	0.06	0.10	0.04	0.01	0.01	0.01
	26	0.01	0.02	0.25	0.05	0.08	0.23	0.01
0.06% sprinkle, shorn	1	0.23	0.04	0.06	0.01	0.41	0.01	0.03
	15	0.12	0.14	0.11	0.04	0.01	0.04	0.09
	26	0.07	0.07	0.01	0.03	0.03	0.04	0.01
Untreated, not shorn	26	0.10	0.01	0.03	0.01	0.01	0.02	0.03
Untreated, shorn	26	0.06	0.02	0.03	0.03	0.41	0.07	0.04

Table LIX. *Diazinon residues in pheasant and pigeon tissues* (BUNYAN *et al.* 1969).

Time of feeding (days)	Residue (p.p.m.) in			
	Pheasant		Pigeon	
	Fat	Liver	Fat	Liver
14	0.1	1	15	1
14	1	< 0.1	57	< 0.1
28	< 0.1	< 0.1	0.4	10
28	0.5	< 0.1	0.2	5
42	2	0.4	< 0.1	< 0.1
42	1.6	0.1	< 0.1	< 0.1

16. DIMEFOX. — Bis(dimethylamido) phosphoryl fluoride

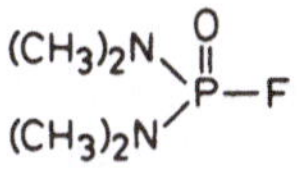

Alternate names: Pestox 14, Terra Systam, CR 409, DIFO, DMF, BEPO.
Application: Systemic insecticide of the phosphoroamide group on plants with long residual effect. No application in veterinary medicine.
Toxicity: See Table LX. The effective substance had as cholinergic effect which attacked predominantly on the periphery and showed tendency for cumulation after repeated application (OKINAKA *et al.* 1954).

Table LX. *Acute toxicities of dimefox for various animals.*

Animal species	Mode of application	LD_{50} (mg./kg.)	Reference
Mouse	*i.p.*	1.2	HOLMSTEDT (1959)
Mouse	*i.p.*	1.4	OKINAKA *et al.* (1954)
Rat	*per os*	5	MARTIN (1961)
Rat	*per os*	7.5	OKINAKA *et al.* (1954)
Rat	*i.p.*	5	MARTIN (1961)
Rat	*i.p.*	5	OKINAKA *et al.* (1954)
Guinea pig	*i.p.*	2.5	OKINAKA *et al.* (1954)
Dog	*i.v.*	5–10	OKINAKA *et al.* (1954)

Table LXI. *Residues in rat tissues after P^{32}-dimefox application* (ARTHUR and CASIDA 1958 a).

Tissue	Residue		
	s.c. 10 µg./g. after 5–6 min. = death [p.p.m. (equiv.)]	*per os* 2.5 µg./g. after 5 days	
		Hydrolysis (%)	(p.p.m.)
Brain	7.48	8	0.18
Blood	7.94	8	0.15
Heart	1.96	20	—
Intestine	5.38	4	0.32
Kidney	13.26	12	—
Liver	7.83	25	0.98
Muscle	2.56	8	—
Nerves	6.79	0	0.25
Pancreas	6.95	6	—
Salivary gland	4.62	9	—
Skin	4.22	2	—
Spleen	11.93	16	—
Stomach	1.68	10	—
Testicle	3.70	11	—

Metabolism and residues: Dimefox was turned into a strong ChE inhibitor by (rat) liver homogenate, while other tissues such as kidney, brain, duodenum, ileum, colon, skeleton muscles, heart muscle, thyroid gland, and suprarenal gland did not show an obvious effect (FEUWICK *et al.* 1957, ARTHUR and CASIDA 1958 a). OKINAKA *et al.* (1954), in their tests with liver homogenate, could not establish this activation. These tests, showed that the decontamination took place through hydrolysis at the fluorophosphate bond (OKINAKA *et al.* 1954) and led to hydrogen fluoride and bis-(dimethylamino) phosphate.

After *i.p.* injection of dimefox, the blood level for rats after 15 minutes was 6.8 µg./ml., after 30 minutes 5.4 µg./ml., and after 60 minutes 3.4 µg./ml. (OKINAKA *et al.* 1954).

After *i.v.* infusion of seven mg. of dimefox/kg. body wt., 0.5 to 1.2 percent of the total quantity appeared in the urine of dogs; 0.7 percent was excreted with the urine of rats during the first six hours after application and, in contrast, only 0.2 percent in 18 hours. Twelve hours after treatment neither dimefox nor its chloroform-soluble metabolites were excreted (OKINAKA *et al.* 1954).

Detailed reports about the excretion of dimefox by rats are found in ARTHUR and CASIDA (1958 a and b). Within five days 24 percent of the applied radioactive material was excreted with the urine, whereby 23 percent was reached after 24 hours. At the end of the second day completely water-soluble metabolites were the only ones present. Excretion with the feces reached about 13 percent within five days. The distributions in the tissues of rats are in Table LXI.

Reports about residues in meat of edible domestic animals could not be found.

17. DIMETHOATE. — O,O-Dimethyl-*S*-(*N*-monomethyl)-carbamoylmethyl dithiophosphate

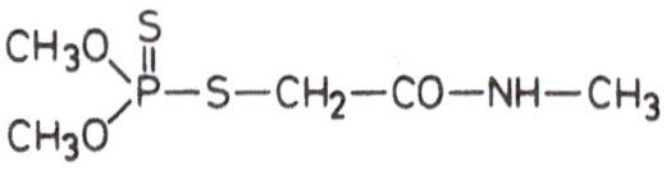

Alternate names: Dimethoate, Rogor, Roxion.
Application: Systemic insecticide and acaricide in plant protection, fly control (CHENG *et al.* 1961). Systemic control of bot-fly larvae on cattle; control of screw worms and ticks by oral, intramuscular, and dermal treatment (DRUMMOND 1959). The dosage was ten mg./kg. for *i.m.* injection, the concentration in feed (during ten days) two mg./kg. (MARQUARDT and LOVELACE 1961) or ten to 40 mg./kg., respectively, *per os* as a single application (DAUTERMANN *et al.* 1959), and 0.75 to 1.0 percent as spray.
Toxicity: See Table LXII.

DAUTERMANN *et al.* (1959), however, reported the *per os* LD_{50} for dimethoate and derivatives in rats as in Table LXIII.

Table LXII. *Acute oral toxicities of dimethoate for various animals after oral application.*

Animal species	Sex	LD_{50} (mg./kg.)	Remarks	Reference
Mouse	—	140	—	HOLMSTEDT (1959)
Rat	—	245	—	MARTIN (1961)
Rat	—	425	tech.	BRADY *et al.* (1960)
Rat	♂	186	a.i.	KLOTZSCHE (1961)
Rat	♂	200	40%	KLOTZSCHE (1964)
Rat	♂	224	25%	KLOTZSCHE (1961)
Rat	♀	190	25%	KLOTZSCHE (1961)
Rat	—	215–250	tech.	CASIDA & SANDERSON (1963)
Rat	♂	350	purified	CASIDA & SANDERSON (1963)
Rat	♀	650	purified	CASIDA & SANDERSON (1963)
Hen	—	50	purified	CASIDA & SANDERSON (1963)
Hen	—	25–40	tech.	CASIDA & SANDERSON (1963)

Table LXIII. *Acute oral toxicities of dimethoate and derivatives for the rat* (DAUTERMANN *et al.* 1959).

Compound	LD_{50} (mg./kg.)
Dimethoate	600
Dimethoate-P=O	55
Desmethyl [a]	1,500–2,000
Carboxy	2,500–3,000
O,O,*S*-Trimethylphosphorodithioate	900–1,100

[a] Impure sample containing some potassium O,O-dimethyl phosphorodithioate.

The compatibility of dimethoate was considerably dependent on formulation and purity. No poisonous symptom were recognized in human beings after *per os* treatment of 0.04 mg./kg. body wt. over four weeks; 0.13 to 0.26 mg./kg. body wt. did not cause a ChE inhibition in 21 days (SANDERSON and EDSON 1963). The metabolic products of dimethoate were 40 times more toxic than dimethoate itself, and the starting substance together with the metabolite had a greater toxic effect than the metabolite alone (RADELEFF 1960) (cf. CASIDA and SANDERSON 1963).

Tolerances: In the U.S.A., two p.p.m. in plants and fruit (FREAR and FRIEDMANN 1968).

Detection: Colorimetric method according to STENERSEN (1967) with 2,6-dibromobenzoquinone-4-chloroimide and according to SHERMAN and CHANG (1967) a microcolorimetric method according to DUGGAN *et al.* (1967).

Metabolism and residues: Dimethoate was hydrolyzed by half-hour cooking in plant tissue homogenate 22 to 39 percent (potato) and 44 to 52 percent (cabbage) (ASKEW *et al.* 1968). Dimethoate was not hydrolyzed by the rumen fluid (AHMED *et al.* 1958). It was resorbed well by the digestive tract (KAPLANIS *et al.* 1959 b).

Because of the rapid metabolism and excretion from the body, BÄR (1964 a) considered only short waiting times as being necessary before slaughtering. Dimethoate was tolerated in long-duration feeding by hens (SHERMAN *et al.* 1963) and cattle (MARQUARDT and LOVELACE 1961). From 0.28 to 0.56 mg./kg. were without influence on the ChE activity of the blood (HARDEE *et al.* 1963). With *in vitro* studies, UCHIDA *et al.* (1964) proved that dimethoate was predominantly decomposed in the liver and faster there than in other tissues, but different for different animal species: rabbits > sheep > dogs > rats > cattle > chickens > guinea pigs > mice > pigs. Among the liver metabolic products were dimethoate acid (sheep, rat, mouse) and O,O-dimethylphosphorothioate (guinea pig, rat, mouse). The metabolism of rats and cattle showed similarities (DAUTERMANN *et al.* 1959).

Dimethoate offered four possibilities of hydrolysis (BRADY and ARTHUR 1963): (1) hydrolysis of the O-methyl ester to desmethyldimethoate, (2) hydrolysis of the P–S–C bond to O,O-dimethyl thiophosphoric acid, (3) hydrolysis of the P–S–C bond to O,O-dimethyl dithiophosphoric acid, and (4) hydrolysis at the carbamoyl group to form the carboxy derivative.

In contrast, DAUTERMANN *et al.* (1959) reported five products (Fig. 9).

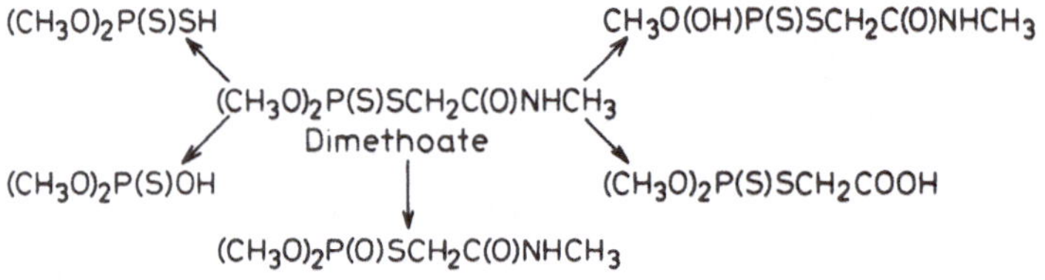

Fig. 9. Proposed initial sites of metabolic attack of the dimethoate molecule (DAUTERMANN *et al.* 1959).

The most important position of attack was the C–N bond, since 20 to 40 percent of the urine constituents were still carboxy derivatives. DAUTERMANN *et al.* (1959) established that the P–O isomer of dimethoate was not found in excretion products, tissues, or in blood.

On the contrary, CHAMBERLAIN *et al.* (1961) pointed to the higher P–O-dimethoate content in blood after *per os* intake, while the metabolism of dimethoate after *i.m.* treatment was similar for rats, sheep, and cattle, and WESTLAKE *et al.* (1960) pointed to the similarity of processes in plants and animals. The P–O compound was approximately 40 times more effective against stable flies than dimethoate (ROBERTS *et al.* 1958, PLAPP *et al.* 1960 b).

CHAMBERLAIN *et al.* (1961) considered the pathways of dimethoate metabolism in Figure 10 for sheep as being possible, whereby the cleavage of the C–N bond, as mentioned above, apparently prevailed since it was recognized from the enrichment of carboxy compounds in the urine.

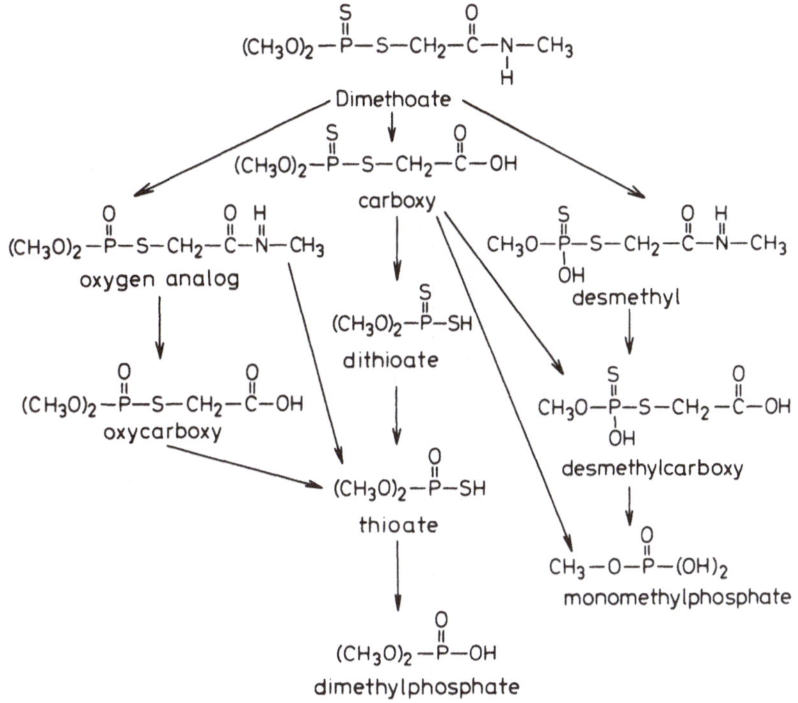

Fig. 10. Proposed metabolic pathway for dimethoate in sheep (Chamberlain *et al.* 1961).

Rat: After 100 mg. of dimethoate/kg. *per os*, male rats excreted 90 percent and female rats 55 percent with the urine within 48 hours, with the feces three and ten percent, respectively (Dautermann *et al.* 1959).

Dautermann *et al.* (1959) identified five out of seven metabolites in the urine of rats, which were present as hydrolysis products. The scheme in Figure 11 results (O'Brien 1960).

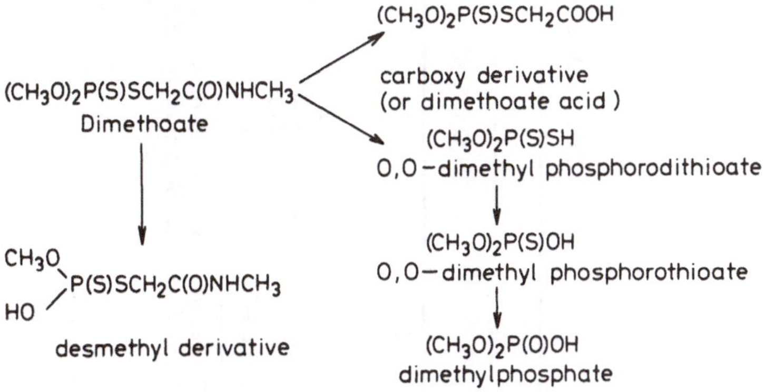

Fig. 11. Hydrolytic pathway of dimethoate (O'Brien 1960).

Table LXIV. *Natures of P^{32}-dimethoate metabolites in rat* [a] *urine* (Dautermann *et al.* 1959).

Hours after administration	Various hydrolysis products in the urine (%)						
	$(CH_3O)_2P(O)OH$	Carboxy	Carboxy + $(CH_3O)_2P(S)OH$	$(CH_3O)_2P(S)OH$	Desmethyl	$(CH_3O)_2P(S)OH$	Unknowns A + B
2	6.2	32.4	—	20.5	12.0	23.4	5.5
4	19.6	21.1	—	25.8	5.2	18.3	10.0
12	11.4	42.4	—	20.4	1.2	21.4	3.2
18	12.4	—	63.9 [b]	—	1.2	21.0	1.5
24	17.6	35.2	—	26.6	1.8	17.2	1.6
48	21.7	22.0	—	32.7	5.5	17.4	0.7
Composite 0–168 hr.	12.5	—	63.4 [b]	—	2.7	19.2	2.2

[a] Treated *per os* with 100 mg. of dimethoate/kg.
[b] The resolution was inadequate to differentiate the carboxy and $(CH_3O)_2P(S)OH$ fractions.

DAUTERMANN *et al.* (1959) treated rats with P^{32}-dimethoate (100 mg./kg.) *per os*. Male rats excreted 81 percent of the radioactive material within 24 hours. The fractionation results are seen in Table LXIV.

Rats decomposed dimethoate 50 to 75 times faster than insects; after 24 hours less than ten percent of the starting material was found in the urine and feces, after *per os* treatment or after dermal application. According to BRADY and ARTHUR (1963), who worked with P^{32}-dimethoate, the excretion data in Table LXV were found for rats, more than 95 percent of which were hydrolysis products.

Table LXV. *P^{32}-equivalents of dimethoate in rat excreta* (BRADY and ARTHUR 1963).

Mode of application	Residue in 72 hours (%)	
	Urine	Feces
Oral	45	5.8
Dermal	30.6	6.5

The derivatives which were either chloroform- or water-soluble are listed in Table LXVI.

Table LXVI. *P^{32}-dimethoate metabolites in rat excreta following oral or dermal treatment* (BRADY and ARTHUR 1963).

Compound	Residue as P^{32} equivalent (%) in							
	Oral [a] treatment, after				Dermal [b] treatment, after			
	Urine		Feces		Urine		Feces	
	6 hr.	24 hr.	72 hr.	0–72 hr.	6 hr.	24 h.	72 hr.	0–72 hr.
Dimethoate	<1	<1	<1	<1	<1	<1	<1	1
Oxygen analog	4	4	1	<1	5	2	1	<1
Carboxy derivative	32	12	16	4	37	27	6	11
Unknowns (silica gel)	2	3	3	3	3	1	4	1
O,O-Dimethyl-phosphoric acid	15	20	25	37	14	18	18	30
O,O-Dimethyl-phosphorothioic acid	19	18	18	10	<1	10	14	7
Desmethyl derivative	10	13	11	26	20	17	14	41
O,O-Dimethyl-phosphorodithioic acid	13	11	9	9	10	8	22	2
Unknowns [c]	4	19	17	2	<1	16	20	4

[a] 50 mg./kg.
[b] 100 mg./kg.
[c] By ion-exchange chromatography.

Residues in rat tissues after *per os* treatment with P^{32}-dimethoate show the highest persistent values in skin, liver, and bones, while the initially high value in kidney tissue decreases rapidly (Table LXVII).

Table LXVII. *Tissue residues of P^{32}-dimethoate after oral administration* [a] *of dimethoate to male rats* (Dautermann *et al.* 1959).

Tissue	Dimethoate equivalent (p.p.m.) after				
	24 hr.	72 hr.	168 hr.	336 hr.	672 hr.
Liver	10.1	2.0	1.2	0.58	0.53
Heart	2.1	0.08	0.12	0.22	0.07
Kidney	5.6	0.61	0.38	0.20	0.03
Brain	1.1	0.26	0.49	0.14	0.16
Fat	2.0	0.32	0.30	0.11	< 0.01
Muscle	1.6	0.25	0.29	0.08	0.09
Skin	5.9	4.1	1.8	2.1	0.32
Blood	2.8	0.11	0.14	—	0.02
Bone	2.8	1.80	1.8	—	—

[a] 100 mg./kg.

Cattle: After *per os* application of dimethoate, the level in blood of cattle reached maximum within three hours (6.4 p.p.m. after nine or ten mg./kg. body wt.); the radioactivity of chloroform-soluble substances reached maximum with 1.5 p.p.m. (after nine or ten mg./kg. body wt.) after two hours; after 48 hours, the blood value was under 0.05 p.p.m. (Dautermann *et al.* 1959). Plapp *et al.* (1960 b) found in the blood of cattle, after *per os* treatment of nine to ten mg. of P^{32}-dimethoate, 1.5 p.p.m. after two hours and 1.0 to 2.3 p.p.m. after three-to-six hours. After *i.m.* injection of ten mg./kg. body wt., the blood level reached 4.9 p.p.m. after one hour.

After *per os* treatment with nine, ten, and 40 mg. of dimethoate/kg., 73, 72, and 55.3 percent were excreted with the urine of cattle within 24 hours, and 2.4, 3.2, and 2.4 percent, respectively, with the feces.

Dimethoate was eliminated from the blood of cattle within 24 hours (Roberts *et al.* 1958) and elimination was more rapid after parenteral than after oral treatment.

The hydrolysis products occurring in the urine are reported in Table LXVIII; for cattle, dimethoate acid prevailed with 74 percent, which decreased during one day, while the amount of dimethylphosphate increased. Shortly after treatment the carboxy derivatives of dimethoate dominated as hydrolysis products; after 288 hours the following hydrolysis products were found in the urine of a cow (Dautermann *et al.* 1959): O,O-dimethyl-*S*-carboxymethyl phosphorodithioate, O,O-dimethylphosphoric acid, O,O-dimethylthiophosphoric acid, O,O-dimethyldithiophosphoric acid, and O-methyl *S* – CN-methylcarbamoyl-methyldithiophosphoric acid. Of the total radioactivity 3.7 percent was found in a sample of cattle feces, 0.015

Table LXVIII. *Dimethoate metabolites in the urine of a male steer* [a] (DAUTERMANN *et al.* 1959).

Hours after administration	Hydrolysis products in the urine (%)						
	$(CH_3O)_2P(O)OH$	Carboxy	Carboxy + $(CH_3O)_2P(S)OH$	$(CH_3O)_2P(S)OH$	Desmethyl	$(CH_3O)_2P(S)SH$	Unknowns A + B
1.2	2.1	74.0	—	9.0	2.1	11.6	1.2
2.3	4.3	—	84.5 [b]	—	2.1	6.2	2.9
4.2	11.9	—	61.0 [b]	—	8.1	15.1	3.9
6.1	28.0	22.9	—	28.9	10.3	8.0	1.9
12.3	4.4	11.1	—	25.8	8.3	6.9	3.5
19.6	56.3	—	31.0 [b]	—	2.7	7.4	2.6
30.1	45.7	18.3	—	12.5	3.9	17.4	2.2
Composite [c] of 0 to 30 hr.	32.6±2.1	24.8 [d]	45.8±0.67	21.0 [d]	7.1±1.1	12.6±4.0	1.9±1.7

[a] 100 mg./kg. *per os.*
[b] The resolution was inadequate to differentiate the carboxy and $(CH_3O)_2P(S)OH$ fractions.
[c] Variability from three values.
[d] Average of two values.

Table LXIX. *Excretion of dimethoate in the feces and urine of cattle* (Plapp *et al.* 1960 b).

Mode of application [a]	Blood max. (hours)	Duration of detection (hours)	Metabolites	90% excretion in	
				Urine (hours)	Feces
Per os	2.8	24	dimethoate + O-analog	24	traces
i.m.	1.0	—	dimethoate + O-analog	9	traces

[a] 10 mg./kg.

Table LXX. *P^{32}-dimethoate residues in tissues after oral administration to dairy cattle* (Dautermann *et al.* 1959).

Tissue	Dimethoate equivalents (p.p.m.) after		
	9.0 mg./kg.	10.0 mg./kg.	40.0 mg./kg.
	288 hr.	144 hr.	144 hr.
Bile	0.07	0.12	8.82
Bone marrow	0.00	0.05	0.16
Fat			
Kidney	< 0.01	0.02	0.09
Mesenteric	< 0.01	0.01	0.22
Gall bladder	0.10	0.01	—
Gland			
Adrenal	—	0.58	2.16
Mammary	0.17	0.32	1.15
Parotid	0.14	0.12	0.92
Thyroid	0.13	0.40	1.38
Intestine, small	0.16	0.30	2.16
Lung	0.29	0.86	1.40
Lymph node			
Mammary	0.25	—	0.68
Mesenteric	0.15	0.26	0.86
Subiliac	0.26	0.30	0.92
Submaxillary	0.13	0.55	2.00
Muscle, rear leg	0.10	0.14	0.37
Pancreas	0.34	0.43	1.20
Spinal cord	0.07	0.07	0.41
Spleen	0.24	0.23	1.10
Stomach			
Abomasum	0.20	0.22	0.62
Omasum	0.11	0.19	0.72
Reticulum	0.09	0.21	1.34
Rumen	0.15	0.15	2.50
Sublingual parotid	0.52	2.30	0.92
Skin	0.02	0.06	0.33
Tongue	0.11	0.22	0.26
Urinary bladder	0.09	0.11	0.33
Uterine horn	0.08	0.20	0.57

Table LXXI. *Natures of tissue residues in P^{32}-dimethoate-treated cattle* (DAUTERMANN *et al.* 1959).

Tissue	Dimethoate equivalents (p.p.m.) 9.0 mg./kg., after 288 hr.			10.0 mg./kg. after 144 hr.			40.0 mg./kg. after 144 hr.		% Recovery [a]
	Total	$CHCl_3$-soluble	Dimethoate	Total	$CHCl_3$-soluble	Dimethoate	Total	$CHCl_3$-soluble	
Liver	2.10	0.23	0.03	4.40	0.45	0.08	5.00	0.62	69.8 ± 2.9
Heart	0.17	0.05	trace	0.24	0.08	0.01	0.93	0.35	59.6 ± 6.2
Kidney	0.26	0.14	0.01	0.55	0.19	0.10	1.70	0.25	63.5 ± 4.6
Brain	0.13	0.08	trace	0.15	0.10	0.01	1.80	0.91	51.6 ± 6.5
Fat, subcutaneous	0.01	0.01	trace	0.01	0.01	trace	0.22	0.00	74.4 ± 5.0
Muscle loin	0.10	0.01	trace	0.22	0.01	trace	0.35	0.05	65.3 ± 4.4

[a] The percent recovery was determined by adding four p.p.m. of radioactive dimethoate initially to the tissues and immediately proceeding with the normal extraction procedure.

percent of which was chloroform-soluble; only 0.0015 percent of the radioactive compounds corresponded to dimethoate (DAUTERMANN 1959).

The data of PLAPP *et al.* (1960 b) serve as comparative values (Table LXIX).

Dimethoate remained in the bodies of cattle only a short time after oral application; it was rapidly metabolized and excreted. The residues in cattle tissues are reported in Table LXX. Maximum (equivalent) P^{32}-dimethoate in *s.c.* fat as well as in blood was reached three hours after application; the radioactivity of the chloroform-soluble fraction decreased from 0.95 p.p.m. after three hours to <0.1 p.p.m. after eight hours. After 12 hours only traces were found in the tissues (Table LXXI).

CLABORN and RADELEFF (1960) reported the residue data in Table LXXII for P^{32}-dimethoate applications to cattle and sheep.

Table LXXII. *Tissue residues after P^{32}-dimethoate application to cattle and sheep* (CLABORN and RADELEFF 1960).

Animal species	Mode of application	Dosage (mg./kg.)	Slaughtering after days	Residue (p.p.m.) in					
				Omental fat	Renal	Muscle	Liver	Kidney	Heart
Cattle	*per os*	10	7	0.012	0	0.03	1.13	0.99	0.27
Cattle	*i.m.*	10	7	0	0	0.02	0.30	0.18	0.06
Sheep	*i.m.*	25	14	0	—	trace	0.01	trace	trace
						trace	0.02	0.01	0.01
Sheep	*i.m.*	25	28	0	—	trace	trace	0.01	0.01
						0.01	0.02	0.01	0.02

After an oral treatment with ten mg./kg. body wt., PLAPP *et al.* (1960 b) reported residues in fat of cattle obtained by bioptic sampling as three p.p.m. after three hours, and 0.1 p.p.m. after eight hours; 14 days after oral intake the values in all tissues had dropped to <0.1 p.p.m. Shortly after treatment with P^{32}-dimethoate, high blood values were observed for cattle, which reached their maximum after one hour for *i.m.* treatment and after three to six hours for *per os* treatment. Similar time values were found by ROBERTS *et al.* (1958) with the help of biological tests *(Stomoxys calcitrans)*; their values from *i.v.* application are only a few minutes. From 87 to 98 percent of the radioactive material exhibited the R_f-value of dimethoate, while about 12 percent remained unknown (KAPLANIS *et al.* 1959).

On the contrary, simultaneously with a very rapid decrease of dimethoate concentration there was an increase of an unknown substance (ROBERTS *et al.* 1958) which was 40 times more toxic for stable flies than the starting substance (KAPLANIS *et al.* 1959, ROBERTS *et al.* 1958), and which exhibited a 365 times stronger ChE inhibition. The magnitude of toxicity changed in combination with varying quantities of dimethoate (ROBERTS *et al.* 1958).

During the very rapid decomposition of dimethoate, the metabolic products in the calf appeared predominantly in the urine, 87 to 90 percent within 24 hours after *per os* and within nine hours after *i.m.* treatment; only 0.2 percent was chloroform extractable in the alkaline range (KAPLANIS *et al.* 1959). With radioactive material 3.7 to 5.0 percent appeared in the feces after *per os* intake and 1.1 percent after *i.m.* injection. The metabolic products in the urine were dimethylphosphate, dimethylthiophosphate, a little dimethyldithiophosphate, and unknown substances. Only traces of dimethoate could be found. Of the metabolic products in the feces between six and 36 hours after *per os* application 68.8 percent were unknown substances, while 31.2 percent was dimethoate. After *i.m.* injection, the larger part was identified as dimethoate, and only traces came from unknown substances (KAPLANIS *et al.* 1959). The analysis of tissues two weeks

Table LXXIII. *Radioactive compounds in calf tissues two weeks after administration* [a] *of* P^{32}*-dimethoate* (KAPLANIS *et al.* 1959).

Tissue	Residue (μg.-equiv./g. of tissue) [b]	
	Total [c]	Chloroform-extractable [d]
Liver	1.72	0.02
Kidney	0.17	0.00
Spleen	0.15	0.00
Brain	0.31	0.07
Spinal cord	0.09	0.00
Testes	0.18	0.02
Lung	0.27	0.02
Heart	0.09	0.00
Tongue	0.08	0.00
Gullet	0.09	0.00
Muscle		
Loin	0.11	0.00
Round	0.09	0.00
Shoulder	0.10	0.00
Blood	0.03	0.00
Gall	0.00	—
Bone		
Spongy	2.01	—
Compact	0.04	—
Fat		
Subcutaneous	—	0.00
Omental	—	0.00
Perirenal	—	0.00
Marrow	—	0.00

[a] 10 mg./kg.
[b] Based on wet wt. except bone.
[c] As determined from tissue homogenates; significant sensitivity 0.034 μg.-equiv./g.
[d] Significant sensitivity for fat 0.007 μg.-equiv./g.; for the remainder of the tissue, 0.015 μg.-equiv./g.

after *i.m.* injection gave the concentrations reported in Table LXIII. Marrow bones and liver contained the largest quantities of radioactive substances. Water-soluble radioactive substances were found only in liver and muscles. The total residue quantity was low.

Sheep: The maximum blood level of P^{32}-dimethoate after *i.m.* injection was reached between one-half and one hour (<12 μg.-equiv./ml.). After three days only 0.1 p.p.m. of dimethoate equivalents were detectable. The products, which were soluble in organic solvents such as methylene chloride, varied between 5.4 and 20.7 percent. After 12 hours they were under 0.1 percent. Also, after *per os* treatment maximum concentration in blood was reached after one-half to one hour; however, the relations of the residues which were soluble in organic solvents were different from those after *i.m.* injection. The dimethoate concentration decreased rapidly in blood, while the concentration of its O-analog increased correspondingly (CHAMBERLAIN *et al.* 1961). The excretion of dimethoate for sheep after *i.m.* injection was 80 percent in 72 hours, predominantly with the urine and with maximum excretion between one and six hours for both male and female animals. After feeding of a single offering it peaked in the urine after six hours. The concentration of radioactive material was three to five times higher for female than for male animals. Eleven or 12 compounds were established in the urine, of which only six were identified (Tables LXXIV and LXXV). The carboxy derivatives prevailed for one-half to three hours; during their decrease dimethylphosphoric acid and an unknown substance, of which male animals excreted four times more than female, increased. Further metabolites were dimethylthiophosphoric acid and small amounts of dimethyldithiophosphoric acid, the O-analog of dimethoate, and dimethoate

Table LXXIV. *Metabolic products in urine of four sheep* [a] *treated i.m. with P^{28}-dimethoate* [b] (CHAMBERLAIN *et al.* 1961).

Metabolite and R_f value	Percentages (av.) after					
	1 hr.	3 hr.	6 hr.	12 hr.	24 hr.	48 hr.
Unknown A 0.00	0.22	0.30	0.72	0.78	1.16	7.96
Unknown B 0.03	0.00	0.00	0.02	0.60	1.15	0.00
Unknown C 0.06	0.28	2.94	6.24	2.62	2.38	1.26
Unknown D 0.10	2.02	5.99	20.94	12.06	19.56	18.61
Dimethylphosphoric acid 0.17	1.73	7.35	26.26	47.21	52.96	50.55
Unknown E 0.25	1.39	0.85	1.17	2.64	2.17	2.1
Dimethylphosphorothioic acid 0.35	4.21	8.58	8.04	11.46	7.05	7.68
Dimethylphosphorodithioic acid 0.40	1.63	2.04	2.68	0.60	2.53	0.41
Carboxy derivative 0.51	86	68	30	17	6.88	4.26
Unknown F 0.64	2.52	2.31	1.35	3.50	4.25	4.65
Oxygen analog 0.74	0.12	0.43	0.65	1.02	0.11	0.00
Dimethoate 0.91	0.18	0.02	0.01	0.32	0.04	1.70

[a] Two males and two females.

[b] Analyses by an 80:20 $CH_3CN:H_2O$ paper chromatography system.

Table LXXV. *Metabolic products in urine of sheep fed*[a] *P^{32}-dimethoate in cracked grain* (Chamberlain *et al.* 1961).

Metabolite and R_f value	Percentages after						
	3 hr.	6 hr.	15 hr.	18 hr.	24 hr.	48 hr.	72 hr.
Unknown A 0.00	0.4	0.2	0.7	1.25	7.0	2.2	18.2
Unknown B 0.03	0.0	0.0	0.0	0.0	0.0	2.8	0.0
Unknown C 0.06	3.1	2.0	5.7	4.7	8.7	6.8	13.8
Unknown D 0.10	22	13	5.1	27	43	60 [b]	68 [b]
Dimethylphosphoric acid 0.17	17	28	63	44	21		
Unknown E 0.25	1.4	0.9	0.0	0.2	0.8	0.0	0.0
Dimethylphosphorothioic acid 0.35	14	17	17	11	12	12	0.0
Dimethylphosphorodithioic acid 0.40	5.7	3.9	3.2	5.9	3.4	9.3	0.0
Carboxy derivative 0.51	34	29	5.1	5.9	1.3	5.0	0.0
Unknown F 0.64	2.1	4.1	0.0	0.3	2.4	2.0	0.0
Oxygen analog 0.74	0.3	0.0	0.0	0.35	0.5	0.0	0.0
Dimethoate 0.91	0.1	0.2	0.1	0.0	0.0	0.0	0.0

[a] Single dose of 3.0 mc.
[b] Combination of unknown D and dimethylphosphoric acid.

itself (Chamberlain *et al.* 1961). Only a small quantity of radioactivity appeared in the feces after *i.m.* injection with an excretion maximum of 12 to 24 hours; after *per os* intake maximum excretion was reached between six and ten hours, with 3.2 percent of the total radioactivity (Chamberlain *et al.* 1961).

Four weeks after *i.m.* injection the residue maximum in the tissues was 0.021 p.p.m. In heart and muscle the values were 0.02 and 0.01 p.p.m., respectively. Of these residues 15 to 20 percent were phospholipids (Chamberlain *et al.* 1961).

Poultry: The microcolorimetric method used by Sherman and Chang (1967) did not allow the detection of the O-analog of dimethoate and of metabolites which did not have the thiono group. Even after an one-year application of dimethoate (30 p.p.m. in water), only negligible residues remained in the tissues of hens. After feeding of technical dimethoate 0.12 to 0.21 p.p.m. could be found at slaughter and seven days later in some animals, but not in all of them.

Table LXXVI. *Residues of dimethoate in pheasants and pigeons*[a] (Bunyan *et al.* 1969).

Animal species	Duration of feeding (days)	Residues (p.p.m.) in	
		Liver	Fat
Pheasant	42	0.5, 0.4	3.8, 4.5
Pigeon	14	0.4, 1.2	— —

[a] 100 p.p.m. of dimethoate in feed; two birds for each test.

For pheasants and pigeons BUNYAN *et al.* (1969) established the residues in Table LXXVI after feeding times of 14 and 42 days with 100 p.p.m. of dimethoate.

18. DIOXATHION. — *p*-Dioxane-2,3-diyl ethyl phosphorodithioate

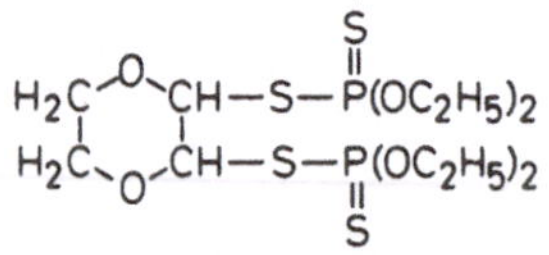

Alternate names: Delnav, Navadel, Hercules AC 528. The technical product consisted of 70 percent *cis*- and *trans*-isomers, and 30 percent related insecticidal compounds (FRAWLEY *et al.* 1963). ARTHUR and CASIDA (1959) found a total of eight fractions. It is an insecticide and acaricide.
Veterinary application: Tick control; 0.15 percent effective against lice, horn flies, etc. with long residual effect.
Toxicity: See Table LXXVII. The *cis*-isomer was more toxic than the *trans*-isomer (ARTHUR and CASIDA 1959). For the human being, 0.075 mg./kg. body wt. showed no toxic effect (FRAWLEY *et al.* 1963).

Table LXXVII. *Acute toxicities of dioxathion for various animals after oral and s.c. application.*

Animal species	Mode of application	Toxic dosage (mg./kg.)	LD_{50} (mg./kg.)	Remarks	Reference
Mouse	*per os*	—	176	—	FRAWLEY *et al.* (1963)
Rat	*per os*	—	23–118	— [a]	FRAWLEY *et al.* (1963)
Rat [b]	*per os*	—	110	—	MARTIN (1961)
Rat	*s.c.*	—	95	in oil	ARTHUR & CASIDA (1959)
Dog	*per os*	—	10–40	—	FRAWLEY *et al.* (1963)
Calf	*per os*	max. nontox. 5	—	1–2 weeks	RADELEFF & BUSHLAND (1960)

[a] Dependent on solvents and strain of animal.
[b] Male.

Detection: See DUGGAN *et al.* (1967).
Tolerances and restrictions: Tolerance in the U.S.A., one p.p.m. for fat and meat of cattle, goats, pigs, and sheep (compare for plants: 2.1 to 4.9 p.p.m.) (FREAR and FRIEDMAN 1968).
Metabolism and residues: Dioxathion residues were found neither after feeding nor after spraying in the muscles of test animals (DANGSCHAT 1965). For rats, the excretion after *per os* treatment was mainly with the urine, of which more than 98 percent was hydrolysis products (ARTHUR and CASIDA 1959). PLAPP *et al.* (1960 a) proved in studies with mice that there was no difference in hydrolysis when dioxathion was applied *per os*, dermally, or *s.c.* After *per os* application of one to five mg./kg. of P^{32}-

Table LXXVIII. *Dioxathion residues in the tissues of various animals.*

Animal species	Mode of application	Days after treatment	Residues (p.p.m.) in					Reference
			Kidney	Liver	Muscle	Kidney fat	Omental fat	
Bull	spray 0.25%	2	0.06	0.13	0.08	1.4	1.4	JACKSON *et al.* (1962)
Goat	spray 0.25%	2	—	0.0	0.02	0.53	0.56	JACKSON *et al.* (1962)
Calf	spray 16.2 mg./kg. (P^{32})	7	0.07	0.20	0.0	1.07	1.51	CLABORN *et al.* (1960 a)
Bull	spray 8.8 mg./kg. (P^{32})	7	0.42	2.60	< 0.5	0.24	0.26	PLAPP *et al.* (1960 a)
	spray (Chem-Best)	7	0.25	1.97	0.02	< 0.01	< 0.01	PLAPP *et al.* (1960 a)
Sheep	spray 16 mg./kg.	7	0.06	0.16	0.0	0.86	1.25	CLABORN & RADELEFF (1960)
Sheep	spray 0.25%	2	0.15	0.24	0.14 [a]	0.42	—	ANONYMOUS 28 [b]
Bull	spray 0.25%	2	0.13	0.06	0.08	1.44	1.44	ANONYMOUS 28
Pig	spray 0.25%	1	0.07	0.05	0.01	0.0	—	ANONYMOUS 28
		2	0.01	0.03	0.04	0.0	—	ANONYMOUS 28

[a] Extracted with *n*-hexane; 0.0 when extracted with 2:1 *n*-hexane:isopropyl alcohol.

[b] Comparative data with respect to analyses which were conducted at the same time by Hercules in Kerrville and Corvallis or comparisons between colorimetric and isotope methods show only negligible deviations.

Table LXXIX. *Dioxathion residues in omental biopsy fat after Delnav spray* [a] (JACKSON *et al.* 1962).

Animal species	Group spray (%)	No. of animals	Residues (p.p.m.) after [b]										
			Control value	1 day	2 days	5 days	7 days	10 days	14 days	17 days	21 days	22 days	28 days
Sheep	0.00	3	0.19	0.24	—	—	0.35	—	0.12	—	0.24	—	—
	0.25	3	0.17	0.32	—	—	0.44	—	0.39	—	0.36	—	—
	0.15	6	0.19	0.28	0.48	0.39	0.39	0.29	0.20	0.51	0.25	0.27	—
Angora goats	0.00	3	0.09	—	—	0.06	—	—	—	—	—	—	0.07
	0.25	3	0.00	—	—	1.31	—	—	—	—	—	—	0.11
	0.15	3	0.01	—	—	0.59	—	—	—	—	—	—	0.00
Cows	0.00	3	0.10	—	0.14	—	0.08	—	0.12	—	0.16	—	—
	0.25	3	0.12	—	1.05	—	0.57	—	0.11	—	0.23	—	—
	0.15	3	0.08	—	0.73	—	0.33	—	0.03	—	0.00	—	—
Pigs	0.00	5	—	0.17	0.17	—	0.02	—	0.00	—	0.03	—	—
	0.25	3	—	0.16	0.16	—	0.06	—	0.1	—	0.10	—	—

[a] EC.

[b] One animal each slaughtered for each test day.

dioxathion over ten days, rats excreted about 45 percent with the urine and 20 percent with the feces (ARTHUR and CASIDA 1959). After feeding of this compound, fatty tissue showed only a slight tendency to accumulate it; however, it decreased rapidly after discontinuation of feeding (ARTHUR and CASIDA 1959). After a single application *per os* of five mg./kg., 0.4 p.p.m. of P^{32}-compounds was found after 24 hours in the fat.

After *per os* application of 25 mg./kg. of the *trans*-compound, which ARTHUR and CASIDA (1959) found in Delnav, two p.p.m. was found in the liver after 48 hours, one p.p.m. in fat and kidneys, and $<$one p.p.m. each in muscle, brain, and heart. The corresponding values after treatment with the *cis*- compound were four p.p.m. in liver, one p.p.m. in kidneys, and $<$one p.p.m. for each of the other tissues. The residues in the tissues were $>$90 percent water-soluble, and the ones in fat more than half hexane-soluble.

The results of quantitative residue determinations for various domestic animals are summarized in Tables LXXVIII, and LXXIX.

The common application dosage was 0.15 percent Delnav; however, for higher dosages the residues also remained low, especially in muscle tissue. The cumulation in fatty tissues is shown in Table LXXIX. Ninety-seven percent of the benzene-soluble residues in fat consisted of unchanged dioxathion, two percent were salts of diethylphosphoric and diethylthiophosphoric acid. No oxidation products with phosphate or thiophosphate structure were found of the well-known active ChE inhibitor type (ANONYMOUS 28).

The highest residue values were found in fat and reached their maximum between the second and seventh day after treatment. Similar values for cattle fat after colorimetric determination were reported (ANONYMOUS 28). Two days after a single spray with Delnav of 0.15 percent or 0.25 percent EC the residues in fat were 0.7 and 1 p.p.m., respectively, concentrations which fell under 0.1 p.p.m. within two or three weeks, respectively. CLABORN and RADELEFF (1960) noted the residues in fat two days after 0.25 percent spray application with the following p.p.m. values: pigs 0.05, cattle 1.64, sheep 0.12, and goats 0.3. For an application concentration of 0.15 percent, the residues remained below one p.p.m. Also, after several repeated 0.15 percent sprays with 14-day intervals, the highest residue values for cattle were 0.25 p.p.m. after the fourth treatment and thus remained under one p.p.m. (JACKSON *et al.* 1960, CLABORN and RADELEFF 1960); after a single feeding of 0.4 mg. of Delnav/kg. body wt. only 0.08 p.p.m. residues were found in the cattle fat (ANONYMOUS 28).

After *per os* treatment with Delnav, which is only very slowly atacked by the rumen fluid (AHMED *et al.* 1958), the highest P^{32}-count for the bull was reached after 12 hours (CHAMBERLAIN *et al.* 1960 [18]); after dermal application the maximum approximately three hours. Also, PLAPP *et al.*

[18] CHAMBERLAIN worked for the *per os* study with purified dioxathion which had 62.8 percent of *cis*- and *trans*- isomers.

(1960 a) found, for only a short time, merely traces of dioxathion and its metabolites in the blood of bulls after spray treatment. In their tests the P^{32} could not be measured any more after 36 hours, and in those of Chamberlain *et al.* (1960) not after one week. Excretion tooke place mainly with the urine with maximum after 12 hours (Plapp *et al.* 1960 a), or six hours after dermal and nine hours after *per os* treatment, respectively (Chamberlain *et al.* 1960); to a very slight degree excretion fraction in the feces was four with maximum after 24 hours. The excretion fraction in the feces was four times lower after dermal treatment than after *per os* application (Chamberlain *et al.* 1960). Excretion products in the urine and feces were insoluble in organic solvents or only soluble in traces. Cleavage of the P – S, or also the S – C bond, and oxidation before and after hydrolysis (Arthur and Casida 1959) were apparent from the main urine excretion product: diethylthiophosphoric acid. Furthermore, there were diethylphosphoric acid, diethyldithiophosphoric acid, and a few unknown metabolites present. Dioxathion was decomposed in a few hours to nontoxic compounds in cattle blood (Chamberlain *et al.* 1960); this proved the poor systemic effect of this compound, indeed.

19. DURSBAN. — Phosphorothioic acid, O,O-diethyl O-(3,5,6-trichloro-2-pyridyl) ester

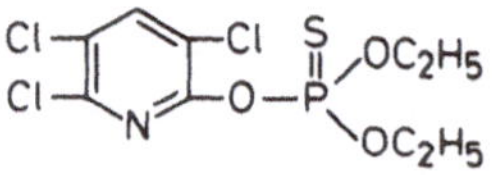

Alternate names: ENT 27311.
Application: Wide-range insecticide in plant protection (Kenaga *et al.* 1965); as spray for mosquito control; effective against animal parasites, especially ticks. There was also a good effect against *Neoschongastia americana* on turkeys (Dishburger *et al.* 1969).
Toxicity: See Table LXXX.

Table LXXX. *Acute oral toxicities of Dursban for various animals* (Frear 1965).

Animal species	LD_{50} (mg./kg.)
Rat [a]	135
Rat [b]	160
Rabbit	1,000–2,000
Guinea pig	500

[a] Female.
[b] Male.

The O-analog of dursban is the actual ChE inhibitor (Smith *et al.* 1967).
Detection: See Smith and Fischer (1967), Claborn *et al.* (1968), and Hunt *et al.* (1969).

Table LXXXI. *Dursban and related residues in rat tissues after per os treatment* [a] (SMITH *et al.* 1967).

Elapsed hours	Residue (millimoles/kg.) in									
	Kidney	Liver	Lung	Fat	Heart	Skin	Spleen	Testicle	Bone	Muscle
4	0.09240	0.06900	0.04060	0.03170	0.02880	0.02430	0.02130	0.01580	0.01020	0.00930
72	0.00177	0.00110	0.00210	0.00452	0.00140	—	0.00089	0.00177	—	0.00072
168	0.00043	0.00026	0.00026	0.00275	0.00013	0.00083	0.00022	0.00026	0.00029	0.00019
240	0.00010	0.00026	0.00010	0.00119	0.00010	0.00079	0.00020	0.00006	0.0028	0.00009
480	0.00020	0.00016	0.00016	0.00013	0.00016	0.00077	0.00008	0.00019	0.00013	0.00019

[a] 10 mg./300 g. body wt.

Table LXXXII. *Dursban residues in cattle tissues* (CLABORN *et al.* 1969).

Treatment and concentration	Weeks after treatment	Residue (p.p.m.)								
		Omental fat	Renal fat	Subcuta-neous fat	Muscle	Brain	Liver	Heart	Kidney	Spleen
Spray, 0.25%	1	0.60	0.67	0.71	0.01	trace	trace	trace	trace	—
Spray, 0.05%	1	0.19	0.20	0.19	—	—	—	—	—	—
Dip, 0.05%	1	0.38 [a]	0.38 [a]	0.37 [a]	trace	trace	trace	trace	trace	trace
Dip, 3×0.05% at	2	0.15 [b]	0.13 [b]	0.15 [b]	—	—	—	—	—	—
2-week intervals	1	2.07 [a]	1.85 [a]	2.19 [a]	0.03 [a]	0.01 [a]	trace	trace	0.01 [a]	trace

[a] Average of two values.
[b] Average of three values.

Metabolism and residues: SMITH *et al.* (1967) investigated the metabolism of Cl^{36}-Dursban in rats. The largest quantity, 89 percent of radioactive substances, was eliminated with the urine; 11 percent was excreted with the feces; 81 and nine percent, respectively, were reached after 26 hours. The metabolic products consisted 75 to 80 percent of 3,5,6-trichloro-2-pyridyl-phosphate and 15 to 20 percent of 3,5,6-trichloro-2-pyridinol. Furthermore, there were persistent traces of Dursban, which was cumulated in the tissues and stored in the fat, from which it was slowly eliminated. The distribution in the organs of rats after *per os* intake of the labeled substance is shown in Table LXXXI, reported as millimoles of radioactive components/kg. of body tissue.

Dursban was not decomposed by the rumen fluid (GUTENMANN *et al.* 1968). Of the applied dosage of five p.p.m. of Dursban in a daily ratio of 50 lb. over four days, 1.7 percent appeared in the feces of cattle during the last three days of treatment and the following day, but none later. Dursban could not be detected in the urine; however, two metabolites were present identified as the methyl esters of diethylthiophosphate and diethylphosphate and which represent 35.9 and 26.8 percent, respectively, of the total applied dosage (GUTENMANN *et al.* 1968).

Residues in tissues of cattle after external application are reported in Table LXXXII. They were present mainly in fat tissue. The concentrations in fat were about twice as high after a dip than after a spray, and after several dips about six times higher than after a single dip. The O-analog of Dursban in fat samples was about one percent of the residues; it was not present in the other tissues.

Five weeks after a spray and a single treatment, the residue concentration in fat decreased to negligible values. After several dip treatments residues were eliminated within ten weeks (CLABORN *et al.* 1968).

Residues of Dursban in turkey tissues were insignificant when their enclosures had been treated with different formulations of Dursban (EC, WP, or granular) (DISHBURGER *et al.* 1969). In Table LXXXIII the average values are summarized. Values in skin and fat were somewhat higher after

Table LXXXIII. *Residue data in turkey*[a] *tissues after use of Dursban in their enclosures* (DISHBURGER *et al.* 1969).

Formulation	Dosage (lb. a.i./acre soil)	Days after treatment	Residue (p.p.m.) in			
			Skin	Fat	Muscle	Liver
EC (M-2838)	4.5	7	0.02	0.01	< 0.01	< 0.01
	4.5	14	0.01	< 0.01	< 0.01	< 0.01
Granular (M-3119)	4.5	7	0.01	~ 0.01	< 0.01	< 0.01
	4.5	14	0.02	~ < 0.01	< 0.01	< 0.01
WP (TF-137)	4.5	7	0.06	0.02	< 0.01	< 0.01
	4.5	14	0.03	0.02	< 0.01	< 0.01

[a] Three birds/test.

WP treatment than for the other formulations. HUNT *et al.* (1969) established residues only in skin and fat of turkeys after dusting.

SMITH *et al.* (1966) reported investigations with C^{14}-Dursban on fish, which are able to take in the substance from the water, for instance, after a mosquito control action. Fish ingested Dursban only in slight amounts and rapidly metabolized it. The largest intake with 50 p.p.m. Dursban was during the first eight to ten hours of exposure in the water; the maximum was reached in 12 hours. It was established from the radioactivity that the largest residues were present in the viscera. After one day of exposure, they contained 0.08 mmol./kg., the head 0.07 mmol./kg., the skin 0.004 mmol. per kg., and meat 0.003 mmol./kg. The radioactivity decreased rapidly within one to two days. Metabolic products were predominantly acetone-soluble after 30 hours exposure and consisted of Dursban plus hydrolysis products: 3,5,6-trichloro-2-pyridylphosphate, 3,5,6-trichloro-2-pyridinol, and ethyl O-(3,5,6-trichloro-2-pyridyl) thiophosphate (Table LXXXIV).

LXXXIV. *Distribution of radioactivity in fish exposed to water containing 50 p.p.m. of C^{14}-Dursban* (SMITH *et al.* 1966).

Tissue	Radioactive residue (mmoles/kg. tissue) after					
	30 hours			9 days		
	Acetone extract	Water extract	Tissue residue	Acetone extract	Water extract	Tissue residue
Head	0.072	0.001	trace	0.009	0.001	trace
Skin	0.045	0.001	trace	0.006	0.002	trace
Meat	0.058	0.001	trace	0.009	0.001	trace
Viscera	0.013	0.070	0.003	0.017	0.026	0.001

The distribution and change of concentration depending on time as well as the type of metabolites are seen in this table. After nine days only one-third of the residues was still soluble in acetone. After 48 hours the following products plus Dursban were identified in the tissues by SMITH *et al.* (1966), when the concentration in water had ben 300 p.p.m. of Dursban: ethyl O-(3,5,6-trichloro-2-pyridyl) thiophosphate, ethyl O-(3,5,6-trichloro-2-pyridyl) phosphate, 3,5,6-trichloro-2-pyridyl-phosphate, and 3,5,6-trichloro-2-pyridinol. None of these substances inhibited ChE. The last-mentioned metabolite was mostly present in the end, and apparently was slowly decomposed by dehalogenation and by cleavage of the ring (SMITH *et al.* 1966).

20. EPN. — Phosphonothioic acid, phenyl-, O-ethyl O-*p*-nitrophenyl ester

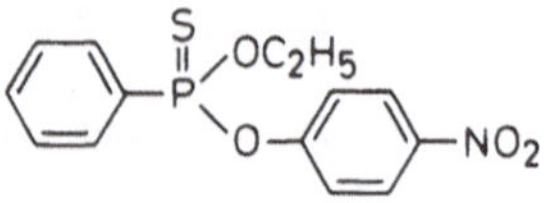

Alternate name: EPN 300.
Application: Plant protection against insects and mites as WP or EC and as granules and dusts.
Toxicity: See Table LXXXV. There was a fast resorption through the skin. The ChE inhibiting effect was activated in the liver by conversion to the O-analog (NEAL and DU BOIS 1965, HODGE *et al.* 1954). In chronic feeding tests over a period of two years 75 p.p.m. were tolerated by female rats and 150 p.p.m. by male rats without showing symptoms. However, PERKOW (1956) pointed out that 25 p.p.m. in rat food created cumulative effects. Dogs did not show any damage after two mg./kg. body wt. over one year (HODGE *et al.* 1954).

Table LXXXV. *Acute toxicities of EPN to rats and rabbits after different applications.*

Animal species	Mode of application	Sex	Toxic dosage (mg./kg.)	LD_{50} (mg./kg.)	Reference
Rat	*per os* [a]	♂	—	42	HODGE *et al.* (1954)
Rat	*per os* [a]	♀	—	14	HODGE *et al.* (1954)
Rat	*per os*	♂	—	35–45	MARTIN (1961)
Rat	*per os*	♀	—	9–15	MARTIN (1961)
Rat	*per os*	♂	—	91	FRAWLEY *et al.* (1952)
Rat	*per os*	♀	—	14.5	FRAWLEY *et al.* (1952)
Rat	*i.p.* [b]	♂	—	64	HOLMSTEDT (1959)
Rat	*i.p.* [b]	♀	—	48	HOLMSTEDT (1959)
Rat	percutan.	♂	—	230	ANONYMOUS 18
Rat	percutan.	♀	—	25	ANONYMOUS 18
Rabbit	percutan.	♂	30–50	—	ANONYMOUS 18
Rabbit	percutan.	♀	90–150	—	ANONYMOUS 18

[a] Crystalline substance.
[b] Technical product.

Detection: GUNTHER and BLINN (1955), DUGGAN *et al.* (1967); compare also glc method in plant tissues (KIRKLAND and PEASE 1967).
Tolerances: In the U.S.A., 0.5 to 3.0 p.p.m. in certain plants (FREAR and FRIEDMANN 1968, ANONYMOUS 18).
Metabolism and residues: In a two-year study with rats, HODGE *et al.* (1954) established only a low and varying residue which was idependent of the EPN content of the food. The residue content was increased in some tissues for the highest fed EPN dosage, but without showing a cumulative effect (Table LXXXVI).

The desulfuration of the EPN molecule is not a necessary presupposition for subsequent hydrolysis in the organism (compare data for parathion), the endpoint of which is *p*-nitrophenol. From 500 p.p.m. of EPN in the rumen fluid there were recovered in 24 hours 1.8 percent amino-EPN, aside from hydrolysis products (AHMED *et al.* 1958).

A combination of EPN and malathion leads to potentiation. The metabolic processes in this regard deal chiefly with malathion (see malathion);

Table LXXXVI. *Ranges of EPN residues in rat tissues after two years on diets shown* (HODGE *et al.* 1954).

Tissue	Residues (p.p.m.)			
	Male		Female	
	50–150 p.p.m. in diet	450 p.p.m. in diet	25–75 p.p.m. in diet	225 p.p.m. in diet
Liver	0–5	4–7	0–9	5–7
Kidney	0–2	2–3	0–3	2–5
Perirenal fat	0–2	2–4	0–4	3
Brain	0–7	4–6	0–6	3–12
Spleen	0–6	5–9	0–22	5–31

they are reported by KNAAK and O'BRIEN (1960). No data could be found for tissue levels in domestic animals.

21. FAMPHUR. — Phosphorothioic acid, O,O-dimethyl O-*p*-(dimethylsulfamoyl) phenyl ester

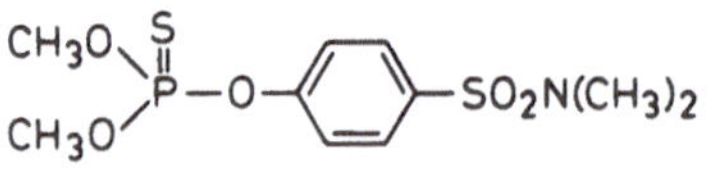

Alternate names: Warbex, Famophos, ENT 25644, 38023.

Application: Effective against lice, flies, and bot-fly attack, as well as against stomach and intestinal worms of ruminants (DRUDGE and SZANTO 1963). It was applicable for the control of bot-fly larvae dermally and *per os* as well as by injection (SUPPERER *et al.* 1954). The injection dosage for cattle was reported as seven to 15 mg./kg. body wt. (KOHLER and ROGOFF 1962). KUTZER (1966) injected *s.c.* or *i.m.* 14 mg./kg. of a 35 percent solution; TURNER *et al.* (1962) treated with 15 mg./kg.

Toxicity: See Table LXXXVII.

Metabolites of famphur were, with the exception of the O-analog, considerably less toxic than famphur itself (GATTERDAM *et al.* 1967). The ChE

Table LXXXVII. *Acute toxicities of famphur for various animals.*

Animal species	Mode of application	Toxic dosage (mg./kg.)	LD_{50} (mg./kg.)	Reference
Mouse	*per os*	—	27 (18) [a]	GATTERDAM *et al.* (1967)
Mouse	*i.p.*	—	11.6 (5.8) [a]	O'BRIEN *et al.* (1965)
Rat	*per os*	—	35	ANONYMOUS 29
Cattle	*i.m.*	25 tolerated	—	RADELEFF (1964)

[a] Famoxon.

[b] In propylene glycol.

activity regenerated rapidly after a decrease from treatment with famphur (ZACHERL *et al.* 1965). Famphur inhibited the erythrocyte ChE 100 times less than famoxon (O'BRIEN *et al.* 1965).

Restrictions and tolerances: In the U.S.A., 0.1 p.p.m. in fat, meat, and meat products of cattle (not milk cows) (FREAR *et al.* 1969).

Detection: By glc (PARASELA *et al.* 1967).

Metabolism and residues: Mice decomposed famphur very rapidly. One hour after an *i.p.* injection of one mg./kg. H^3-famphur in propylene glycol, 8.11 percent of the totally applied radioactivity was present in a toluene extract from the mice, while the famoxon part was 0.22 percent and desmethylfamphur was 0.01 percent (O'BRIEN *et al.* 1965). GATTERDAM *et al.* (1967) gave a scheme for the degradation of famphur in mammals (Fig. 12).

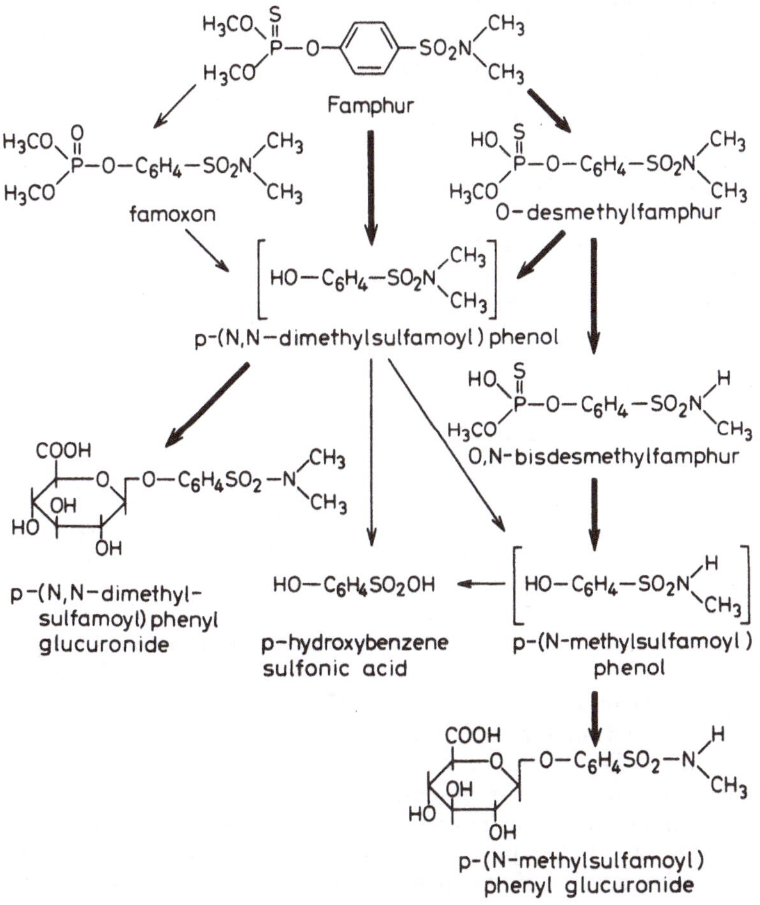

Fig. 12. Proposed metabolic scheme for famphur in mammals (GATTERDAM *et al.* 1967)

The decontamination of famphur in sheep was mainly through hydrolysis of the P – O-phenyl and P – O-methyl as well as the N-methyl bond (GATTERDAM *et al.* 1967). After P^{32}-injection *(i.m.)*, famoxon, O-desmethylfamphur, mono- and dimethylphosphoric acid, and dimethylthiophosphoric acid were identified as metabolites in the urine (BOURNE [19] cited from GATTERDAM *et al.* 1967).

ZACHERL *et al.* (1965) used the iodide-acid reaction for the detection of residues up to 0.7 p.p.m. on a chromatogram, which showed a blue fluorescence. After *i.m.* treatment with 18 mg./kg. body wt. famphur *(a.i.)*, no effective substance was found in the blood of cattle. With double the dosage a positive reaction was obtained after two hours, which again disappeared after four hours. Also the three-fold dosage exceeded the detection limit after only one and two hours. It also became negative after four hours. After oral intake of 18 mg./kg. body wt., a positive reaction occured only sporadically between 18 and 24 hours. The detection reactions were predominantly positive between six and 72 hours after intake of double the oral dosage. The values then were >0.7 p.p.m. (LITSCHAUER 1964). After 96 hours they were again below the detection limit.

A detailed report about levels in blood can be found in the paper by GATTERDAM *et al.* (1967) (Table LXXXVIII). It can be seen that for sheep

Table LXXXVIII. *Plasma levels of famphur and famoxon in sheep and a calf by extraction with carbon tetrachloride and chromatography* (GATTERDAM *et al.* 1967).

Animal species	Dosage (mg./kg.)	Route	Vehicle	Time of sampling (hours)	Fraction		Residue (p.p.m.)	
					Organophilic (%)	Water-soluble (%)	Famphur	Famoxon
Sheep	22.3	*i.v.*	dimethyl-	2	27.0	< 70	0.60	5.60
			formamide	24	2.8	—	trace	0.01
Sheep	55.1	*i.m.*	diethyl-	2	21.0	—	0.90	0.10
			succinate	72	5.6	—	0.06	0.01
Calf	60.7	*i.m.*	diethyl-	4	41.0	—	0.40	0.00
			succinate	72	20.2	—	0.18	0.05

already after two hours >70 percent of the radioactive substance present as water-soluble metabolites. The famoxon fraction was higher from *i.v.* injection than after *i.m.* treatment. The hydrolytic cleavage obviously proceeded slower in the calf, since 72 hours after *i.m.* application still 20 percent of the activity which was present in the plasma consisted of famphur and famoxon. The absolute values appear low; after *i.m.* application they reached their maximum in the calf after 24 hours with 0.61 p.p.m. for famphur, and 0.05 p.p.m. for famoxon between 48 and 72 hours. Fifty percent of *i.v.* applied H^3-famphur was excreted by sheep after six hours,

[19] The paper by J. R. BOURNE, M. S. thesis, Auburn Univ., Auburn, Ala. (1963) was not available here.

Table LXXXIX. *Radiometabolites in urine of sheep and calf following administration of H^3-famphur* (GATTERDAM *et al.* 1967).

Animal and application	Hours posttreatment	H^3-famphur equivalents (p.p.m.)					
		O-desmethyl famphur	O,*N*-bisdes-methyl famphur	*N*,*N*-dimethyl-sulfamoylphenyl glucuronide	*N*-methyl-sulfamoylphenyl glucuronide	*p*-Hydroxy-benzenesulfonic acid	Unknowns
Sheep (*i.v.*)	0–6	825	1956	2035	904	92	299
	6–12	229	779	525	292	trace	45
	12–24	42	159	166	94	trace	6
Sheep (*i.m.*)	0–6	310	430	650	85	98	149
	6–24	330	575	522	139	24	27
	24–48	513	487	420	152	trace	20
Calf (*i.m.*)	0–4	303	122	226	43	19	—
	4–24	262	159	384	29	trace	—
	24–48	103	65	232	16	trace	—
	48–72	28	5	80	5	trace	—

Table XC. *Average residue values in cattle tissue after oral famphur application* (PASARELA *et al.* 1967).

No. of animals	Dosage (mg./lb.)	Days after treatment	Residue (p.p.m.) in							
			Muscle		Fat		Liver		Kidney	
			Famphur	O-Analog	Famphur	O-Analog	Famphur	O-Analog	Famphur	O-Analog
1	0 [a]	0	0.02	0.02	0.04	0.02	0.02	0.02	0.03	0.01
3	1.5	0	< 0.05	< 0.05	0.28	< 0.05	0.43	~ 0.107	< 0.05	< 0.11
1	0 [a]	1	0.01	0.02	0.01	0.03	0.03	0.01	0.02	0.01
3	1.5	1	< 0.05	< 0.05	< 0.24	< 0.05	< 0.05	< 0.05	< 0.05	< 0.05
1	0 [a]	0	0.03	0.03	0.03	0.04	0.03	0.02	0.05	0.04
3	4.5	0	0.17	< 0.05	1.24	< 0.11	3.10	0.42	0.33	0.16
1	0 [a]	1	0.03	0.05	0.03	0.04	0.05	0.02	0.01	0.03
3	4.5	1	< 0.05	< 0.05	0.14	< 0.05	0.08	< 0.05	< 0.05	< 0.05

[a] Control.

and 98 percent after 48 hours. Only three percent appeared in the feces; the major part was in the urine, and less than one percent of its radioactivity was soluble in carbon tetrachloride. This means that no famphur or famoxon was excreted with the urine. The excretion was slower after *i.m.* treatment; 64 percent of the applied dosage was regained in 72 hours (GATTERDAM *et al.* 1967).

The phenolic metabolites were excreted mainly as glucuronide compounds with the urine. The distribution of metabolites in the urine is explained in Table LXXXIX.

The above-described metabolic data give only an indication of the short-lived occurrance of the effective substance and its metabolites, but they tell a little about the effective residues. PASARELA *et al.* (1967). reported residues after feeding famphur to cattle. When 1.5 or 4.5 mg./kg body wt. were applied, all tissues were free of famphur and famoxon after two to four days, showing values of <0.05 p.p.m. Average values are in Table XC; however, the experimental dosages were lower than the ones recommended for practical use.

GATTERDAM *et al.* (1967) reported residue values in tissues of sheep, calculated as equivalents from the H^3-radioactivity. The higher concentration in the muscle tissue at the site of injection after *i.m.* application was obvious here, and also the tissue residues were higher than after *i.v.* application, although the level in blood for a smaller dosage was higher there. Kidney and bile showed the highest values (Table XCI).

Table XCI. *Residual radioactivity in sheep tissues following i.v. and i.m. administration of H^3famphur* [a] (GATTERDAM *et al.* 1967).

Tissue	Famphur equiv. based on initial specific activity (p.p.m.)	
	Sheep [b] (sacrificed at 72 hr.)	Sheep [c] (sacrificed at 96 hr.)
Kidney	8.0	0.30
Bile	6.6	0.05
Fat	5.0	0.02
Muscle (injection site)	15.0	—
Liver	2.3	0.30
Spleen	1.7	0.30
Lung	1.6	0.40
Blood	2.0	1.40
Brain	0.9	0.10
Muscle (thigh)	0.7	0.03
Cerebrospinal fluid	0.7	0.60

[a] Famphur 25%; *i.v.* = 22.3 mg./kg., *i.m.* = 55.1 mg./kg.
[b] Intramuscular administration.
[c] Intravenous administration.

22. FENCHLORPHOS. — Phosphorothioic acid, O,O-dimethyl O-2,4,5-trichlorophenyl ester

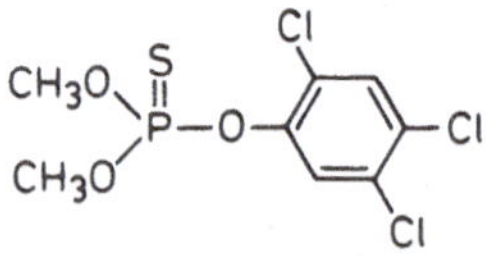

Alternate names: Trolene, Dow ET-14, Dow ET-57, Korlan, Nankor, ronnel. *Application:* Systemic insecticide with effect against *Diptera,* especially against bot-fly attack (French *et al.* 1958, Jones 1959, Jones and Matsushima 1959, McGregor and Bushland 1957, Neel 1958). Effective against *Dermatobia hominis,* screw worms, face flies, and horn flies (Graham *et al.* 1959, Wallace and Turner 1964, and others). A wide application range is possible for practically all domestic animals such as cattle, sheep, goats, and pigs. Cows should not be lactating at the time if possible (cf. Frear *et al.* 1969).

There are many application methods. The substance dosage for drench application against stomach worms in ruminants was 100 mg./kg. body wt. (Schad *et al.* 1958, Herlich and Porter 1958). Jones and Matsushima (1959) also treated with 100 to 110 mg./kg. against bot-fly attack on cattle; Raun and Herbick (1960) gave 15 to 25 mg./kg. daily as feed additive, and Rich (1960) ten to 15 mg./kg. but a total of 180 to 250 mg./kg., or Rich and Iveland (1959) eight to ten mg./kg. over a 25-day period. De Foliart *et al.* (1958) gave a *per os* dosage of 55 mg./kg. for two days and Weintraub *et al.* (1959 a) and Weintraub *et al.* (1959 b) applied 110 mg./kg. as bolus or drench (see also Weintraub and Thompson 1961). Medley *et al.* worked with low-level dosages. Long duration dosages for "self treatment" in mineral salt were given by Rogoff and Kohler (1959) and Knapp *et al.* (1967). Control of face-fly larvae was possible with a five percent mineral salt mixture (Wallace and Turner 1964). External application was done with a 2.5 percent spray (Roth and Eddy 1957). Drummond and Moore (1959) used a concentration of 0.75 percent for repeated spraying. For screw worm control 0.5 to one percent spray was necessary (Graham *et al.* 1959). Burns *et al.* (1959) investigated the application with back rubber. Marquardt and Hawkins (1958) used 150 to 200 mg./kg. body wt. for the treatment of fly strike.

Toxicity: See Table XCII. Skin resorption was negligible; cattle, calves, and sheep tolerated 2.5 percent sprays and dips, and ten percent powder (Radeleff *et al.* 1963). Fifteen mg./kg. daily for rats and ten or 25 mg./kg. daily for dogs were nontoxic in long duration tests (McCollister *et al.* 1959).

Detection: See Duggan *et al.* (1967), Claborn and Ivey (1964), Smith and Thiegs (1962), and Webley (1961). Claborn and Ivey (1965) described a very sensitive glc detection method which determined 0.0005 p.p.m. in meat. The enzyme-inhibiting method, acording to Cook (1954), corre-

Table XCII. *Acute oral toxicities of fenchlorphos for various animal species.*

Animal species	Special remarks	Toxic dosage (mg./kg.)	LD_{50} (mg./kg.)	Author
Mouse	—	—	2,000	SCHRADER (1963)
Rat	—	—	1,740	MARTIN (1961)
Rat	♂	—	1,250	GAINES (1960)
Rat	♀	—	2,630	GAINES (1960)
Dog	—	—	~ 500	SCHRADER (1963)
Sheep	—	max. nontox. 400 min. tox. 250	—	RADELEFF & BUSHLAND (1960)
Calf	1–2 weeks	max. nontox. 100 min. tox. 125	—	RADELEFF & BUSHLAND (1960)
Cattle	—	max. nontox. 100 min. tox. 125	—	RADELEFF & BUSHLAND (1960)
Cattle	—	125 [a]	—	RADELEFF & WOODARD (1957 b)
Cattle	—	100–110 [b]	—	RICH (1960), RICH & IVELAND (1959), WEINTRAUB *et al.* (1959 a and b), JONES & MATSUSHIMA (1959)

[a] Light symptoms.
[b] Sometimes light symptoms.

sponded to only four percent of the sensitivity of diazinon (MILLAR 1964), because fenchlorphos was a weak ChE inhibitor (WESTLAKE *et al.* 1960).
Tolerances and restrictions: In the U.S.A., zero tolerance in and on meat or meat products of cattle and in milk and 0.5 p.p.m. in bananas (FREAR *et al.* 1969). BÄR (1964 a) reported a waiting time of 60 days for fenchlorphos. This corresponds to a report in a fenchlorphos petition (§ 121209) at FDA of 60 days' waiting time before slaughtering after a *per os* treatment of 0.0018 lb./100 lb. body wt. for seven days, or 28 days' waiting period after 0.00078 lb./100 lb. over a 14-day period (ANONYMOUS 32) (cf. PLAPP *et al.* 1960 b).

The Feed Additive Compendium for 1967 (ANONYMOUS 6) specified the following waiting times before slaughtering: for 14 days' feeding (0.35 g./lb.) = 28 days, for 7 days' feeding (0.82 g./lb.) = 60 days, and for continuous feeding = 21 days.
Metabolism and residues: PLAPP and CASIDA (1958 a) proved similar metabolic pathways for rats and cattle. Hydrolysis started either at the methylphosphate or at the phenylphosphate bond. The degradation went to phosphoric acid (Fig. 13).

After *per os* treatment with P^{32}-fenchlorphos maximum radioactivity in rat tissues was reached after 12 hours; it remained for 12 days. Fenchlorphos as well as its oxon were found in the tissues. There was an especially high concentration in the skin (Table XCIII).

Excretion for rats in form of hydrolysis products was mainly with urine and to a slighter degree with the feces. Total excretion was approximately 70 percent of the applied *per os* dosage. The high content of phenyl-

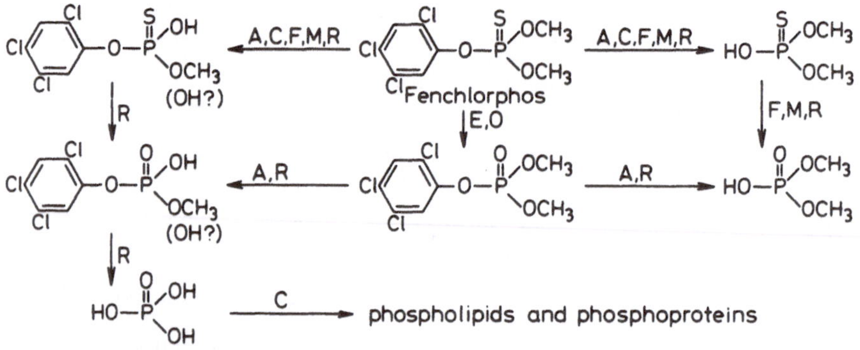

Fig. 13. Proposed metabolic pathway for fenchlorphos and its oxygen analog (PLAPP and CASIDA 1958 a): *A*=alkaline hydrolysis, *C*=cow, *E*=enzyme inhibition, *F*=housefly, *M*=bovine rumen fluid, *O*=chemical oxidation, and *R*=rats.

Table XCIII. *P^{32}-fenchlorphos and derivatives in rat tissues seven days after oral administration* [a] *of fenchlorphos and its oxygen analog* (PLAPP and CASIDA 1958 a).

Tissue	Total radioactivity (p.p.m.)	
	Fenchlorphos	Oxygen analog
Fat	6.8±2.7	1.7±0.6
Mesenteric fat	2.7±0.6	1.7±0.5
Liver	5.6±2.1	10.4±1.9
Spleen	0.8±0.3	2.9±0.7
Kidney	5.1±2.0	5.4±1.2
Brain	2.9±1.7	5.6±1.5
Skin	53.4±6.0	86.0±17.7

[a] 100 mg./kg.

phosphoric acid and thiophosphoric acid in the excretions in the beginning decreased steadily in favor of the correspondingly increasing content of dimethylphosphoric acid compounds (Table XCIV).

The influence of the rumen flora and rumen fluid on the effective substance is of interest in cattle after *per os* intake. According to AHMED *et al.* (1958) fenchlorphos was only slightly attacked within 24 hours. PLAPP and CASIDA (1958 a) reported that there was no formation of the oxygen analog of fenchlorphos through the influence of the rumen fluid. Hydrolysis attacked predominantly the O-methyl group leading to phenylphosphoric acid. Small quantities of dimethylphosphoric acid and dimethylthiophosphoric acid were formed, pointing to an oxidative degradation. Decomposition and excretion of fenchlorphos were slower in the bodies of cattle than of rats (PLAPP and CASIDA 1958 a). After an oral application of 100 mg./kg. body wt. of P^{32}-ronnel, PLAPP *et al.* (1960 b) detected in the blood of cattle

Table XCIV. *Hydrolysis products of fenchlorphos and derivatives based on ion-exchange chromatography* (PLAPP and CASIDA 1958 a).

Compound [a]	Treatment [b] (hours)	Hydrolysis products (%)				
		$(HO)_2P(O)OH$	$(CH_3O)_2P(O)OH$	$(CH_3O)_2P(S)OH$	Phenyl phosphates	Unidentified
$(CH_3O)_2P(S)O\phi Cl_3$	0–12	0	20	8	72	0
	12–24	0	42	8	50	0
	24–48	0	57	26	17	0
	48–168	0	65	25	10	0
	0–168 (total)	—	33	11	56	0
$(CH_3O)_2P(O)O\phi Cl_3$	0–168	0	46	—	54	0
	0–12	0	28	—	72	0
	12–24	0	36	—	64	0
	24–48	0	52	—	44	4
	48–168	0	58	—	36	6
	0–168 (total)	0	44	—	53	3
$(CH_3O(HO)P(S)O\phi Cl_3$	0–72	12	—	—	88	0
$(CH_3O)_2P(O)OH$	0–72	0	100	—	—	0

[a] ϕ = phenyl ring.
[b] Estimated dosage of 250 mg./kg.

1.4 p.p.m. after eight hours and 3.1 p.p.m. after 12 hours. Maximum radioactivity in blood after 100 mg./kg. fenchlorphos was reached with 25 p.p.m. fenchlorphos equivalents. This value decreased within seven days to five p.p.m. Skellysolve-B-soluble fenchlorphos decreased in 24 hours to 0.24 p.p.m. and in seven days to 0.05 p.p.m. (PLAPP and CASIDA 1958 a). According to KAPLANIS *et al.* (1956) (unpublished data, cited from PLAPP *et al.* 1960 b) maximum concentration in blood of cattle was reached within eight hours. The substances in the blood were fenchlorphos and its oxygen analog.

According to KAPLANIS *et al.* (1956), 74 percent of *per os* applied P^{32}-fenchlorphos was excreted with the urine of cattle in three days. Two percent was in the feces. PLAPP and CASIDA (1958 a), in comparison, regained 49 percent of a single dosage with an excretion maximum between 18 and 38 hours (approx. 1,800 p.p.m. equivalents of 100 mg./kg. of Trolene), preponderantly as O-methyl-O-hydrogen-O-(2,4,5-trichlorophenyl) thiophosphate. The quantitative recovery of the total radioactive substances was achieved within 11 days (KAPLANIS *et al.* 1956, cited from PLAPP *et al.* 1960 b); moreover, no intact fenchlorphos was found. On the contrary, traces of nonmetabolized fenchlorphos were found in the feces. PLAPP and CASIDA (1958 a) found seven percent of the dosage in the feces, one-seventh of which was soluble in Skellysolve B and was fenchlorphos; the concentration decreased from 24 p.p.m. after 24 hours to 2.3 p.p.m. after 70 hours and reached 0.1 p.p.m. after 120 hours.

Tissue residues of fenchlorphos and its metabolites in cattle were higher seven days after application than the corresponding values which were found one day after treatment in rats tissues. The concentration-distribution of fenchlorphos and its metabolites, seven days after *per os* application, are in Table XCVI.

The largest residue was 80 p.p.m. in kidneys; the highest level of Skellysolve-B-soluble fenchlorphos appeared in fat, kidney, and lung tissues. More than 95 percent of the radioactive substances of these extracts behaved like fenchlorphos on a chromatogram.

Fourteen days after *per os* treatment with 100 mg./kg. PLAPP *et al.* (1960 b) established the highest P^{32}-residue values in brain, liver, and kidney of cattle. The analytical values were from nine to 12 p.p.m., of which only slight amounts were not composed of metabolites. The insecticidal residues in meat were <0.05 p.p.m., while fat samples still contained seven p.p.m. after two weeks. McLAUGHLIN (1969) established, after a single spray treatment with 7.57 l. of a 0.1 percent fenchlorphos preparation, a maximum of 2.63 p.p.m. in omental fat four days later, and a minimum of 0.09 p.p.m. 16 days after treatment in perirenal fat. After complete deposition, the omental fat contained more residue than the perirenal fat.

After application of back rubbers, no fenchlorphos appeared in the feces of cattle; the low P^{32}-fractions in the urine were hydrolysis products, since only slight amounts were soluble in chloroform (KNOWLES and ARTHUR 1966 a). IVEY *et al.* (1967) found after back rubber application predominantly fenchlorphos residues in fatty tissues of cattle, using the glc method

Table XCVI. *Fenchlorphos and derivatives in tissues seven days after oral administration* [a] *to a cow* (PLAPP and CASIDA 1958 a).

Tissue	Residue (p.p.m.) [b]			
	Total	Fenchlorphos	Water-soluble	Skellysolve-B-soluble
Subcutaneous fat	44.3±7.7	8.2±5.1	19.1±1.0	18.0±5.0
Mesenteric fat	23.1±3.5	1.0±0.2	13.2±2.7	8.9±2.5
Loin muscle	18.2±1.1	3.2 [c]	10.8 [c]	4.2 [c]
Neck muscle	7.5±1.0	3.6±0.8	2.0±1.0	1.9±1.0
Liver	31.9±6.7	6.8±1.1	23.3±1.1	1.8±0.4
Spleen	11.6±2.1	0.3±0.5	10.3±0.5	1.0±0.4
Kidney	80.0±16.5	21.9±3.9	48.7±7.4	9.4±3.9
Lung	45.6±6.7	8.0±1.5	28.4±2.8	9.2±1.5
Heart	25.4±2.8	5.5±2.0	18.2±1.6	1.7±1.2
Brain	13.8±1.2	1.0 [d]	10.9 [d]	1.9 [d]
Spinal cord	6.2±0.8	0.3 [d]	3.7 [d]	2.2 [d]
Tongue	9.7±0.1	3.2±0.9	5.8±1.0	0.7±0.1
Hide	9.6±1.5	3.7±0.6	3.9±2.1	2.0±1.5
Diaphragm	11.3±2.2	4.8±0.3	1.6±0.8	4.9±0.7
Rumen wall	8.0±0.7	1.6±0.2	3.6±1.5	2.8±1.3
Rumen contents	8.3±2.8	0.9±0.4	5.8±0.9	1.6±0.8
Small intestine and contents	32.6±7.7	0.8±0.2	28.9±1.1	2.9±1.0
Bone (rib)	14.4±0.9	—	—	—
Ovary	27.7±1.4	—	—	—

[a] 100 mg./kg.
[b] Three replicates each.
[c] Two replicates.
[d] One replicate.

of CLABORN and IVEY (1965) which determined as little as 0.0005 p.p.m in the tissue. The residues in the other tissues were approximately proportional to the fat content. Here, it is striking that with increasing duration of treatment (two weeks/four weeks) the residue decreased, the highest concentration being reached with 0.06 p.p.m. in kidney fat after 14 days back-rubber treatment (two percent compound). The decrease may possibly have external reasons as, for instance, decrease of insecticide in the back rubber. In any case, the very low residues were zero two weeks after discontinuation of treatment (Table XCVII).

There were also differences with regard to residues from the types of application, according to how the effective substance was dropped onto the body cover. Altogether, the values for tank-type back rubber were higher than for cable-type. In the test of IVEY *et al.* (1967), the residues after one percent fenchlorphos were higher than after two percent treatment. The maximum value appeared with 0.12 p.p.m. after four weeks' continuous treatment with two percent fenchlorphos (Table XCVIII).

Meat of cattle treated with fenchlorphos did not give changes in taste in comparison to the meat of control animals (BROGDON *et al.* 1962). MILLAR

Table XCVII. *Fenchlorphos in cattle tissues using cable-type back rubbers* (IVEY *et al.* 1967).

Fenchlorphos conc. (%)	Residue (p.p.m.) [a] in								
	Omental fat	Renal fat	Sub-cutaneous fat	Muscle	Liver	Kidney	Heart	Brain	Spleen
				Pre- and posttreatment					
Controls	0	0	0	0	0	0	0	0	0
				1 week of treatment					
1.0	0.012	0.008	0.008	0	0	0.001	0	0	0
1.0	0.007	0.005	0.003	0	0	0.001	0	0.001	0
2.0	0.031	0.031	0.016	0.002	0.001	0	0	0.001	0
2.0	0.005	0.005	0.004	0.001	0	0.001	0	0	0
				2 weeks of treatment					
1.0	0.023	0.009	0.014	0.001	0	0.001	0	0	0.001
1.0	0.003	0.001	0.001	0.001	0	0	0	0	0.001
2.0	0.061	0.064	0.048	0.004	0.001	0.001	0.002	0.001	0.001
2.0	0.007	0.014	0.005	0.001	0	0.001	0	0	0.001
				4 weeks of treatment					
1.0	0	0	0	0	0	0	0	0	0
1.0	0.001	0	0	0	0	0	0	0	0
2.0	0.001	0	0.001	0	0	0	0	0	0
2.0	0.005	0.004	0.005	0	0	0	0	0	0
				1 week posttreatment					
1.0	0	0	0	—	—	—	—	—	—
1.0	0	0	0	—	—	—	—	—	—
2.0	0	0	0	—	—	—	—	—	—
2.0	0.004	0.001	0.003	—	—	—	—	—	—
				2 weeks posttreatment					
1.0	0	0	0	—	—	—	—	—	—
1.0	0	0	0	—	—	—	—	—	—
2.0	0	0	0	—	—	—	—	—	—
2.0	0	0	0	—	—	—	—	—	—

[a] 0 = < 0.0005 p.p.m.

Table XCVIII. *Fenchlorphos in fat of cattle exposed to tank-type back rubbers* (IVEY *et al.* 1967).

Fenchlorphos conc. (%) [b]	Residue (p.p.m.) [a] in	
	Omental fat	Renal fat
	Pre- and posttreatment	
Controls	0	0
	2 weeks of treatment	
1	0.035	0.038
1	0.028	0.028
2	0.013	0.007
2	0.027	0.028
	4 weeks of treatment	
1	0.011	0.010
1	0.033	0.033
2	0.091	0.110
2	0.112	0.121
	2 weeks posttreatment	
1	0	0
1	0	0
2	0.001	0.001
2	0	0
	3 weeks posttreatment	
1	0	0
1	0	0
2	0	0
2	0	0

[a] 0 = < 0.0005 p.p.m.
[b] In oil solution.

(1964) worked with P^{32}-fenchlorphos on sheep. After oral application of 50 mg./kg., maximum concentration in blood appeared with 7.5 µg./g. after four hours, as unchanged fenchlorphos in hexane extract. The remainder contained, after protein precipitation, degradation products such as O-methyl-O-hydrogen-O-(2,4,5-trichlorophenyl) thiophosphate, dimethylphosphate, and dimethylthiophosphate. The oxygen analog of fenchlorphos was not present. Within 48 hours a considerable decrease in concentration took place. Excretion was preponderantly with the urine; the maximum was reached after 20 hours and 58 percent was excreted (after 50 mg./kg.) in two days and 68 to 72 percent (after 100 mg./kg.) within 21 days. Maximum excretion with the feces likewise was 20 hours after application: in two days 4.9 percent was excreted with 7.1 to 7.7 percent in 21 days. The feces contained merely traces of unchanged fenchlorphos. There was no fenchlorphos in the urine; the total radioactivity was attributed to the previously-mentioned metabolic products, where O-methyl-O-hydrogen-O-(2,4,5-trichlorophenyl) thiophosphate prevailed during the first two days.

Tissue residues two days after *per os* treatment with 50 mg./kg. body wt. are in Table XCIX.

Table XCIX. *P^{32}-fenchlorphos residues in the tissues of sheep two days after per os treatment* [a] (MILLAR 1964).

Tissue	Fenchlorphos equivalent (µg./g.)		Substance
	Radio-chemical method	ChE inhibition method	
Kidney	7.45	0.38	preponderantly metabolites
Brain	1.40	—	
Liver	1.94	0.34	
Spleen	0.42	0.68	
Adrenals	1.78	0.85	
Hind leg muscle	1.84	0.79	
Perirenal fat	32.95	37.25	preponderantly fenchlorphos
Subcutaneous fat	18.50	20.83	
Omental fat	29.05	24.63	

[a] 50 mg./kg.

After application of 100 mg. of compound/kg. body wt., 29.9 to 32.2 p.p.m. were are found after seven days, 8.4 to 10.5 p.p.m. after 16 days, and 0.2 to 0.6 p.p.m. after 40 days, especially in the *s.c.* fatty tissue, part of which was identified by chromatography as unchanged fenchlorphos.

It is of interest that with spray treatment of 0.2 to 0.4 percent fenchlorphos less than one p.p.m. of active insecticide adhered to the wool (*Lucilia* larvae test) while two to eight p.p.m. were extracted with hexane 60 days after the spray.

After 0.2 to 0.4 percent spray treatment no activity was found in *s.c.* fatty tissue after 21 days, but after 14 days 0.01 to 0.04 p.p.m., and after seven days 0.03 to 0.35 p.p.m. No ChE inhibition was established in the tissues of poisoned animals. The equivalent fenchlorphos concentrations after nine, 16, and 21 days were 0.08, 0.06, and 0.11 p.p.m. in the kidneys; 0.04, 0.03, and 0.19 p.p.m. in the liver; and 0.02, 0.02, and zero p.p.m. in the back thigh muscles. Furthermore, MILLAR (1965) reported in another work that 15 days after a 0.2 to 0.4 percent fenchlorphos spray 0.35 p.p.m. residue was present in the sheep fat.

23. FENTHION. — Phosphorothioic acid, O,O-dimethyl O-(4-methylthio)-*m*-tolyl) ester

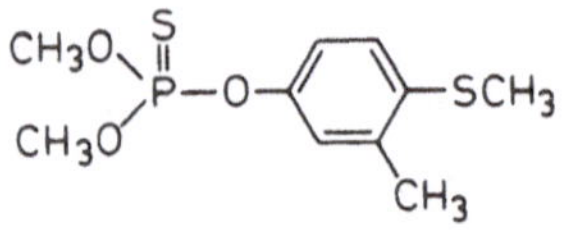

Alternate names: Entex, Baytex, Lebaycid, Tiguvon, Bayer 29493, Bayer 29/493, S-1752, ENT 25540, mercaptophos.
Application: Acaricide and insecticide; application in the hygiene sector against flies, chinches, roaches, etc. with long residual effect (JUNG *et al.* 1960); systemic insecticide for bot larvae control (UNWIN 1965, ANONYMOUS 9); against horn flies, aphids, etc. (COX *et al.* 1967).

Table C. *Acute toxicities of fenthion for various animals.*

Animal species	Mode of application	Toxic dosage (mg./kg.)	LD_{50} (mg./kg.)	Reference
Rat	*per os*	—	175–375	SCHRADER (1960)
Rat [a]	*per os*	—	190	DU BOIS & KINOSHITA (1964)
Rat [b]	*per os*	—	310	DU BOIS & KINOSHITA (1964)
Rat	dermal	—	345–410	ANONYMOUS 9
Guinea pig	*per os*	> 100 p.p.m.	—	DRUMMOND (1960)
Guinea pig	*per os*	> 100 p.p.m.	—	DRUMMOND (1960)
Chicken	*per os*	—	~ 15	DU BOIS & KINOSHITA (1964)

[a] Male.
[b] Female.

Application on the animal: Two percent oil solution for pour-on treatment, 5.0 to 10.0 mg./kg.; as spray; as feed additive (COX *et al.* 1967, NELSON *et al.* 1967); 1.0 mg./kg. for three days or 2.5 mg./kg. for two days for cattle *per os* (ROSENBERGER 1967).
Toxicity: See Table C. This substance penetrated easily through the skin. The toxicities of possible metabolites are listed in Table CI.

Toxicity increased for the oxidative metabolic products; SCHRADER (1960) reported the fenthion oral LD_{50} for rats was 250 mg./kg., and for the sulfoxide and sulfone was 125 mg./kg. Rats tolerated daily oral applications of ten mg./kg. body wt. over a 60-days period (DU BOIS and KINOSHITA 1964); the toxicity varied for other mammals and was thus dependent on the animal species. The LD_{50} for fenthion in oil was 40 mg./kg. body wt. for *i.m.* injection; under these conditions horses tolerated 70 mg./kg. body wt. (NELSON *et al.* 1967).
Tolerances and restrictions: In the U.S.A, use in milk cow barns and animal and chicken houses is prohibited; otherwise there is "zero tolerance" or "no residue" (Group IV according to FREAR *et al.* 1969).
Detection: See also MCDOUGALL 1964. The detection of fenthion was possible in a biological test with *Diptera* (UNTERSTENHÖFER 1960). NIESSEN *et al.* (1962) used paper chromatography and made the spots visible with $PdCl_2$ and HCl in water. SCHRADER (1960) described IR spectrocopy in the range of 700 to 5,000 $cm.^{-1}$, as well as the absorption curve in the UV range. IRUDAYASAMY and NATARAJAN (1964) detected fenthion after hydrolysis by using the UV absorption curve of 4-methyl-mercapto-3-methylphenol, or after coupling with diazotized sulfanilic acid; HIRANO and

TAMURA (1964) used a color reaction of the acyl residue with 4-aminoantipyrine. SCHRADER (1963) oxcidized fenthion to its sulfoxide and determined this stronger ChE inhibitor by enzyme reaction, or used the phosphorus-molybdenum reaction according to LAWS and WEBLEY (1961) [20]. MÖLLHOFF (1967 and 1968) mentioned colorimetric and glc methods; ANDERSON *et al.* (1966 c) described a specific glc method for fenthion and five of its metabolites in animal tissue.

Metabolism and residues: A small cumulation of fenthion was mentioned in a general report (ANONYMOUS 9): eight days after treatment a maximum of 0.3 p.p.m. was found, especially in animal fat.

According to MÖLLHOFF (1967), fenthion was either hydrolyzed in the organism to less toxic substances or it was oxidized; the oxidation products could again be hydrolyzed. The possible structures are:

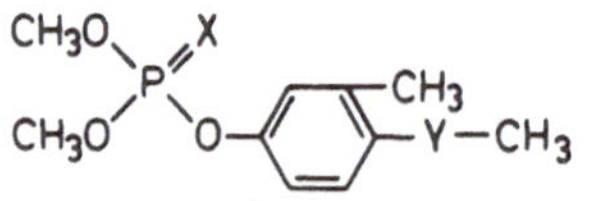

$X = S, Y = S$
$X = S, Y = SO$
$X = S, Y = SO_2$
$X = O, Y = SO$
$X = O, Y = SO_2$

The hydrolysis of the P – O-aryl bond of fenthion and its oxidation products included about 90 percent of the hydrolyzed metabolites as dimethylthiophosphate and dimethylphosphate (KNOWLES and ARTHUR 1966 b).

BRADY and ARTHUR (1961) conducted excretion and residue studies on rats with P^{32}-fenthion. After a ten-times repeated *i.p.* injection, 79.5 percent of the applied quantity was excreted with the urine and feces within 20 days after the first injection. There was less radioactive substance in the feces than in the urine. The concentration remained lower for this application mode than after *per os* treatment. After *per os* application, 86.2 percent of the radioactivity was eliminated with the urine and feces within seven days. The feces contained more P^{32}-substances after oral application than after *i.p.* injection. Of the excretion products in rat urine after *per os* treatment 96 to 99 percent were hydrolysis products. O,O-Dimethylphosphoric acid prevailed in the feces, and O,O-dimethylthiophosphoric acid in the urine. Two further nonidentified substances occurred after *i.p.* injection (BRADY and ARTHUR 1961).

Residues in the tissues of test animals after *i.p.* and *per os* application are in Table CII. The high residue in bones is obvious. According to BRADY and ARTHUR (1961) this is a sign for rapid degradation. There was no clear cumulation of fenthion and its oxidative metabolites in the tissues, even

[20] Cited by SCHRADER (1963).

Table CI. *Possible metabolites of fenthion and their toxicities* (Du Bois and Kinoshita 1964).

Substance	Structure	$\sim LD_{50}$ per os, rats (mg./kg.)
S-Methyl-isomer	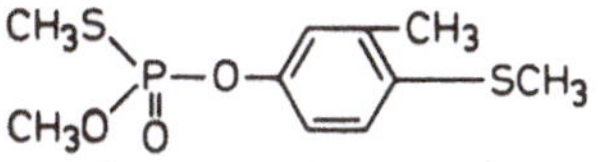 CH_3S, CH_3O–P(=O)–O–⟨ ⟩–CH_3, –SCH_3	55
Sulfoxide	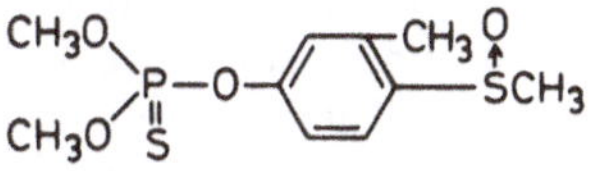 CH_3O, CH_3O–P(=S)–O–⟨ ⟩–CH_3, –S(→O)CH_3	250
Sulfone	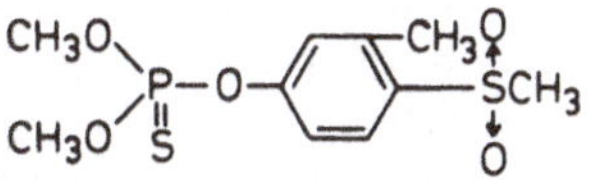 CH_3O, CH_3O–P(=S)–O–⟨ ⟩–CH_3, –S(→O)(↓O)CH_3	250
Oxygen-analog	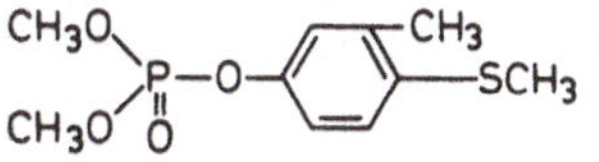 CH_3O, CH_3O–P(=O)–O–⟨ ⟩–CH_3, –SCH_3	26
Oxygen-analog-sulfoxide	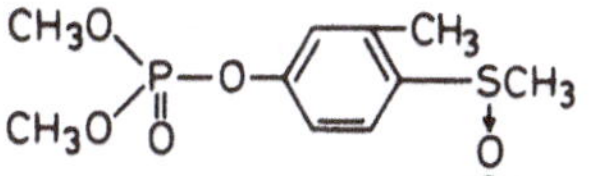 CH_3O, CH_3O–P(=O)–O–⟨ ⟩–CH_3, –S(↓O)CH_3	22
Oxygen-analog-sulfone	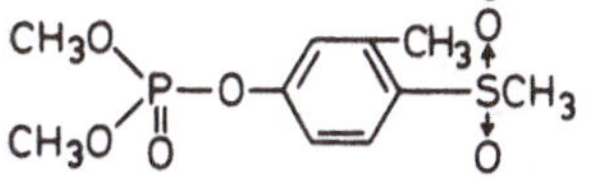 CH_3O, CH_3O–P(=O)–O–⟨ ⟩–CH_3, –S(→O)(↓O)CH_3	9

Table CII. *Fenthion equivalents in rat tissues treated i.p. or per os* (Brady and Arthur 1961).

Dosage and time after treatment	Fenthion equivalents (p.p.m.) in					
	Liver	Kidney	Bone	Muscle	Skin	Heart
10 mg./kg./day for 10 days *i.p.* [a]						
3 days	12.7	7.2	14.8	1.4	4.5	3.0
7 days	14.5	12.9	13.3	5.5	6.3	5.9
10 days	12.4	9.4	60	4.2	6.3	6.6
13 days	12.6	10.3	50	6.7	4.9	8.6
20 days	4.1	2.9	51.4	3.4	2.1	3.2
200 mg./kg. single *i.p.* [b]						
1.5 hours	124	92	22	53	25	21
100 mg./kg. single oral [b]						
3 days	34	25	—	12.1	12.1	13.1
7 days	12.4	8.3	—	6.9	3.8	6.3

[a] Averaged from three rats at each time interval.
[b] Averaged from two rats at each time interval.

after repeated treatment. There was no cumulation of effective substance or its O-analog. The amount of acetonitrile-soluble residues after several injections was below the detection limit (>0.05 p.p.m.) of the method.

BRADY and ARTHUR (1961) established acetonitrile-soluble residues after a single injection of 200 mg./kg. *i.p.* only 1.5 hours later. These calculated, equivalent fractions for both *i.p.* and oral treatments are in Table CIII. Blood, brain, and fat contained no detectable acetonitrile-soluble residues three to seven days after the oral treatment.

MÖLLHOFF (1967) determined, on the basis of phosphorus, the total quantity of remaining effective substance and its metabolites in cattle after pour-on treatment. He found residues mainly in the fatty tissue, with a maximum of 1.3 p.p.m. after two days. The highest value in muscle was 0.5 p.p.m. Twelve to 13 days after treatment, 0.1 p.p.m. was reached in all tissues. Fenthion had a long persistence in the body because of its low polarity (MÖLLHOFF 1967) (Table CIV).

Further detailed analytical data about the behaviour of P^{32}-fenthion in cows after *i.m.* injection or pour-on application are in the paper by KNOWLES and ARTHUR (1966 b). The highest level in blood was reached within 24 hours. Ten to 38 percent of the radioactive substances in blood were soluble in chloroform, the rest were hydrolysis products. After seven

Table CIII. *Fenthion in rat tissues* (BRADY and ARTHUR 1961).

Mode of application	*i.p.*	*per os*
mg./kg.	200	100
Time of killing	1.5 hours	3 days
Extracting solvent	acetonitrile	chloroform
Tissue	Residue (p.p.m.)	
Liver	30	0.2
Muscle	9.6	< 0.01
Skin	6.1	
Kidney	27	
Heart	9.6	

Table CIV. *Fenthion in meat and fat after treatment of cattle* [a] *with ten p.p.m. based on body weight* (MÖLLHOFF 1967).

Wt. of animal kg.	318	268	237	275	216
Time of killing (days)	2	8	10	12	13
Tissue	Residue (p.p.m.) [b]				
Back muscle	0.5	0.3	0.3	< 0.1	n.d.
Back thigh muscle	0.4	n.d.	0.2	n.d.	< 0.1
Diagonally lying front muscle	0.2	n.d	0.2	0.2	n.d.
Omental fat	1.3	0.3	0.2	0.1	n.d.
Kidney fat	1.2	0.3	0.1	< 0.1	0.1
Liver	0.1	n.d.	0.1	n.d.	< 0.1
Kidney	< 0.1	n.d.	0.2	< 0.1	—

[a] Two percent pour-on.
[b] < 0.1 = that it is only qualitatively detectable (until about 0.05 p.p.m.);

days no chloroform-soluble P^{32} was present in the blood. Fenthion, which was rapidly decomposed to phosphoric acid derivatives, was excreted mainly with the urine and a small amount with the feces. Maximum excretion in urine after pour-on and *i.m.* injection was reached the first day after treatment. After injection the level decreased from 33 p.p.m. on the first day to 1.6 p.p.m. on the twenty-first day, but more than 95 percent of the chloroform-soluble substances was hydrolysis products; fenthion and its O-analog as well as fenthion sulfoxide were present in small amounts in the chloroform extract; more than 70 percent corresponded to fenthion sulfone and/or the sulfone of its O-analog. Dimethylphosphate, dimethylthiophosphate, and an unknown metabolite, which might be a desmethyl derivative, were in the aqueous phase. Excretion in the feces, calculated as P^{32}-activity, reached 5.8 p.p.m. two days after *i.m.* and 2.3 p.p.m. after pour-on application. Maximum acetonitrile-soluble substances in feces were reached one day after *i.m.* application and three days after dermal application. More than 50 percent of these substances was fenthion, while 65 percent of the radioactive substances in the aqueous phase consisted of dimethylthiophosphate. Residue concentrations in tissues 14 and 21 days after fenthion application are in Table CV. The highest residue quantity appeared in the liver. After dermal application of one quart/animal of a 0.5-percent emulsion, none of the edible tissues contained acetonitrile-soluble radioactive substances after 14 days; however, after *i.m.* injection (3.5 g./cow), the extracts still contained 50 percent fenthion 21 days afterwards. It was ob-

Table CV. *Total and acetonitrile-soluble P^{32}-fenthion equivalents in cattle tissues* (KNOWLES and ARTHUR 1966 b).

Tissue [b]	Method of treatment [a]			
	Dermal		Intramuscular	
	Total (p.p.m.)	CH_3CN-soluble (p.p.m.)	Total (p.p.m.)	CH_3CN-soluble (p.p.m.)
Round steak (R)	0.04	trace	0.11	0.03
(L)	0.03	trace	1.03	0.38
Sirloin steak (R)	0.03	trace	0.17	0.02
(L)	0.04	trace	0.80	0.27
Subcut. fat (R)	0.01	—	0.16	0.08
(L)	0.05	—	0.30	0.20
T-bone steak	0.04	trace	0.16	0.05
Omental fat	0.04	trace	0.56	0.15
Liver	0.44	trace	3.34	0.76
Skin	0.49	0.08	—	—
Injection site	—	—	163	77

[a] Cows treated dermally killed 14 days after treatment; cows treated *i.m.* killed 21 days after treatment.
[b] R and L indicate right and left sides of the cows.

vious that the tissues after the injection showed more radioactive residues than those from the dermal treatment.

Supplement: During a human fenthion poisoning CLARMANN *et al.* (1966) found insecticide-effective stomach contents with biological testing (Drosophila). Uncleaved effective substance and, after alkaline hydrolysis, aromatic cleavage products (3-methyl-4-methylmercaptophenol) were found with TLC. The urine of the victim contained approximately 40 μg.-percent 3-methyl-4-methylmercaptophenol, but no dimethylthiophosphoric acid.

24. FORMOTHION. — Phosphorodithioic acid, O,O-dimethyl *S*-(*N*-formyl-2-mercapto-*N*-methylacetamide) ester

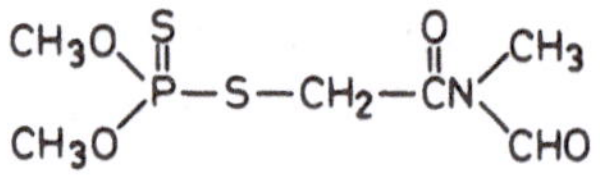

Alternate names: Authio, Aflix (25% formulation).

Application: Systemic insecticide and acaricide in plant protection (WOOD and TYSON 1965).

Toxicity: See Table CVI.

Table CVI. *Acute toxicities of formothion for rats and chickens.*

Animal species	Sex	Mode of application	LD_{50} (mg./kg.)	Remarks	Reference
Rat	♂	*per os*	330	effective subst.	KLOTZSCHE (1961)
Rat	♂	*per os*	375	25% form.	KLOTZSCHE (1961)
Rat	♀	*per os*	350	25% form.	KLOTZSCHE (1961)
Rat	♂	*per os*	250	25% form.	KLOTZSCHE (1964)
Rat	♂	*per os*	370–400	tech.	KLOTZSCHE (1966)
Rat	♀	*per os*	500–540	tech.	KLOTZSCHE (1966)
Rat	—	dermal acute	1,490–1,800	—	WOOD & TYSON (1965)
Rat	♂	dermal acute	700–1,500	—	KLOTZSCHE (1966)
Chicken	—	*i.v.*	*ca.* 20	tech.	KLOTZSCHE (1966)

In a semichronic test dogs tolerated 16 to 32 mg./kg. *per os* (KLOTZSCHE 1966). After 35 mg./kg. a slight loss in weight was observed. Formothion is not a strong ChE inhibitor; there also seemed to exist a kind of habituation (KLOTZSCHE 1966).

Metabolism and residues: WOOD and TYSON (1965) emphasized that there is no danger of accumulation of residues in plant and animal tissues (without report of numbers).

25. GARDONA. — Phosphoric acid, O,O-dimethyl-O-[2-chloro-1-(2,4,5-trichlorophenyl)vinyl] ester

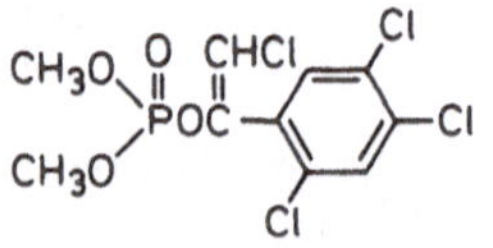

Alternate name: SD 8447.
Application: Plant-protection insecticide, also for animal barns and chicken houses, effective against bot-fly attack (pour-on method).
Toxicity: See Table CVII. Rats tolerated 15 to 10,800 p.p.m. *s.c.* daily over

Table CVII. *Acute toxicities of gardona for various animals.*

Animal species	Mode of application	LD_{50} (mg./kg.)	Reference
Rat [a]	*per os*	4,000–5,000	WHETSTONE *et al.* (1966)
Mouse [a]	*per os*	> 5,000	WHETSTONE *et al.* (1966)
Rabbit	dermal	> 2,500	WHETSTONE *et al.* (1966)

[a] Male.

a two-week period without obvious pathological changes; >1,200 p.p.m. gave a light increase in weight. Low dosages (<400 p.p.m. for two weeks) did not lead to significant ChE inhibition in rats; there was a fast regeneration within three to four days after discontinuation. Increasing ChE inhibition was observed after >0.1 mg./kg. *i.v.* of Gardona in dimethylsulfoxide, and a slowly increasing inhibition after application in aqueous alkaline solution with >0.26 mg./kg. in two to 24 hours, and after *s.c.* injection in 24 to 48 hours.
Metabolism and residues: Gardona was extraordinarily rapidly metabolized and excreted. The largest excreted amounts after *per os* application were found in the urine: after one day 55 to 73 percent and within seven days 61 to 82 percent. Corresponding values were established by WHETSTONE *et al.* (1966) with P^{32}-Gardona, which also demonstrated metabolites. No more Gardona was observed in the urine; the radioactivity present came from the metabolites dimethyl-hydrogenphosphate, methyl-dihydrogenphosphate, and the desmethyl derivative of Gardona.

It can be deduced indirectly that metabolites were present only for a short time in tissues. Their low solubility limited penetration and transport in mammal tissue, where they were decomposed without toxic effects. AKINTONWA and HUTSON (1967) supplemented reports about Gardona metabolism in rats using C^{14}-vinyl labelled substance. Of these C^{14}-substances 95 percent was excreted within four days, mainly through the urine pathways (78 percent) and partially with the feces (16.5 percent). The largest quantity appeared within the first 24 hours in the urine and varied from 44 to 78 percent. There was practically no difference in the urine excretion rate for C^{14}- or P^{32}-labelling.

Metabolic investigations for the dog revealed that 92 percent of the radioactive material was excreted with the urine and feces within four days after *per os* treatment (AKINTONWA and HUTSON 1967).

Unchanged insecticide was not found in the urine of rats or of dogs (AKINTONWA and HUTSON 1967). The following metabolites appeared for rats and dogs (reported in percent of dosage):

(1) 2,4,5-trichlorophenylethanediol glucuronide (eight and 12 percent),
(2) 1-(2,4,5-trichlorophenyl)ethyl glucuronide [22] (35 and zero percent),
(3) 2,4,5-trichlorophenylglycolic acid (24 and 22 percent),
(4) 2-chloro-1-(2,4,5-trichlorophenyl)vinylmethyl hydrogenphosphate (four and 46 percent),
(5) 2,4,5-trichlorophenylethanediol (2.5 and four percent), and
(6) 1-(2,4,5-trichlorophenyl)-ethanol (two and zero percent).

The metabolic pathway possibly follows Figure 14.

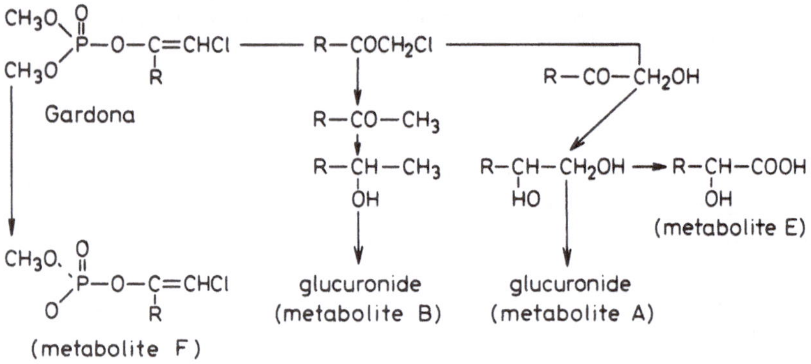

Fig. 14. Possible routes of metabolism of Gardona in animals (AKINTONWA and HUTSON 1967): $R =$ 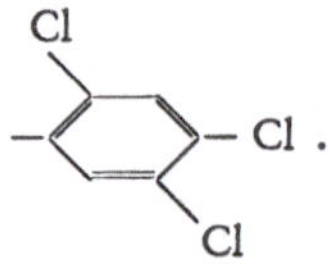 .

Quantitative reports concerning residue values in meat of domestic mammals exist only for cattle sprayed with Gardona (IVEY *et al.* 1968). No residues could be found by glc in tissues three weeks after treatment with a 0.25 percent spray, and two weeks after treatment with a 0.125 percent spray; liver and kidney were free of residues at each time-point. Table CVIII contains a shortened survey of residue values which do not exceed a 0.1 p.p.m. maximum.

When the straw or dust baths in chicken houses were treated with 450 g. of three percent Gardona or 45 g. of a 75 percent WP Gardona, the chickens contained — after four weeks continuous exposure and one week after discontinuation of treatment — a maximum in the back skin of 0.06 p.p.m., and four weeks after discontinuation 0.05 p.p.m. Gardona in fat. Other tissues such as meat and liver were practically free of residues after one week (IVEY *et al.* 1969).

[22] (β-D-glucopyranoside) uronic acid.

Table CVIII. *Gardona residues in tissues after spray treatment of cattle* (IVEY *et al.* 1968).

No. of animals	Spray conc. (%)	Sprayed quantity (ml.)	Days after treatment	Residue (p.p.m.) [a] in						
				Omental fat	Renal fat	Subcuta-neous fat	Muscle	Heart	Spleen	Brain
1	0.125	3,785	7	0.008	0.008	0.010	0	0	0	0
1	—	—	—	0.002	0	0	0	0	0	0
1	—	—	—	0.003	0.002	0.003	0	0	0	0
3	0.123	3,785	14	0	0	0	0	0	0	0
1	0.25	3,785	7	0.019	0.016	0.012	0	0.002	0	0.006
1	0.5	—	—	0.108	0.091	0.097	0.003	0.002	0.005	0.002
1	0.25	7,570	7	0.005	0.004	0.01	0	0	0	0
1	—	—	—	0.035	0.016	0.02	0	0	0	0
1	—	—	—	0.044	0.060	0.103	0	0	0	0
1	—	—	—	0.088	0.081	0.097	0	0	0	0
3	0.25	7,570	14	0.002	0	0	0	0	0	0
1	—	—	—	0.002	0	0	0	0	0	0
12	0.25	7,570	21	0	0	0	0	0	0	0

[a] 0 = < 0.002 p.p.m.

26. GS-13005. — Dithiophosphoric acid, O,O-dimethyl-*S*-[2-methoxy-1,3,4-thiadiazol-5(4H) onyl-(4)-methyl] ester

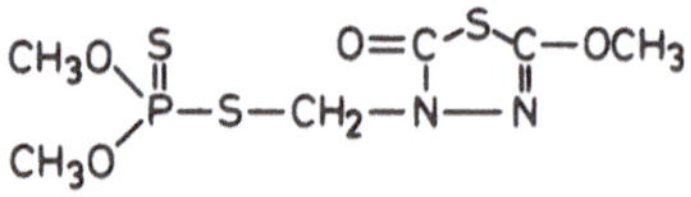

Alternate name: Supracide.
Application: For plant protection with special usefulness for the stages before and after blooming; grain-worm control.
Toxicity: See Table CIX.

Table CIX. *Acute toxicities of GS-13005 for various animals.*

Animal species	Mode of application	LD_{50} (mg./kg.)	Reference
Rat	*per os*	25–48	GROB *et al.* (1965)
Rat	dermal [a]	150	GROB *et al.* (1965)
Rat	dermal [b]	400	GROB *et al.* (1965)
Rabbit	*per os*	80	GROB *et al.* (1965)
Chicken	*per os*	80	GROB *et al.* (1965)

[a] Pure substance.
[b] Technical formulation.

Detection: By colorimetry (sulfide method), glc, and TLC (EBERLE *et al.* 1967, MATTSON *et al.* 1969, CASSIDY *et al.* 1969). Reference points for purposes of comparison were shown by ESSER and MÜLLER (1966) on rats with GS-13005 C^{14}-labelled in the 5-position in the heterocyclic ring.
Metabolism and residues: This compound was completely decomposed by rats: the ring C^{14}-carbonyl group was converted to CO_2 (ESSER and MÜLLER 1966, BULL 1968). Radioactive GS-13005 or its labelled metabolites were 68 percent excreted within a day, 40 percent with the urine, 28 percent with the breath, and 0.63 percent with the feces. Within 96 hours, 80.5 percent of the radioactivity was eliminated. Maximum radioactivity in blood plasma and in the cellular blood fractions was achieved one-half hour after *per os* application of the effective substance. The maximum in the liver was 1.84 percent after one-half hour; in kidneys, lungs, and testicles it was 0.42, 0.34, and 0.69 percent, respectively, after three hours. The concentration in muscle tissue increased from 9.64 percent after one-half hour to 17.4 percent after eight hours; it was 3.17 percent after 24 hours, and 0.25 percent after 48 hours. Radioactivity in body fat decreased from 3.48 percent after one-half hour to 3.26 percent after three hours, to 2.54 percent after eight hours, and to 0.65 percent after 24 hours. After 48 hours, the radioactivity in all organs with the exception of muscles amounted to 0.05 percent or less of the starting activity.

CASSIDY *et al.* (1969) investigated the tissue residues of a milk cow with regard to the intake of GS-13005 with the food, *i.e.*, especially with lucerne, after a daily dosage of one mg./kg. body wt. for five days. The GS-13005 was labelled as 5-carbonyl-C^{14}. The blood level reached maximum on the last day of intake, during with the radioactivity measured corresponded to 0.2 p.p.m. of GS-13005. After ten days the level decreased to 0.02 p.p.m. Of the total applied radioactivity about 24 percent was regained with the urine and about 34 percent with the feces; maximum in the urine was reached on the third day after application, in the feces on the fourth day. Eighty-five percent of the urine radioactivity was due to polar metabolites which corresponded neither to GS-13005 nor to its O-analog nor to 2-methoxy-Δ^2-1,2,4-thiadiazolin-5-one. Sixteen percent of the residues in the feces was extracted with acetone-methanol; predominantly polar metabolites were established.

Tissue residues for cows were low. Ten days after treatment the radioactivity corresponded to 0.11 p.p.m. in the liver, 0.04 p.p.m. in the kidneys, 0.03 p.p.m. in the spleen, and 0.02 p.p.m. each in heart, muscle, and brain. The equivalent concentration in fat was 0.02 to 0.03 p.p.m. The types of metabolites in the cow were not determined.

Young bulls (average 145 kg.) received daily zero, 0.5, 1.0, and 2.0 mg. per kg. body wt. in capsules over a ten-week period; one animal each died after 12, 33, and 34 days after the highest dosage. The erythrocyte ChE was linearly inhibited in dependence on the dosage. Residues in tissues were low. No O-analog was found. No residues could be established in the tissues after one mg./kg. body wt. Ten weeks after 2.0 mg./kg. body wt. dosage 0.04 p.p.m. was found in omental fat and brain (sensitivity of the method 0.01 p.p.m.); the other tissues were essentially free. Five weeks after discontinuation of the test the perirenal fat of one bull contained 0.02 p.p.m. GS-13005. One animal which lived longer than two weeks had 0.73 p.p.m. in the omental fat, 0.03 p.p.m. each in perirenal tissue, brain, and heart; the kidneys contained 0.02 p.p.m. after 14 days treatment while muscle, liver, and spleen were free of residues (POLAN *et al.* 1969).

27. HALOXON. — Phosphoric acid, O,O-di-(2-chloroethyl)-O-(3-chloro-4-methylcumarin-7-yl) ester

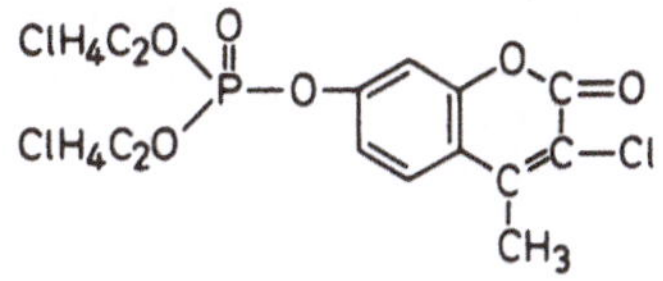

Alternate name: Eustidil.
Veterinary application: Wide-range anthelmintic (NUNNS *et al.* 1964) for application on ruminants, poultry, and horses.
Application dosage on the animal: 30 to 50 mg./kg. body wt.
Toxicity: See Table CX.

Table CX. *Acute toxicities of Haloxon for various animals.*

Animal species	Mode of application	Toxic dosage (mg./kg.)	LD_{50} (mg./kg.)	Remarks	Reference
Rat	*per os*	—	2,040	—	Harbour (1963)
Rat	dermal	> 3,000	—	—	Harbour (1963)
Rat	*per os*	—	2,042	WP 75%	Harbour (1963)
Rat	*per os*	—	896	in glycerin-formaldehyde	Malone (1964)
Sheep	*per os*	—	1,378	WP 75%	Malone (1964)
Goose	*per os*	500	—	—	Lee & Pickering (1967)
Duck	*per os*	1,500	—	—	Lee & Pickering (1967)
Chicken	—	5,000	—	symptoms	Lee & Pickering (1967)

Residues: Haloxon is a phosphoric acid ester of good compatibility; however, an LD_{50} of 3,645 mg./kg. for poultry and of 687 mg./kg. for sheep led to neurotoxic symptoms. ChE inhibition was low. Therefore, residues of P^{32}-Haloxon in tissues seven days after application can be neglected (Malone 1964).

28. IMIDAN. — Phosphorodithioic acid, O,O-dimethyl ester, *S*-ester with *N*-(mercaptomethyl) phthalimide

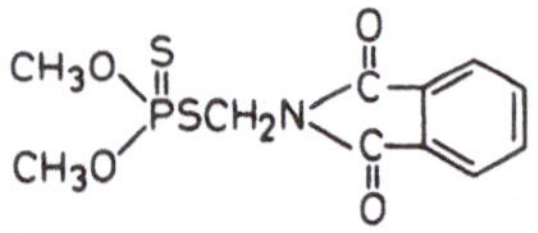

Alternate names: Prolate; Stauffer R-1,504; R-1,504.
Application: Systemic insecticide and acaricide against ticks, bot-flies, and *Haematobia* as 0.375 to 0.5 percent spray, with 250 ml. of a two percent preparation for pour-on treatment, or 50 mg./kg. *per os.*
Toxicity: [23] See Table CXI. The dermal resorption of imidan is good.
Tolerances and restrictions: In the U.S.A., earlier "zero tolerance" or "no

Table CXI. *Acute toxicities of Imidan for rats and rabbits.*

Animal species	Mode of application	LD_{50} (mg./kg.)	Reference
Rat	oral	147	Eichler (1965)
Rat	oral [a]	216	Frear (1965)
Rabbit	dermal [a]	3,160	Frear (1965)

[a] Technical product.

[23] Rogoff *et al.* (1967) mentioned a report on toxicity by Younger *et al.* (1967) as being in press, but which did not appear in the journal cited.

residue" [see Group IV in Pesticide Handbook-Entoma (FREAR *et al.* 1969)].

Detection: See ACKERMANN (1967) and ACKERMANN *et al.* (1969).

Metabolism and residues: Imidan was rapidly metabolized to water-soluble substances in the mammal (Fig. 15).

Excretion with 78 percent of the applied dosage in the urine reached its maximum in 24 hours. After oral intake not more than 0.04 percent of the dosage was excreted in the urine as Imidan or Imidoxon by rats. After benzene extraction the aqueous fraction contained 98.9 percent of the C^{14}-Imidan metabolites of the urine. Excreted metabolites were distributed as 40.7 percent phthalamidic acid, 21 percent phthalic acid, 10.9 percent as five metabolites of the phthaloyl type which are present in small amounts, and 5.5 percent unknown substances. The benzene extract contained 1.1 percent of the urine C^{14}-Imidan metabolites (McBAIN *et al.* 1968). Within 30 hours 11.4 percent of the applied C^{14}-Imidan dosage was isolated from the feces in the aqueous phase (McBAIN *et al.* 1968).

Comparable data for rats by FORD *et al.* (1966) signified that after *per os* doses of Imidan its metabolites were 78 percent eliminated in the urine and 19 percent in the feces 120 hours after application. Imidan or Imidoxon [N-(mercaptomethyl)phthalimide-S-(O,O-dimethylphosphorothiolate)], was present in the urine <1.0 percent. There was no relative cumulation in the tissues and the residue was about 2.6 percent of the applied radioactivity (C^{14}). Calculated as absolute values, the average residue in the entire body of the rat was 0.71 p.p.m. (C^{14}-Imidan equivalent) 72 hours after treatment, and 0.41 p.p.m. after 120 hours, which is only 58 percent of the 72-hour value. Rat tissues contained the values in Table CXII.

Table CXII. *Imidan residues in rat tissues* (FORD *et al.* 1966).

Tissue	Imidan equivalent (p.p.m.)			
	After 72 hours		After 120 hours	
	Av.	Range	Av.	Range
Fat	0.23	0.17–0.33	0.1	0.09–0.1
Brain	0.43	0.36–0.49	0.25	0.24–0.26
Heart	0.48	0.41–0.58	0.3	0.26–0.35
Liver	0.65	0.41–0.91	0.32	—
Lung	0.53	0.41–0.60	0.46	0.23–0.69
Muscle	0.86	0.75–1.04	0.56	0.50–0.63
Kidney	1.25	1.09–1.55	0.60	0.56–0.65

The distribution of Imidan for pregnant animals is noteworthy. After application of 20 mg. of Imidan/kg. body wt. to pregnant rats, 215 ng./g. were found after 30 minutes in the liver tissue of the mother animal, and 380 ng./g. in the liver of the fetus, 120 ng./g. in its muscles, and 60 ng./g. in its brain tissue. The P–O-analog of Imidan was not established (ACKERMANN and ENGST 1970).

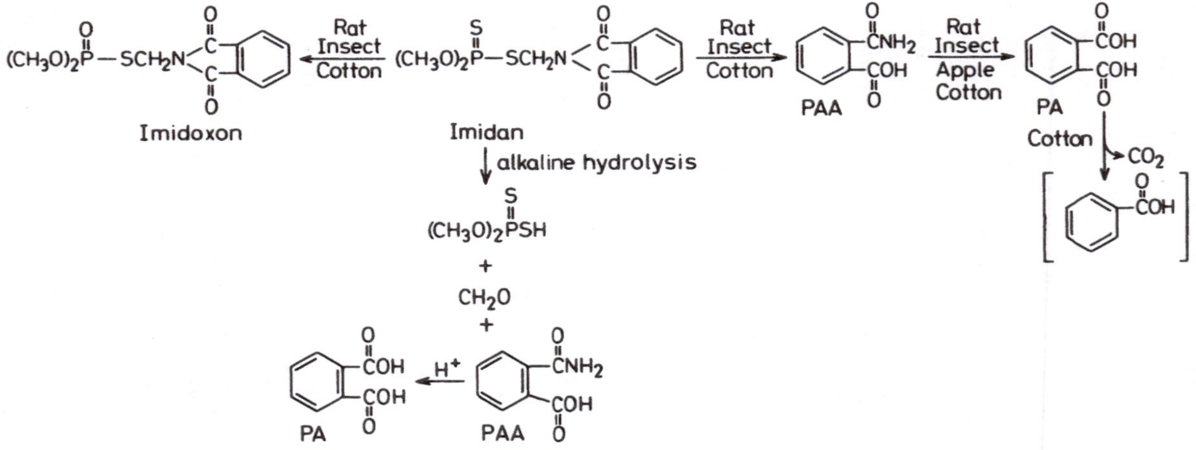

Fig. 15. Proposed pathways of Imidan degradation in mammals (rat), insects (cockroach), plants [apple (BATCHELDER and WISE 1963) and cotton], and in alkaline solution (McBAIN *et al.* 1968).

Chamberlain (1965) investigated Imidan C^{14}-labelled in one of the carbonyl groups after spraying of a bull with a specially prepared emulsion mixture; 4.76 g. of Imidan was applied to the animal. The resorbed quantities were low. Resorption and metabolism were rapid. Radioactivity in blood reached its maximum with very low concentrations six to nine hours after application. From blood <2.0 percent was soluble in benzene. In the urine there was maximum excretion of radioactive substances after six hours, but the level was not high. Approximately eight percent of the totally applied dosage was excreted with the urine in seven days, of which 0.01 percent was benzene-soluble. Maximum excretion in the feces lay between nine and 24 hours after treatment; the excretion rate was 1.7 percent of the applied dosage. It was demonstrated with chromatography and electrophoresis that degradation of Imidan in cattle occurred primarily at the N-atom. The metabolites in the urine were phthalic acid and phthalamidic acid, while the detection of benzoic acid was not convincingly possible.

Rogoff *et al.* (1967) confirmed the rapid decrease of measurable Imidan residues in cattle. After treatment with a 0.25 percent spray, measurable residues appeared only in fat, liver, and muscle tissue. With regard to the percent recovery of 58.7 percent, and the sensitivity of the phosphorus molybdate method used, the detection limit of which was 0.2 p.p.m., the residues in omental fat three days after treatment were 0.4 p.p.m., in perirenal fat 0.6 p.p.m., and in subcutaneous fat 0.7 p.p.m. All the tests at later times up to the fifty-ninth day after treatment gave values which were below the detection limit. The residue values in muscle tissue and in liver were determined with the anthranillic acid method, with a detection limit of 0.04 p.p.m.; a corrected content of 0.06 p.p.m. was found in the muscle three days after treatment. The values in liver fell from 0.10 p.p.m. on the third day to 0.09 p.p.m. on the seventh, 0.08 p.p.m. on the fourteenth, and 0.06 p.p.m. on the twenty-eighth day after slaughter. These values were no longer significant in comparison to the control (0.08 p.p.m.) (Rogoff *et al.* 1967). McBain *et al.* (1968) had this optimistic conclusion: "Consequently Imidan represents, by virtue of its rapid metabolism and elimination, a biodegradable pesticide which is not likely to have toxic residues in the environment."

29. MALATHION. — Succinic acid, mercaptodiethyl ester, *S*-ester with O,O-dimethyl phosphorodithioate

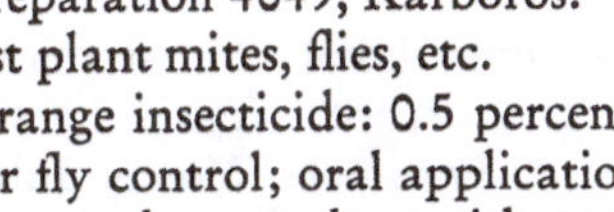

Alternate names: Malathon, preparation 4049, Karbofos.
Application: Insecticide against plant mites, flies, etc.
Veterinary application: Wide range insecticide: 0.5 percent against lice and mite attack; spray and dust for fly control; oral application for larvae control in the feces; ectoparasite control on poultry with one to three percent

spray (Furmann and Weinmann 1956). For general information about the importance of insect control with malathion see Lindquist (1959).

Toxicity: See Table CXIII. The oxidation product of malathion, malaoxon, is the actual toxic substance. Toxicity was dependent on age and sex. Generally, malathion and malaoxon were more toxic for female than for male animals; older animals decontaminated more rapidly. This difference in toxicity was explained by the increasing enzyme activity (Brodeur and Du Bois 1967). The low toxicity for mammals corresponded to a low ChE inhibition (Hazleton 1955). Even a long duration treatment was possible without damage. Rats tolerated 1,000 p.p.m. (tech.) *per os* over a 92-week period (Martin 1961).

Detection: See Sutherland (1964) and Duggan *et al.* (1967); with glc in fish tissues (Ragab 1968) and in fat (Corley and Beroza 1968); paper chromatography and TLC (König *et al.* 1966). The Norris *et al.* (1954) method is, according to Hazleton (1955), not adequate for residue determinations in animal tissue; however, the later colorimetric method (Norris *et al.* 1958) appeared suitable. The original Norris method (1954) was criticized because certain carbon tetrachloride-soluble excretion products also gave a positive color reaction and therefore by some ether extraction was preferred (Mattson and Sedlack 1959).

Restrictions and tolerances: In the U.S.A., malathion received a tolerance of four p.p.m. in meat, meat products of horses, cattle, goats, sheep, and pigs, as well as in poultry (Radeleff and Bushland 1960, Frear *et al.* 1969). Lucerne, clover, grass, and grass hay may contain up to 135 p.p.m.

Metabolism and residues: Malathion was rapidly hydrolyzed by the rumen fluid (Ahmed *et al.* 1958). Various enzyme systems of the body took part in the degradation of malathion, for instance, phosphatases, and — predominantly in mice — carboxylase (Krueger and O'Brien 1959 b, March *et al.* 1956 a, Matsumura and Boush 1966, Bourke *et al.* 1968).

The balance between the oxidation of malathion to malaoxon and its hydrolysis caused the great compatability ratio for mammals. Malaoxon was a stronger ChE inhibitor than malathion (O'Brien 1957, Krueger and O'Brien 1959 b). Malathion and malaoxon were decomposed to a high degree by the liver tissue of mammals *in vitro* (Murphey 1966).

The liver microsomes, DPNH, Mg^{++}, and nicotinamide seemed to be of importance for the activation of malathion to malaoxon in mouse (mammal) liver by oxidative desulfuration $(>\underset{\underset{O}{\|}}{P}-S-)$ (Brodeur and Du Bois 1967). The corresponding transformation in heart and testicle tissue occured to a lesser degree (O'Brien 1957).

Hydrolysis of malaoxon took place predominantly in liver, kidney, and lung; the carboxyl ester bond of malathion and malaoxon was attacked (O'Brien 1957). The decontamination activity by carboxyesterases was influenced by the sex hormones. Young animals did not decontaminate as well as adults; accordingly, testosterone increased the enzyme activity in

Table CXIII. *Acute toxicities of malathion and malaoxon for various animals.*

Substance	Animal species	Special factors	Mode of application	Toxic dosage (mg./kg. or conc.)	LD_{50} (mg./kg.)	Reference
Malathion	Mouse	—	*per os*	—	930	Perkow (1956)
	Mouse	—	*per os*	—	450–5,800	Holmstedt (1959)
	Mouse	♂	*per os*	—	4,059	Hazleton & Holland (1953)
	Mouse	—	*i.p.*	—	1,590	Krüger & O'Brien (1959 b)
	Rat	—	*per os* [a]	—	1,400–1,600	Klotzsche (1955)
	Rat	—	*per os*	—	479–1,845	Perkow (1956)
	Rat	—	*per os*	—	450–5,800	Holmstedt (1959)
	Rat	♂	*per os*	—	5,843	Hazleton & Holland (1953)
	Rat	♂	*per os* [b]	—	250	Klotzsche (1964)
	Rat	♂	*per os* [c]	—	1,156	Hazleton & Holland (1953)
	Rat	♀+♂	*per os*	—	1,400	Hazleton (1955)
	Rat	—	*s.c.*	—	1,000	Krüger & Casida (1957)
	Rat	—	*i.p.*	—	750	Holmstedt (1959)
	Chicken	1 week	*per os*	—	370	Sherman & Ross (1959)
	Chicken	—	dip	4% lethal	—	Furmann & Weinmann (1956)
	Calf	1–2 weeks	*per os*	max. nontox. 10 min. tox. 20	—	Radeleff & Bushland (1960)
	Calf	—	dermal	0.5% tolerated	—	Radeleff & Woodard (1957)
	Cattle	juvenile	*per os*	—	80	Eichler (1965)
	Cattle	adult	*per os*	—	560	Eichler (1965)
	Cattle	adult	*per os*	max. nontox. 50 min. tox. 100	—	Radeleff & Bushland (1960)
	Cattle	—	dermal	2% tolerated	—	Radeleff & Woodard (1957)
	Sheep	adult	*per os*	max. nontox. 50 min. tox. 100	—	Radeleff & Bushland (1960)
Malaoxon	Rat	♀	*i.p.*	—	17.5	Brodeur & Du Bois (1967)
	Mouse	♂	*i.p.*	—	25	Brodeur & Du Bois (1967)
		—	*i.p.*	—	75	Krüger & O'Brien (1959 b)

[a] 85 to 95 percent technical product.
[b] 64 percent technical product.
[c] 90 percent technical in propylene glycol.

castrated young male rats (BRODEUR and DU BOIS 1967). The malathion-ase activity was approximately 2.5 times stronger in the liver of males than in the liver of females. After injection of malathion, a rapid degradation through hydrolysis at the acetyl ester bond tooke place in mice, rats, and dogs (KNAAK and O'BRIEN 1960, KRUEGER and O'BRIEN 1959 b).

One-half hour after *i.p.* injection 70 to 80 percent of malathion was already decomposed in mice (KRUEGER and O'BRIEN 1959 b). The resorbed dosage contained 70 percent water-soluble, 20 percent chloroform-soluble, ten percent nonextractable fractions, and 0.13 µg./g. malaoxon. According to KRUEGER and O'BRIEN (1959 b) there were two places of attack for this decomposition:

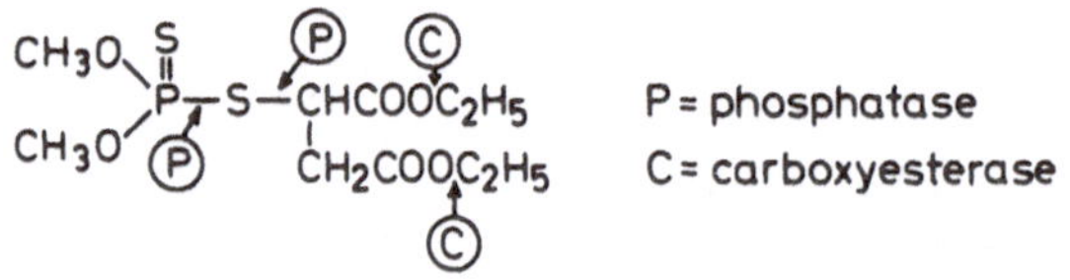

Phosphatases attacked the P–S–C bond, carboxyesterase attacked the $COOC_2H_5$ group.

KRUEGER and O'BRIEN (1959 b) (see also O'BRIEN 1960), 30 minutes after *i.p.* injection of 30 mg./kg. of malathion, identified six metabolites in the aqueous fraction obtained from the whole mouse. These fractions were as shown in Figure 16.

$(CH_3O)_2P(S)SCHCOOC_2H_5$ (with $CH_2COOC_2H_5$) Malathion → $(CH_3O)_2P(S)SCHCOOH$ (with $CH_2COOC_2H_5$) I Malathion-monoacid (68%)

Malathion ↓ $(CH_3O)_2P(S)SH$ II (5%) → $(CH_3O)_2P(S)OH$ III (13%)

III ↓ $(CH_3O)_2P(O)OH$ IV (2.5%)

Unknown: V (1.5%) and VI (10%)

Fig. 16. Metabolites of malathion in the mouse in the yields shown (KRUEGER and O'BRIEN 1959 b).

O'BRIEN (1960) summarized the urine metabolites from his own data and those by KNAAK and O'BRIEN (1960) as in Table CXIV. The differences among the animal species are striking.

The main excretion pathway for the metabolites of malathion was through the kidneys (BOURKE *et al.* 1968), while approximately two percent of $C^{14}O_2$ was exhaled within 24 hours after oral treatment with C^{14}-malathion. In no case was unchanged malathion found in the urine of rats. The

Table CXIV. *Urinary metabolites of malathion in cow, rat, and dog* (O'Brien 1960). [a]

Animal species and dose (mg./kg.)	Urine analysed	Malathion monoacid (%)	Mala-thion diacid (%)	Des-methyl malathion (%)	Dimethyl-phos-phoro-dithioate (%)	Dimethyl-phos-phoro-thioate (%)	Dimethyl-phos-phate (%)
Dog (25)	Av. for 48-hr.	40	21	21	7	7	1
Rat (25)	48-hr. composite	12	48	11	4	10	6
Cow (1.3) for 3 days	1-week composite	63	17	7	trace	11	2

[a] Results are percent of solvent-unextractable metabolites of each compound.

Table CXV. *Percent excretion of radioactivity for rats after oral treatment with C^{14}-malathion* (Bourke *et al.* 1968).

Hours after application	Excretion (%)		
	$C^{14}O_2$ (air)	Urine	Feces
8	1.66	45	0.78
24	2.77	83	5.51

C^{14}-excretion was obtained for rats after oral treatment with 25 mg. of malathion as shown in Table CXV.

According to Mattson and Sedlak (1959) the recovered radioactivity from P^{32}-malathion in the urine of rats averaged 46 percent (20 to 73) within five days after daily *i.p.* injection of 100 mg. of malathion/kg. body wt.; after oxidation with perchloric acid they used ammonium molybdate and aminonaphtholsulfonic acid for the determination of total phosphates extractable from the urine with ether. Ninety-six hours after discontinuation of treatment, the excretion of metabolites decreased 0.25 to 0.53 percent. Only 1.0 percent of the dosage was extracted with carbon tetrachloride as unchanged malathion. Thirteen to 43 percent of the injected dosage or, expressed differently, 66 percent (47 to 78) of purine-specific residues were found in the ether extract. Excretion ratios for low dosages remained at about the same correlation (Mattson and Sedlak 1959).

After oral application of 100 mg./kg. body wt. male and female rats excreted, respectively, 24 and 48 percent in the urine, 31 and 36 percent of which was soluble [24] (Mattson and Sedlak 1959).

The blood concentration for rats which received 25 mg./kg. malathion *i.p.* was 3.3 p.p.m. after one-half hour; 0.52 percent of the substances was chloroform-soluble, 16.4 percent of which, again, was malaoxon. In five to

[24] The recovery of metabolites of malathion was strongly dependent on the solvents utilized. Furthermore, there was a time-dependent transformation after use of carbon tetrachloride or ether (Table CXVI).

Table CXVI. *Solubility of malathion metabolites in human urine* [a] (Mattson and Sedlak 1959).

Time after treatment (accumulative)	Total soluble extractable substances (%) in		
	CCl_4	$CHCl_3$	Ether
2 hr. 50 min.	62.7	22.5	14.7
5 hr. 20 min.	42.5	17.9	39.6
7 hr. 35 min.	18.4	23.0	58.6

[a] After oral treatment with 0.85 mg. of malathion/kg. body wt., 23 percent of the dosage was found within 16.5 hours in the urine; 97 percent of these metabolites had already been excreted with the urine after 7.5 hours.

six hours 39 percent of the applied dosage was excreted, with about 50 percent after 20 hours. The metabolites were distributed as shown in Table CXVII.

The blood level in dogs reached its maximum 2.5 hours after *i.p.* injection of 25 mg. of C^{14}-malathion, with about four p.p.m. malathion-equivalent (Bourke *et al.* 1968). This level decreased rapidly after five to ten hours. The malathion fraction deviated from zero to 2.2 p.p.m.; 51 percent of the total quantity was excreted with the urine within 72 hours. The distribution of these residues in rats is seen in Table CXVIII.

Twenty-four hours after this treatment, only ten percent of the applied dosage was present in the body as radioactive substances. Eight hours after the application lung, heart, and spleen contained less than 0.01 per-

Table CXVII. *Metabolites in rat and dog urine after i.p. injection* [a] *of C^{14}-malathion* (Knaak and O'Brien 1960).

Compound	Metabolite (p.p.m.) after						
	Rat	Dog					
	0–48 hr.	0–2 hr.	4–8 hr.	8–12 hr.	12–24 hr.	24–48 hr.	48–72 hr.
Dimethylphosphate	6	1	1	1	1	1	0
Malathion monoacid	12	56	43	39	28	33	40
Malathion diacid	48	11	18	22	35	20	17
Dimethylphosphorothioate	10	5	7	6	9	10	9
Desmethyl malathion	11	19	22	22	22	22	20
Dimethylphosphorodithioate	4	5	5	6	10	10	8
Total prod. of carboxy-ester cleavage	59	67	61	61	63	53	57
Total prod. of phosphorothiolester cleavage	24	30	35	35	42	43	37
Unknown A	3	0	2	0	1	0	0
Unknown B	0	0	0	0	2	0	0
Total unknowns	3	0	2	0	3	0	0

[a] 25 mg./kg.

Table CXVIII. *Radioactivity in rat excretory products and tissues after 24 mg. C^{14}-malathion per os* (BOURKE *et al.* 1968).

Sample	Radioactivity (%) after	
	8 hours	24 hours
Carbon dioxide	1.66	2.77
Urine	44	83
Feces	0.78	5.51
Tongue	<0.01	<0.01
Heart	<0.01	<0.01
Liver	0.28	0.18
Spleen	<0.01	<0.01
Kidney	0.09	0.05
Gastrointestinal tract	0.3	0.05
Gastrointestinal content	47	7.75
Blood	0.78	0.20

cent, and blood, kidneys, and liver less than 1.0 percent of the applied total dosage.

Malathion was also rapidly excreted by the cow (O'BRIEN *et al.* 1961). For three days the authors applied 1.3 mg./kg. body wt. *per os* of P^{32}-malathion to cattle. The metabolism was similar to that of mice, rats, and dogs, namely hydrolysis at the carboxy ester bond. During the first week 31 percent of the total metabolites from the blood of cows was benzene-acetone soluble. Malathion represented 28 percent and malaoxon 15 percent of this fraction; there were 56 percent nonidentified metabolites and 0.6 percent phospholipids. The metabolites, which appeared quickly in the blood, were excreted mainly with the urine, specifically 69 percent within four days after the first dosage. After seven days 77.2 percent of the applied dosage was regained, of which 69 percent was in the urine, eight percent was in the feces, and 0.2 percent was in the milk, while 22.8 percent seemed to have been built into body tissue. Only 0.00006 to 0.006 percent of the total quantity could be extracted with carbon tetrachloride as malathion or malaoxon: 12 percent of the radioactive material extractable from the feces was malaoxon and 85 percent was malathion.

The major water-soluble metabolites in the feces were dimethylphosphate (47 percent) and O,O-dimethylthiophosphate (29 percent).

The following metabolites were found after one week in the aqueous fraction of urine as percent of total water-soluble metabolites (O'BRIEN *et al.* 1961): malathion monoacid (63), malathion diacid (17), O,O-dimethylthiophosphate (11), desmethyl malathion (7), and dimethylphosphate (2).

O'BRIEN (1960) also treated milk cows with 1.3 mg./kg. body wt. malathion during three consecutive days. The blood level after one hour corresponded to about 18 percent of the applied dosage. The main excretion pathway was in the urine, in which 90 percent of the excreted material was present; 9.7 percent was established in the feces. However, 23 percent of the applied dosage was not excreted within three weeks. This portion was probably present in the phosphorus pool of the organism.

PASARELA *et al.* (1962) established the absence of malathion residues in blood, liver, kidney, heart, muscle, and fat by colorimetry within 14 to 44 days after feeding 200 p.p.m. of malathion (tech. 95 percent) in the total ration; 95 percent of the samples contained <1.0 p.p.m. Only in the liver of cattle which received malathion over a period of 14 days could small but sure malathion residues be established (Table CXIX).

Table CXIX. *Malathion residues in tissues of calves fed 200 p.p.m. in the ration for varying periods* (PASARELA *et al.* 1962).

Calf no.	Days fed malathion	Residue (p.p.m.) [a] in						
		Liver	Heart	Blood	Neck muscle	Thigh muscle	Loin muscle	Fat
1 (control)	0	0.06	0.07	0.02	0.03	0.04	0.08	0.22
2	14	0.64	0.09	0.03	0.07	0.03	0.13	0.13
3	14	0.30	0.09	0.07	0.08	0.09	0.13	0.15
4	41	0.32	0.14	0.00	0.10	0.04	0.00	0.16
5	41	0.16	0.15	0.00	0.09	0.00	0.03	0.08
6	42	0.23	0.09	0.02	0.08	0.09	0.10	0.08
7	42	0.17	0.09	0.00	0.13	0.11	0.14	0.07
8	44	0.18	0.03	0.03	0.01	0.04	0.02	0.12
9	44	0.16	0.00	0.02	0.00	0.00	0.02	0.46

[a] Averages of duplicate portions of the same tissue.

No residues could be established with the method of CONROY (1957) in blood, brain, liver, kidney, and rib meat of slaughtered cattle which earlier had received malathion-treated lucerne hay treated per cow with 0.13 ml. of 57 percent EC daily, or a total of 2.75 ml. (1.65 g.) (SMITH *et al.* 1960).

MARCH *et al.* (1956 b) sprayed two calves twice two weeks apart with P^{32}-malathion in 0.5 percent aqueous emulsion so that each animal received about 50 p.p.m.; they used both radiometric assay and the colorimetric method of NORRIS *et al.* (1954) for residue determinations. After resorption, which was faster and more complete than for chickens, malathion was rapidly metabolized and 96 to 99 percent was excreted with the urine in the form of water-soluble metabolites and degradation products; the highest excretion occurred within 24 hours. Tissue concentrations one and two weeks after the last treatment are in Table CXX.

Total residues in the meat lay between 0.05 and 0.15 p.p.m. Thymus, liver, pancreas, thyroid gland, and bone contents fluctuated from 0.2 to 2.0 p.p.m.; skin contained 3.0 to 18 p.p.m. All tissue residues, with the exception of skin, were present in water-soluble form as metabolites and degradation products. No malathion or chloroform-soluble residues were established (cf. Table CXXI). Only in skin could unchanged malathion or chloroform-soluble metabolites be found two weeks after the last treatment.

Table CXX. *Radiometrically determined malathion and metabolites in tissues of calves given two spray applications each two weeks apart to provide 50 p.p.m. of malathion per animal* (MARCH *et al.* 1956 b).

Tissue	Total P^{32}-malathion and metabolites in tissues (p.p.m.) [a]			
	Calf 1 (sacrificed at one week)		Calf 2 (sacrificed at two weeks)	
	Wet ashed	Dip counted	Wet ashed	Dip counted
Foreleg	0.07	0.06	0.12	0.11
Shoulder rib chops	0.06	0.07	0.13	0.06
Rib chops	0.05	0.05	0.11	0.09
Loin chops	0.05	0.05	0.13	0.08
Breast	0.07	0.05	0.12	0.10
Trimmings	0.06	0.07	0.12	0.10
Rump	0.06	0.06	0.13	0.08
Hind leg	0.07	0.06	0.14	0.11
Tenderloin	0.07	0.06	0.15	0.05
Tail	0.07	—	0.14	—
Tongue	0.17	—	0.18	0.15
Brain	0.08	—	0.12	—
Spinal cord	0.09	—	0.13	—
Thymus	0.44	—	0.57	0.62
Thyroid	0.20	—	—	—
Pancreas	—	—	0.40	—
Kidney	0.18	0.16	0.24	0.26
Liver	1.20	0.99	0.97	1.24
Heart	0.13	—	0.19	0.39
Rumen (tripe)	0.42	—	0.34	—
Suet	—	0.06	—	0.10
Bone	—	0.77	1.37	1.91
Marrow	—	—	0.06	—
Hide	—	—	3.2–18.5	—

[a] Homogenized samples of tissues partitioned between chloroform and water showed no detectable activity in the chloroform phase except in samples of hide, in which a maximum of 2.7 percent of the total activity partitioned into the chloroform.

Similarly, no detectable malathion was found in bioptically obtained fat samples after spray treatment with 0.5 percent malathion of cattle eight days after 16 weekly treatments (CLABORN *et al.* 1956) using the same NORRIS *et al.* (1958) method which could detect 0.5 p.p.m. in tissues for these authors.

ROBERTS *et al.* (1960), using the same colorimetric method, one week after treatment of two pigs with one percent spray found no malathion in one pig and traces in some of the tissues of the second pig. Their residues for sheep and goats are given in Table CXXII.

The metabolic fate of malathion in poultry was investigated by MARCH *et al.* (1956 a) who recognized the compounds in Figure 17 as possible metabolites, of which II, III, and IV represented more polar components, which were the less effective and less toxic, while V was apparently the most im-

Table CXXI. *Colorimetrically determined malathion in tissues of calves given two spray applications each two weeks apart to provide 50 p.p.m. of malathion per animal* (March *et al.* 1956 b).

Sample: Tissue	Sample: Weight (g.)	Vol. extraction solvent (ml.)	Transmittance (%)	Malathion found [a] (µg.)
	Control samples (untreated)			
Fortified solvent blank (324 µg. malathion)	—	200	43.9	324
Fortified rump (324 µg. malathion)	200	400	48.9	275
Fortified foreleg (162 µg. malathion)	200	400	73.5	138
Nonfortified rump (control)	200	400	98.2	None
Nonfortified foreleg (control)	200	400	98.0	None
	Calf No. 1 (sacrificed at one week)			
Foreleg	174	348	98.8	None
	227	454	99.1	None
Hindleg	178	356	98.0	None
	203	406	98.1	None
Rump	224	448	98.0	None
	168	336	98.9	None
	Calf No. 2 (sacrificed at two weeks)			
Foreleg	225	450	96.3	None
	207	414	97.2	None
Hindleg	165	330	97.5	None
	203	406	97.1	None
Rump	212	424	95.5	None
	211	422	98.2	None

[a] None = < 0.2 p.p.m.

portant metabolite [O,O-dimethyl-*S*-(1,2-dicarboethoxy) methylphosphosphorothiolate]. The more polar water-soluble metabolites formed the greater part of metabolites in tissues and feces of poultry; they were relatively nontoxic.

March *et al.* (1956 a) also investigated the fate of P^{32}-malathion in laying hens; 60 percent of the malathion was excreted with the feces within two to four days and 75 percent within five to six days from 100 p.p.m. containd in the feed. Malathion was transformed during the passage through the digestive tract, for only two or three percent of the ingested amount was excreted by hens in unchanged form as chloroform-soluble metabolites. From 97 to 98 percent were water-soluble metabolites and degradation products. The tissues contained < 3.0 percent of the ingested malathion or its metabolites; only small quantities are found in the form of unchanged mala-

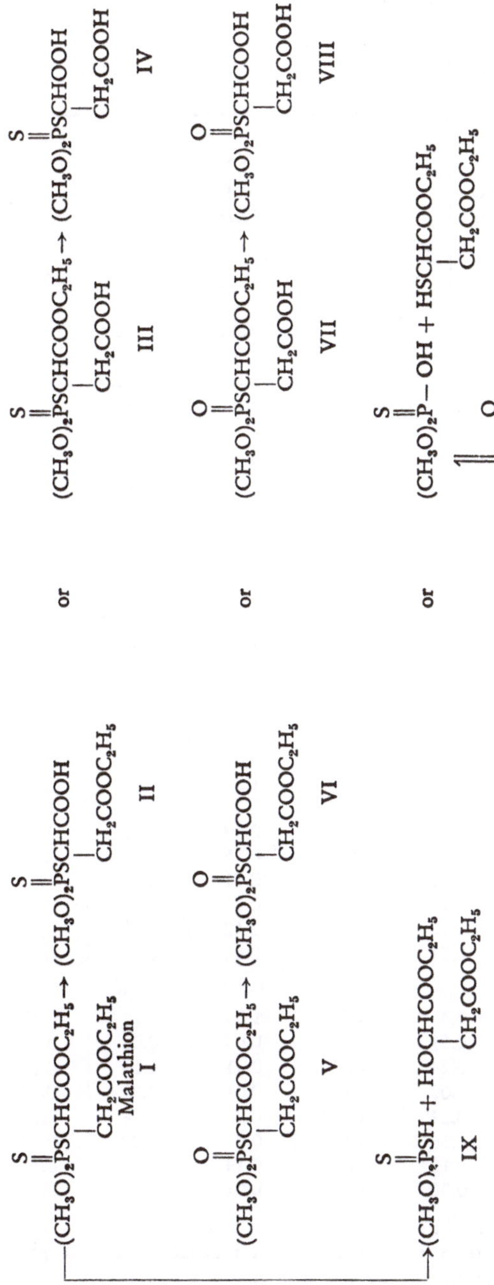

Fig. 17. Metabolites of malathion in poultry (MARCH *et al.* 1956 a).

Table CXXII. *Malathion residues in sheep and goats one week after treatment with one percent spray* (Roberts *et al.* 1960).

Animal	Residue (p.p.m.) in		
	Lean meat	Omental fat	Renal fat
Sheep			
Fleece	0.10	0.07	0
Sheared	0.08 [a]	0.41	0
Control	0.15	0.28	0.72
Goat			
Fur	0.02 [b]	3.20	0
Sheared	0.05 [a]	—	—
Control	0.15	0.20	0.45

[a] *American Cyanamid Co.* reported 0.14 p.p.m.
[b] *American Cyanamid Co.* reported 0.03 p.p.m.

Table CXXIII. *P^{32}-Malathion and metabolites in hen tissues at intervals while being fed radioactive feed and after return to normal feed* (March *et al.* 1956 a).

Days [a]	Fraction [b]	P^{32}-Malathion and metabolites (p.p.m.) in					
		Breast	Drumstick	Liver	Gizzard	Kidney	Blood [c]
		On radioactive feed (100 p.p.m. P^{32}-malathion)					
4	T	0.19	0.21	1.35	0.58	2.08	1.30
	C	0.01	0.02	0.09	0.00	0.01	0.00
5	T	0.16	0.27	1.27	0.52	1.94	1.24
	C	0.01	0.02	0.07	0.00	0.02	0.00
6	T	0.18	0.36	1.44	0.71	2.56	1.48
	C	0.01	0.01	0.06	0.00	0.00	0.00
7	T	0.22	0.41	1.56	0.65	1.94	1.02
	C	0.01	0.02	0.07	0.00	0.03	0.00
11	T	0.34	0.56	2.59	0.77	2.65	1.22
	C	0.02	0.02	0.15	0.03	0.03	0.03
13	T	1.02	0.50	2.71	0.42	1.38	1.08
	C	0.21	0.01	0.01	0.00	0.07	0.02
15	T	1.18	0.33	2.12	0.50	0.93	0.44
	C	0.01	0.02	0.44	0.01	0.00	0.21
		On normal feed					
18	T	0.33	0.34	1.33	0.19	0.53	0.56
	C	0.01	0.02	0.03	0.00	0.06	0.02
20	T	0.24	0.18	0.41	0.11	0.21	0.09
	C	0.00	0.00	0.01	0.00	0.00	0.00
22	T	0.22	0.24	0.76	0.14	0.16	0.07
	C	0.06	0.02	0.27	0.00	0.02	0.00
25	T	0.12	0.10	0.14	0.55	0.12	0.05
	C	0.00	0.00	0.01	0.00	0.06	0.00

[a] Radioactive feed replaced by normal feed after 15 days.
[b] T = maximum total residue P^{32}-malathion and metabolites, C = maximum residue P^{32}-malathion and chloroform-soluble metabolites.
[c] µg./ml. instead of µg./g.

thion and chloroform-soluble metabolites. After discontinuation of feeding with contaminated feed, there was a rapid decrease in concentration of radioactive material in excrement. The blood level remained relatively constant during the feeding period. Highest radioactives were present in liver and kidney. Ten days after discontinuation of contaminated feeding, the tissue concentration reached values which were found in hens after spray treatment (Table CXXIII).

After a 0.5 percent spray (190 mg. P^{32}-malathion/hen), only a small amount of substance was resorbed through the skin, which itself contained relatively high malathion values. The major amount was again excreted within 24 hours; the highest concentration in the feces reached half the value established after feeding. Only two percent of the sprayed dosage was resorbed and excreted within 24 hours, and 12 percent within 32 days in the form of predominantly (90 percent) water-soluble metabolites. The

Table CXXIV. *P^{32}-Malathion and metabolites in hen tissues at intervals after spraying with 0.5 percent emulsifiable P^{32}-malathion at the rate of 190 mg. of P^{32}-malathion/hen* [a] (MARCH *et al.* 1956 a).

Elapsed days	Fraction [b]	P^{32}-Malathion and metabolites (p.p.m.) in							
		Breast	Drum-stick	Liver	Gizzard	Kidney	Blood [c]	Skin (breast)	Feathers
1	T	0.10	0.22	0.54	0.09	0.53	4.8	—	—
	C	0.04	0.08	0.13	0.00	0.01	1.9	—	—
2	T	0.03	0.13	0.32	0.04	0.33	0.11	—	—
	C	0.00	0.00	0.00	0.00	0.00	0.00	—	—
3	T	0.18	0.06	0.51	0.08	0.92	0.13	—	—
	C	0.07	0.05	0.00	0.00	0.00	0.01	—	—
4	T	0.02	0.05	0.22	0.03	0.31	0.04	—	—
	C	0.00	0.02	0.00	0.00	0.00	0.00	—	—
7	T	0.04	0.07	0.23	0.06	0.60	0.06	—	—
	C	0.00	0.06	0.06	0.00	0.00	0.04	—	—
9	T	0.04	0.08	0.11	0.04	0.25	0.04	—	—
	C	—	—	0.03	—	0.12	—	—	—
14	T	0.04	0.05	0.12	0.07	0.24	0.02	—	—
	C	—	—	0.00	0.00	0.00	—	—	—
18	T	0.08	0.05	0.13	0.08	0.21	0.05	9	2,500
	C	0.00	0.00	0.00	0.00	0.00	0.00	—	—
21	T	0.05	0.05	0.04	0.06	0.11	0.00	15	120
	C	0.00	0.00	0.00	0.00	0.00	0.00	—	—
25	T	0.23	0.09	0.16	0.57	0.13	0.24	10	—
	C	0.10	0.00	0.00	0.00	0.00	0.00	—	—
28	T	0.10	0.33	0.17	0.06	0.20	0.03	36	—
	C	—	—	—	—	—	—	—	—
32	T	0.22	0.00	0.00	0.00	0.00	0.00	13	—
	C	—	—	—	—	—	—	—	—

[a] 112 p.p.m. based an average hen weight of 1690 g.
[b] T = maximum total residue P^{32}-malathion and metabolites, C = maximum residue P^{32}-malathion and chloroform-soluble metabolites.
[c] µg./ml. instead of µg./g.

tissue concentrations after spraying were only one-tenth of those obtained after feeding (Table CXXIV).

After *i.p.* injection of P^{32}-malathion into hens, 50 percent of the dosage was excreted after three hours and almost the entire dosage after 24 hours (MARCH *et al.* 1956 a).

During the first hour there were mainly water-soluble metabolites, but during the third hour the highest radioactivity was found in the chloroform fraction of the feces; it was about twice as high as the concentration of water-soluble metabolites. Afterwards the water-soluble products again prevailed to 90 percent. The highest concentrations in the tissues were found in the metabolism and excretion organs such as kidney and liver; all other organs remained under the concentration in the blood (Table CXXV).

Table CXXV. *P^{32}-Malathion and metabolites in hen tissues at intervals after i.p. injection with P^{32}-malathion* (MARCH *et al.* 1956 a).

Hours after injection	Amt. injected/hen		Fraction [b]	P^{32}-Malathion and metabolites in tissues (p.p.m.)						
	ml.	p.p.m. [a]		Breast	Drumstick	Liver	Gizzard	Kidney	Blood [c]	Brain
1.5	0.16	120	T	0.40	0.85	8.60	1.80	7.30	4.50	—
			C	0.00	0.00	0.10	0.00	0.00	0.00	—
5	0.17	140	T	6.00	5.10	56	—	94	17	3.70
			C	—	—		—	—	—	—
17.5	0.20	140	T	0.08	0.09	1.90	0.14	0.65	0.12	—
			C	—	0.00	0.00	0.05	0.07	0.06	—
48	0.25	200	T	0.99	0.62	6.00	—	4.80	1.20	0.87
			C	—	—	—	—	—	—	—

[a] Based on weight of hen.
[b] *T* = maximum total residue P^{32}-malathion and metabolites, *C* = maximum residue P^{32}-malathion and chloroform-soluble metabolites.
[c] µg./ml. instead of µg./g.

BROGDON (1962) did not find a change in taste of meat from malathion-treated animals.

30. METHYL PARATHION and FENITROTHION. — Phosphorothioic acid, O,O-dimethyl O-(*p*-nitrophenyl) ester and phosphorothioic acid, O,O-dimethyl O-(4-nitro-*m*-tolyl) ester

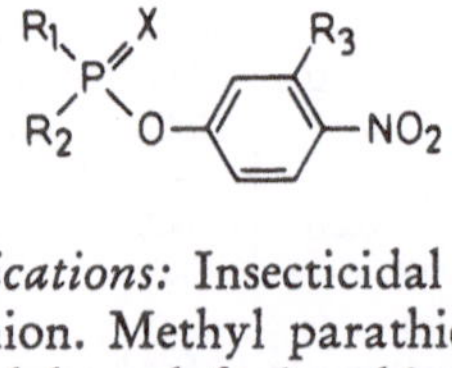

Alternate names and applications: Insecticidal group; application is alone or in mixture with parathion. Methyl parathion is present in Dalf, Metacide, Mikrotox, and Folidal, and fenitrothion (Sumithion) is present in Folithion. Mikrotox is used as an insect powder for domestic animals.
Toxicity: See Tables CXXVI and CXXVII.

Table CXXVI. *Structures and toxicities of methyl parathion, fenitrothion, and their oxons* (HOLLINGWORTH *et al.* 1967 a).

Compound	R_1	R_2	X	R_3	Oral LD_{50} mouse (mg./kg.)	Inhibition of ChE (I_{50}, Molar)	
						Mouse brain	Beef erythrocytes
Methyl parathion	CH_3O	CH_3O	S	H	23	—	—
Fenitrothion	CH_3O	CH_3O	S	CH_3	1,250	—	—
Methyl paroxon	CH_3O	CH_3O	O	H	21	3.3×10^{-7}	1.7×10^{-6}
Fenitrothion oxon [a]	CH_3O	CH_3O	O	CH_3	120	1.9×10^{-6}	7.8×10^{-6}

[a] Sumioxon.

Table CXXVII. *Acute toxicities of methyl parathion and fenitrothion for rodents.*

Compound	Animal species	Mode of application	Toxic dose (mg.-%)	LD_{50} (mg./kg.)	Reference
Methyl parathion	mouse	*s.c.*	50–100	—	MARTIN (1961)
	rat	*per os*	—	25	HOLMSTEDT (1959)
	rat	*s.c.*	—	6	KRUEGER & CASIDA (1957)
Fenitrothion	rat	*per os*	—	500	FREAR (1965)

Table CXXVI allows a comparative survey about toxicity. Certain metabolic processes are of importance for the low toxicity fenitrothion, aside from the *m*-methyl group. More desmethyl compounds are formed during the metabolism of fenitrothion, while more P – O metabolites result from methyl parathion. Negligible clinical symptoms are observed for cattle after two to six mg. of methyl parathion/kg. body wt., and even higher dosages remain without significant consequences (THAMM 1958).

Tolerances: In the U.S.A., a tolerance of 1.0 p.p.m. of methyl parathion is allowed for certain vegetables (FREAR *et al.* 1968).

Detection: ACKERMANN (1967), ACKERMANN *et al.* (1969), FAZEKAS and RENGEI (1965), SCHWERD and SCHMIDT (1952), SCHREIBER (1961), JAGLAN and GUNTHER (1970).

Metabolism and residues [25]: Sumioxon, the most effective metabolic product of fenitrothion, is more rapidly detoxified by liver homogenate than is methyl parathion; it is pharmacologically more effective than methyl parathion. This rapid detoxification is responsible for the low mammalian toxicity of fenitrothion (VARDANIS and CRAWFORD 1964, MIYAMOTO *et al.* 1963). The P – O bond is broken in both substances and free *p*-nitrophenol is formed (ALDRIDGE 1953). The phosphorus-containing metabolic products were excreted mainly through the kidneys whereby maximum excretion was reached within three days (MIYAMOTO *et al.* 1963).

[25] Compare with data in section on parathion.

After oral application methyl paraoxon was decomposed to predominantly dimethylphosphate by mice and, to a slighter degree, to the desmethyl derivative (HOLLINGWORTH 1969).

There was no significant difference in metabolism and rate of excretion of metabolites between methyl parathion and fenitrothion. After application of labelled substances, about 75 percent of the P^{32} was recovered from urine within 24 hours, and 55 percent for an extremely high dosage (850 mg./kg.). The excretion rate in urine and feces together reached 90 percent in 72 hours for fenitrothion and 65 percent for methyl parathion (HOLLINGWORTH *et al.* 1967 b, MIYAMOTO *et al.* 1963). MIYAMOTO *et al.* (1963) established the P^{32}-fractions which remained as residues in the tissues of guinea pigs and rats as being zero after fenitrothion treatment and ten to 15 percent after methyl parathion treament.

After oral application of three mg. of methyl parathion/kg. body wt. to pregnant albino rats, ACKERMANN and ENGST (1970) established 30 minutes after treatment 25 ng./g. in the liver tissues but no methyl paraoxon. They also found 33, 40, and 60 ng./g. of tissue in brain, liver, and muscles, respectively; corresponding values for methyl parathion were 3.5, 2.5, and 1.5 ng./g.

Seven out of eight metabolites which could be identified in mouse urine were hydrolysis and oxidation products: phosphoric acid, methylphosphoric acid, dimethylphosphoric acid (more of which is present after methyl parathion treatment), dimethylthiophosphoric acid, desmethylphosphate, desmethylthiophosphate (more occurred after fenitrothion treatment), and phosphate. There was no indication of reduction of the nitro group; furthermore, there were quantitative differences dependent on the dosage (HOLLINGWORTH *et al.* 1967 b).

Tissue concentrations in blood and brains of guinea pigs and rats reached maxima one-to-three hours after application and the concentrations decreased after 12 hours (MIAMOTO *et al.* 1963). The chloroform extracts of brains and blood contained neither fenitrothion nor methyl paraoxon. Less than three percent of the radioactive material present in urine of guinea pigs was chloroform soluble after treatment with methyl parathion; after fenitrothion treatment, the corresponding values for guinea pigs were 11 percent and for rats 4.5 percent (MIYAMOTO *et al.* 1963).

No literature references could be found concerning residues of methyl parathion and fenitrothion in actual edible animal tissues; these compounds belong to the parathion group (see section on parathion). THAMM (1958)

Table CXXVIII. *Acute toxicities of naphthalophos for rats after oral administration.*

Sex	LD_{50} (mg./kg.)	Reference
—	1,000	ANONYMOUS 8
♂	75	FREAR (1965)
♀	70	FREAR (1965)

established a sweetish-aromatic odor-change in bacon and thigh muscle tissue which still existed six days to six weeks after slaughtering. However, no reports about the possible importance of inert formulation components were made by the authors cited, for they used only a ten percent product (Wolfatox).

31. NAPHTHALOPHOS. — Phosphoric acid, *N*-hydroxynaphthalimide, diethyl ester

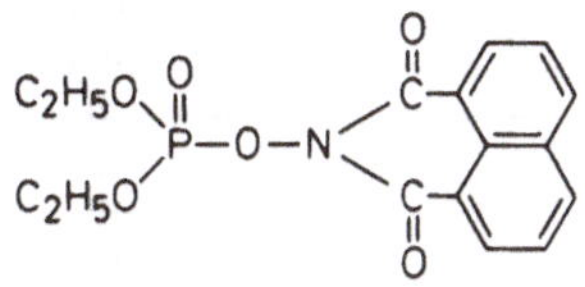

Alternate names: Maretin (Rametin), Bayer 9002, ENT 25567, S 940.
Application: 80 percent powder.
Veterinary application: Internally as suspension against worm attack in stomachs and intestines of ruminants, usually 50 mg./kg. body wt. but for angora goats 15 mg./kg. (ANONYMOUS 8).
Toxicity: See Table CXXVIII. Dosages of 150 mg./kg. *per os* created toxic symptoms for cattle, sheep, and goats; 375 mg./kg. were not lethal for cattle, but 200 mg./kg. was lethal for goats and 250 mg./kg. was lethal for sheep (NELSON *et al.* 1970).
Metabolism and residues: Naphthalophos was resorbed in only slight amounts by the digestive channel and was rapidly decomposed to harmless substances (ANONYMOUS 8). After alkaline hydrolysis the naphthalophos hydrolysis product (naphthostyril) could be detected by fluorometry (ANDERSON *et al.* 1966 b). The same hydrolysis product was found for compound "S-125". The sensitivity of the fluorescence method was 0.1 p.p.m.

No cumulation of naphthalophos was observed in muscle meat nor in organs, neither after double normal application dosage in cattle nor after a three-fold dosage in sheep (ANONYMOUS 8).

32. OMPA. — Pyrophosphoramide, octamethyl

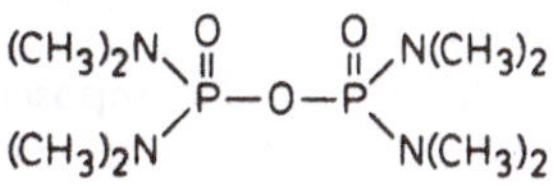

Alternate names: Pestox III, schradan, Systam, octamethyl.
Application: One of the first systemic insecticides, but of little contact effect against insects and mites (HAZLETON 1955); today it is only of historical importance (SCHRADER 1963).
Toxicity: See Table CXXIX.

A *per os* treatment for rats of 50 p.p.m. in feed over a one-year period caused toxic symptoms only in the beginning (BARNES, cited by MARTIN 1961). There was a tendency for cumulation (DU BOIS *et al.* 1950); 0.5 ml.

(60 percent) OMPA *per os* for pigs (McGirr and Papworth 1953), and daily application of one mg./kg. for dogs (Tusing cited by Hazleton 1955), caused toxic symptoms.

Table CXXIX. *Acute toxicities of OMPA for various animal species after different application.*

Animal species	Sex	Mode of application	Toxic dosage (mg./kg.)	LD_{50} (mg./kg.)	Reference
Mouse	♂+♀	*per os*	—	30	Frawley *et al.* (1952)
Mouse	—	*s.c.*	1.5–7	—	Martin (1961)
Mouse	—	*i.p.*	—	17	Du Bois (1950)
Rat	—	*per os*	—	8–10	Holmstedt (1959)
Rat	—	*per os*	18		Martin (1961)
Rat	—	*per os*	—	13.5	Corey *et al.* (1953 a)
Rat	♂	*per os*	—	13.5	Frawley *et al.* (1952)
Rat	♂	*per os*	—	9.7	Du Bois *et al.* (1950)
Rat	♀	*per os*	—	10.0	Du Bois *et al.* (1950)
Rat	♀	*per os*	—	35.5	Frawley *et al.* (1952)
Rat	—	*s.c.*	—	9	Krueger & Casida (1957)
Rat	—	*per os*	—	8–10	Du Bois (1959)
Rat	♂	*i.p.*	—	8.5	Du Bois *et al.* (1950)
Rat	♂	*i.p.*	—	8.0	Du Bois *et al.* (1950)
Rat	♀	*i.p.*	—	8.0	Du Bois (1950)
Rat	♀	*i.p.*	—	8.3	Du Bois (1950)
Guinea pig	—	*i.p.*	—	10	Du Bois *et al.* (1950)
Dog	—	*i.v.*	—	5–10	Du Bois *et al.* (1950)

OMPA was transformed to an active ChE inhibitor in the liver (Du Bois *et al.* 1950, Perkow 1956, Davison 1955, Tsuyuki *et al.* 1955, Gardiner and Kilby 1951). However, the transformation of OMPA differed with the sex, so that male rats formed ChE inhibitors more strongly and more rapidly than females (Aldridge and Barnes 1952), OMPA was nontoxic to mice with experimental hepatectomy (Cheng 1951).

Detection: See Duggan *et al.* (1967).

Tolerances and restrictions: In the U.S.A., in plants (walnuts) 0.75 p.p.m. (Frear and Friedmann 1968).

Metabolism and residues: OMPA was decomposed only a little in 24 hours by the rumen fluid (Ahmed *et al.* 1958). It was rapidly oxidized in the liver to phosphoroamide-N-oxide (Casida *et al.* 1954). Also liver homogenate *in vitro* caused a transformation of OMPA into an active ChE inhibitor (Du Bois *et al.* 1950). The activation apparently tooke place by reaction in the first step, where oxygen was added to the tertiary nitrogen of the dimethylamino group (O'Brien and Spencer 1953). It was observed during metabolism of OMPA in liver homogenate that inactivation was not accompanied by stoichiometric acid formation as, for instance, for TEPP (Fleischer and Jandorf 1952); for the importance of trimethylamino-oxidase, see O'Brien and Spencer (1953).

Tsuyuki *et al.* (1955) and Spencer *et al.* (1957) discussed questions of enzymatic and chemical oxidation of OMPA and considered the following steps as possible:

$$R-N(CH_3)_2 \xrightarrow{\text{oxidation}} R-\overset{\overset{O}{\uparrow}}{N}(CH_3)_2$$

$$R-N(CH_3)(CH_2OH) \longleftarrow \quad \longrightarrow R-NH(CH_3) + HCHO$$

$$R = [(CH_3)_2N]_2\overset{\overset{O}{\parallel}}{P}-O-\overset{\overset{O}{\parallel}}{P}\diagdown_{N(CH_3)_2}$$

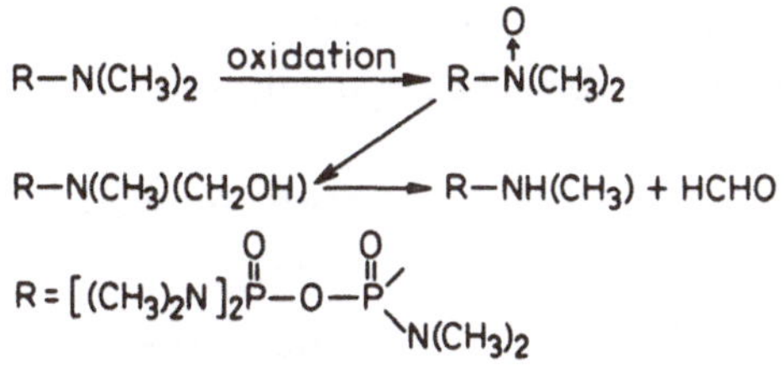

According to Du Bois *et al.* (1950), after a single large dosage OMPA was partially excreted before it became effective through ChE inhibition. Approximately 23 percent was excreted with the urine of rats in 24 hours, and 24 percent in five days; approximately 15 percent went with the feces. At the end of the second day there were exclusively water-soluble hydrolysis products in the urine (Arthur and Casida 1958 a). According to Hofmann-Credner and Siedek (1952) the urine of rats and rabbits contained about five times more radioactivity than the feces after treatment with P^{32}-OMPA. The proportion of chloroform-soluble radioactive substances was only four percent of the water-soluble ones.

Only small dosages (0.5 mg./kg. daily) were tolerated by test animals without cumulative effect. No data are recorded concerning an effective residue measurement for the formation of toxic metabolites in these pharmacological investigations. The active metabolites are chemically unknown (DuBois *et al.* 1950). Quantitative data about tissue residues are found in the older reports about investigations on rats and rabbits by Hofmann-Credner and Siedek (1952). These values give a relative picture, since the radioactive quantities are reported only in measured impulses. It is striking that 38.4 percent of the total P^{32}-activity was contained in the muscle, which thus contained the largest quantities, while the lowest activities were found in the brain. The residues in liver were independent

Table CXXX. *Residues in rat tissues five days after oral treatment* [a] *with OMPA* (Arthur and Casida 1958 a).

Tissue	Equiv. total radioactivity (p.p.m.)
Brain	0.31
Blood	0.27
Intestines	0.24
Liver	0.74
Nerve fiber	0.29

[a] 2.5 µg. of P^{32}-OMPA/g. body weight.

of the mode of application; however, the major part of the OMPA was decomposed. Phosphorus-containing degradation products which were not soluble in chloroform were also excreted with the bile and were found in the urine and feces.

Residue data in rat tissue after P^{32}-OMPA are in Table CXXX.

33. PARATHION and related compounds. —

Parathion

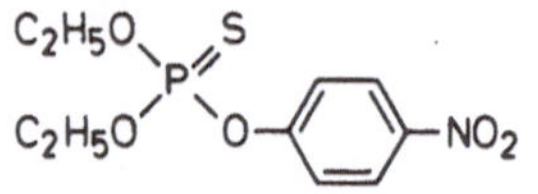

O,O-Diethyl-O-(p-nitrophenyl) thionophosphate (E 605)

Methyl parathion

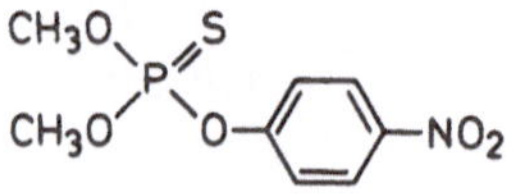

O,O-Dimethyl-O-(p-nitrophenyl) thionophosphate (Dalf)

Chlorthion

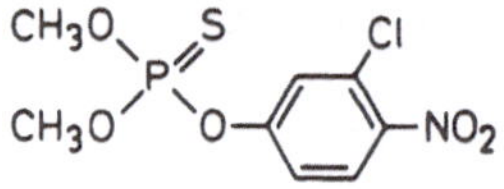

O,O-Dimethyl-O-(3-chloro-4-nitrophenyl) thionophosphate

Isopropyl parathion

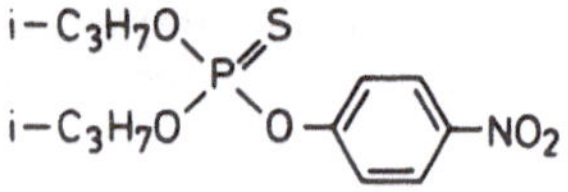

O,O-Diisopropyl-O-(p-nitrophenyl) thionophosphate (Compound 3,456)

Application: Contact insecticide. Parathion is not used in veterinary medicine.

Toxicity: See Table CXXXI. There are many literature reports concerning the toxicity of parathion. Parathion was oxidized *in vivo* to paraoxon, which is the potential inhibitor of the ChE (Ahmed *et al.* 1958). The transformation to paraoxon, which is used as Mintacol in optometry, took place by oxidative desulfuration of P=S to P=O (Diggle and Gage 1951, Davison 1955, Pribilla 1954, Metcalf and March 1953). The oxidation product was not only the stronger ChE inhibitor, it was also absolutely more toxic than parathion. The importance of this toxic reaction can be seen from Table CXXXI.

Parathion was easily resorbed by the skin. There was no sex-dependent difference in sensitivity towards paraoxon (Neal and Du Bois 1965), but there was a difference for parathion. In addition, there obviously was a considerable individual difference in sensitivity towards parathion (Konst and Plummer 1950). The kind of formulation is also of considerable importance. Wilber and Morrison (1955) observed fatalities for goats after eight mg./kg. in a WP formulation, which was applied daily; with EC preparations 16 mg./kg. was survived.

Species sensitivity during repeated treatments has also often been investigated (Table CXXXII). In the feed of rats five p.p.m. of parathion caused inhibition of the erythrocyte ChE after eight weeks (Frawley and Fuyat 1957); the same effects appeared with two p.p.m. in the diet of dogs

Table CXXXI. *Comparative toxicities of parathion and paraoxon* (Hecht and Wirth 1950).

Compound	Frog in lymph sack, in solvent (mg./kg.)	White mouse, *s.c.*			Rat *per os* in water + adhesive cpd.		50% inhibition of horse serum ChE	
		In oil LD_{50} (mg./kg.)	In water and solvent					
			Dose tol. (mg./kg.)	LD_{50} (mg./kg.)	Dose tol. (mg./kg.)	LD_{50} (mg./kg.)	Molar conc.	µg./cm.³
Parathion	200	20	5	10–12.5	1.9	6.4	2.5×10^{-6}	0.73
Paraoxon	30	2	0.1	0.6–0.8	0.8	3	1.3×10^{-8}	0.0036

Table CXXXII. *Acute toxicities of parathion, paraoxon, and isopropyl parathion for various animals after different application.*

Animal species	Sex	Mode of application	Tox. dosage (mg./kg.)	LD_{50} (mg./kg.)	Remarks	Reference
Parathion						
Mouse	—	*per os*	—	25	—	Frawley *et al.* (1952)
Mouse	♂+♀	*per os*	—	6	—	Hazleton & Holland (1950), Kodama *et al.* (1954)
Mouse	♂	*per os*	—	26	in oil, tech.	Konst & Plummer (1950)
Mouse	—	*s.c.*	18–20	—	—	Hecht & Wirth (1950)
Mouse	—	*s.c.*	—	10–13	aqueous	Hecht & Wirth (1950)
Mouse	♂	*i.p.*	—	10	—	Du Bois *et al.* (1949)
Mouse	♀	*i.p.*	—	9–10	—	Du Bois *et al.* (1949)
Rat	—	*per os*	LD_{100} [6]	—	—	Perkow (1956)
Rat	—	*per os*	—	4	—	Ahmed *et al.* (1958)
Rat	—	*per os*	—	7	tech. and in water	Wirth (1949)
Rat	—	*per os*	—	6	—	Hecht & Wirth (1950)
Rat	♂	*per os*	—	5	—	Hazleton & Holland (1950), Kodama *et al.* (1954)
Rat	♂	*per os*	—	22	in oil, tech.	Konst & Plummer (1950)
Rat	♂	*per os*	—	30	—	Frawley *et al.* (1952)
Rat	♂	*per os*	—	15	—	Du Bois *et al.* (1949)
Rat	♂	*per os*	—	13	—	Gaines (1960 a)
Rat	♀	*per os*	—	4	—	Gaines (1960 a)
Rat	♀	—	—	7	in oil, tech.	Konst & Plummer (1950)
Rat	♀	*per os*	—	2	—	Hazleton & Holland (1950), Kodama *et al.* (1954)
Rat	♀	*per os*	—	6	—	Du Bois *et al.* (1949)
Rat	♀	*per os*	—	3	—	Frawley *et al.* (1952)
Rat	♀	*per os*	—	4	—	Deichmann *et al.* (1952), Kodama *et al.* (1954)
Rat	♂	*i.p.*	—	7	—	Du Bois *et al.* (1949)
Rat	♀	*i.p.*	—	4	—	Du Bois *et al.* (1949)
Guinea pig		*per os*	—	32	—	Frawley *et al.* (1952)
	♂	*per os*	—	20	in oil, tech.	Konst & Plummer (1950)
Rabbit	—	parenteral	—	40	—	Hecht & Wirth (1950)
Chicken	—	*per os*	3	—	—	Guarda (1960)
Cat	—	parenteral	—	15	—	Hecht & Wirth (1950)
Cat	—	*i.p.*	—	3–5	—	Du Bois *et al.* (1949)
Dog	—	*i.p.*	—	12–20	—	Du Bois *et al.* (1949)
Dog	—	*per os*	25	—	15% WP	Hazleton & Holland (1950)
Goat	—	*per os*	50	—	—	Wilber & Morrison (1955)
Goat	—	*per os*	20	—	< 7 days	Wilber & Morrison (1955)

Table CXXXII (cont.)

Animal species	Sex	Mode of application	Tox. dosage (mg./kg.)	LD_{50} (mg./kg.)	Remarks	Reference
Goat	—	*i.m.*	20	—	< 8 days	Wilber & Morrison (1955)
Goat	—	*i.m.*	0.5 several times	—	—	Wilber & Morrison (1955)
Sheep	—	*per os*	60 [a]	—	25% WP	Konst & Plummer (1950)
Pig	—	*per os*	0.5 ml.	—	98%	Konst & Plummer (1950)
Pig	—	dermal	50 [b]	—	in oil	Konst & Plummer (1950)
Horse	—	*per os*	3,500 [c]	—	—	Eichler (1965)
Paraoxon						
Mouse	—	*s.c.*	—	0.6–0.8	—	Hecht & Wirth (1950)
Rat	—	*per os*	—	3	—	Hecht & Wirth (1950)
Rat	—	*s.c.*	—	0.5	—	Krueger & Casida (1957)
Rat	—	?	—	0.5	—	Aldridge (1953)
Rat	—	*per os*	—	4	—	Ahmed *et al.* (1958)
Rat	—	*per os*	—	3	—	Wirth (1949)
Pig	—	*per os*	0.5 ml. [d]	—	98%	Weybridge, from McGirr & Papworth (1953)
Isopropyl Parathion						
Mouse	—	*per os*	—	537	—	Camp *et al.* (1969)

[a] 25 at one-week interval.
[b] Fatal in 44 hours, 150 fatal in 32 hours.
[c] The values seems questionable; presumably this is the total dosage per animal.
[d] Strong symptoms.

(Frawley 1957) and the plasma ChE was inhibited with one p.p.m. Five mg./kg. body wt. reduced erythrocyte ChE in calves in nine to 13 days (Venturoli and Tunioli 1959). On the contrary, duration treatments of 0.112 to 0.89 mg./kg. body wt. were tolerated by milk cows without damage over 81 days or four weeks, respectively (Dahm *et al.* 1950 b).

The toxicities of various parathion-related compounds are reported in Table CXXXIII.

Detection: See Gunther and Blinn (1955), Duggan *et al.* 1967), Sutherland (1964), Niessen (1962), Perkow (1956), and others. For understandable reasons detection methods for parathion in tissues are of special interest in forensic medicine or criminology. Therefore there are numerous reports about many different detection methods. Some of the quantitative chemical detection methods are quite old, but they are still mentioned in the following survey for some are still used.

Pribilla (1954) and Schmidt (1954 and 1955) surveyed chemical and biological procedures to those dates. Schreiber (1956) also reviewed and evaluated methods in existence up to 1956, and pointed to the Millon-reactions of [hydrolyzed] phenolic hydroxyl groups as "conclusive" reactions. Arterberg *et al.* (1961) considered the detection of *p*-nitrophenol in the urine as a more sensitive measure of contamination with parathion than the measuement of ChE inhibition. Averell and Norris (1948) detected the nitro group by its

Table CXXXIII. *Tolerated and lethal dosages of parathion-related compounds in an acute test* [a] (Hecht and Wirth 1950).

Compound	White mouse *s.c.*			Rat *per os*	
	In oil LD_{50} (mg./kg.)	In water Dose tol. (mg./kg.)	In solvent LD_{50} (mg./kg.)	In water Dose tol. (mg./kg.)	+adhesive cpd. LD_{50} (mg./kg.)
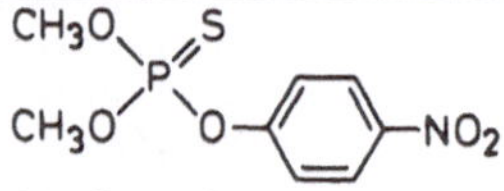 CH_3O–P(=S)(CH_3O)–O–C$_6$H$_4$–NO_2	50–100	10	30	5	15–20
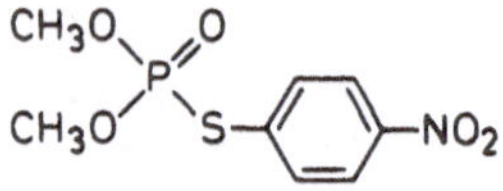 CH_3O–P(=O)(CH_3O)–S–C$_6$H$_4$–NO_2	20–50	2.5	7.5–10	20	45
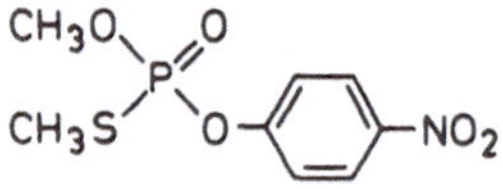 CH_3O–P(=O)(CH_3S)–O–C$_6$H$_4$–NO_2	90–100	5	35	140	200
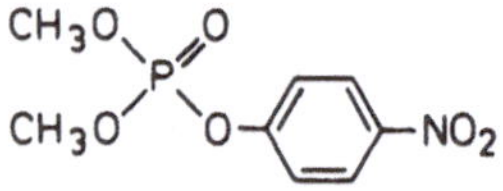 CH_3O–P(=O)(CH_3O)–O–C$_6$H$_4$–NO_2	2.7	0.7	1.4–2.0	1.4	3.4–6.8
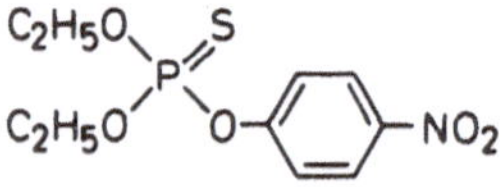 C_2H_5O–P(=S)(C_2H_5O)–O–C$_6$H$_4$–NO_2	20	5	10–12.5	1.9	6.4
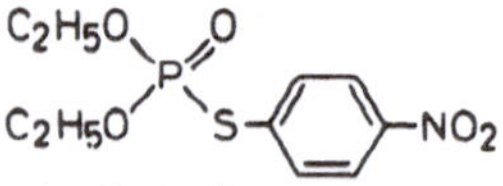 C_2H_5O–P(=O)(C_2H_5O)–S–C$_6$H$_4$–NO_2	2.5–5.0	0.5	1.3	< 2.5	2.5–5.0
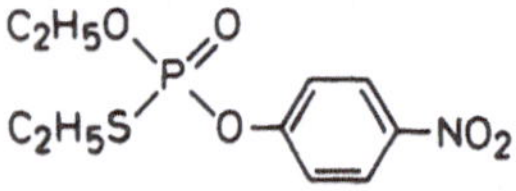 C_2H_5O–P(=O)(C_2H_5S)–O–C$_6$H$_4$–NO_2	25–60	10	20	25	50–100[b]
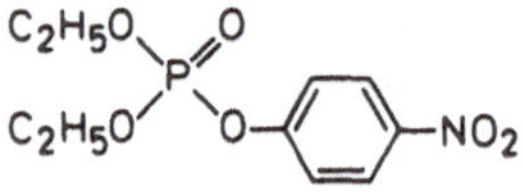 C_2H_5O–P(=O)(C_2H_5O)–O–C$_6$H$_4$–NO_2	2	0.1	0.6–0.8	0.8	3

[a] Values for toxicities were established in part at different times and on different animal material, therefore the deviations.
[b] Twenty-hour old solution.

reduction to the amino group by colorimetry. Weinig *et al.* (1954 and 1955) criticized the method of Averell and Norris (1948) and saw its importance only in the possibility of an exclusion of parathion poisoning, since many other substances give similarly positive reactions. Lieben *et al.* (1953) and von Eicken (1954) determined *p*-nitrophenol. Schwerd and Schmidt (1952) described a "rapid method" by colorimetric detection of the sodium salt of *p*-nitrophenol; this method was modified by Schreiber (1961) using prior alkaline oxidation in order to remove interfering yellow colors and to exclude catalytic-dependent reaction inhibitions of the indophenol reaction utilized. Völksen (1953) mentioned another rapid detection method, which is unspecific, involving layer of concentrated H_2SO_4 under the extract in question to yield a blue-green ring as a positive reaction. Kaiser and Lang

(1953) used an alcohol extract of the organs acidified (after protein removal) with tartaric acid then diazotation and coupling, and colorimetry. Burger (1957) and Hjelt and Mukula (1958) used spectrometric methods. Fretwurst and Naeve (1954 and 1955) utilized the UV absorption curve in benzene extract for the nitrophenol, but nothing was said about the insecticidally effective molecule (Enders 1954 and 1955). Machata (1956) gaves the following scheme, especially for the contents of stomach and intestines:

Steam distillation of test material → preliminary tests:

ether extract (evaporated) ↓ alcohol solution ↓ absorption curve: max. 2725 Å, min. 2350 Å, confirm with indophenol blue reaction, diazo reaction	alkaline test, diazo reaction; odor, appearance (cloudy) → oxidation, phosphate qual. and quant., sulfate qualitative

Szyszko (1965) used polarography. Stenersen (1967) utilized 2,6-dibromobenzoquinone-4-chloroimide (DQC) for detection. Gunther *et al.* (1968) reported oxidation to paraoxon with silver oxide in aqueous solution, followed by automated ChE inhibition. Bäumler and Rippstein (1969) determined parathion by glc with a phosphorus detector.

Restrictions and tolerances: In the U.S.A., 1.0 p.p.m. in lucerne, clover, corn, etc. (Frear *et al.* 1969).

Metabolism and residues: Parathion was not accumulated in the body (Gardoki and Hazleton 1951, Jansen *et al.* 1952). The protein bonding corresponded to that of DFP; affinity to the individual organs such as liver, kidney, and intestines was practically meaningless (Dangschat 1965). Paraoxon was formed by fermentative reaction, and in animal metabolism there was also *p*-aminophenol and *p*-nitrophenol (Westlake *et al.* 1960, Gardoki and Hazleton 1951); *p*-Nitrophenol rapidly colored serum yellow (Aldridge 1953). For hydrolysis products and their ChE inhibition, see Aldridge (1950). Diethylphosphoric acid appeared as another hydrolysis product (Casida 1956). The sulphur which has been cleaved off by oxidation is excreted along with the urine (Hazleton 1955).

Reduction processes to form the amino derivative also occur in decaying organic (corpses) material (Bäumler and Rippstein 1969). Also, the rumen fluid of ruminants transforms parathion to the amino compound (Cook 1957, Ahmed *et al.* 1958). Aside from the reduction processes only hydrolytic reactions took place in the rumen; there was no oxidation, at least down to <0.1 p.p.m. paraoxon (Ahmed *et al.* 1958).

The transformation of parathion in the rumen fluid is dependent on the concentration. For a concentration of two p.p.m. of parathion, 62 percent was found as aminoparathion after two hours *in vitro,* and 25 percent after 2.7 hours for 300 p.p.m. For 500 p.p.m. parathion or paraoxon, respectively, 53 percent and 73 percent, respectively, were recovered as amino compounds after 24 hours (Ahmed *et al.* 1958). More amino derivatives resulted from methyl parathion than from parathion; there was no such transformation for chlorthion. The process *in vitro* was very similar to that *in vivo,* whereby the degradation of parathion *in vivo* was complete within 24 hours.

NEAL and DU BOIS (1965) submitted general data about the metabolism of thiophosphates. They studied the detoxication of cholinergic thiophosphates *in vitro* and established that the livers of adult male rats detoxified tiophosphate compounds down to phenols better than the livers of females or young animals, whereby the major activity was attributed to the liver microsomes (cf. earlier toxicity data).

The detoxication mechanism of thiophosphate compounds such as EPN (*q.v.*) parathion, methyl parathion, and chlorthion follows the pattern of desulfuration to phosphate (P = O), hydrolysis of the phosphate by esterases to phenolic end products, and eventually enzymatic hydrolysis, before the active ChE-inhibiting O-analog is formed. The desulfuration *in vivo* did not seem essential (NEAL and DU BOIS 1965), as seen from the end products which appear in the urine after treatment with these P^{32}-substances (Table CXXXIV).

Table CXXXIV. *Survey of thiophosphate metabolism.*

Compound	Excretion products	Reference
Parathion	O,O-diethylphosphate O,O-diethylthiophosphate	PLAPP & CASIDA (1958 b)
Methyl parathion and chlorthion	O,O-dimethylphosphate O,O-dimethylthiophosphate	BRADY & ARTHUR (1961)

Model schemes for the transformation processes in rats and in ruminants are shown in Figures 18 and 19.

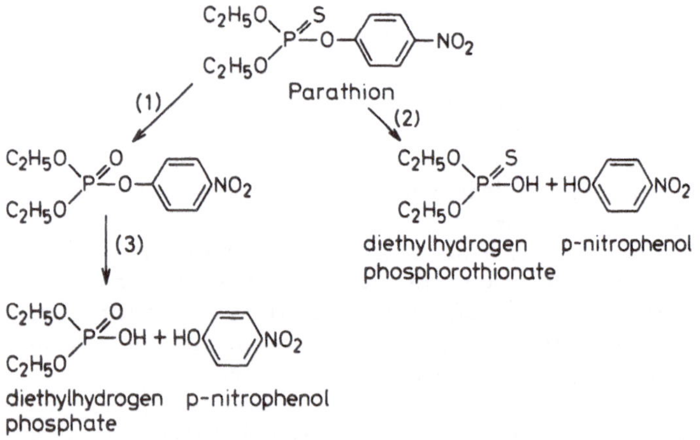

Fig. 18. Metabolic pathway of parathion in rats under the influence of microsomal enzymes (VILLENEUVE *et al.* 1970).

The transformation product from warm-blooded animals and insects was paraoxon (METCALF and MARCH 1953). GAGE (1953) extracted paraoxon as a ChE-inhibiting agent from the liver of a rat which had been

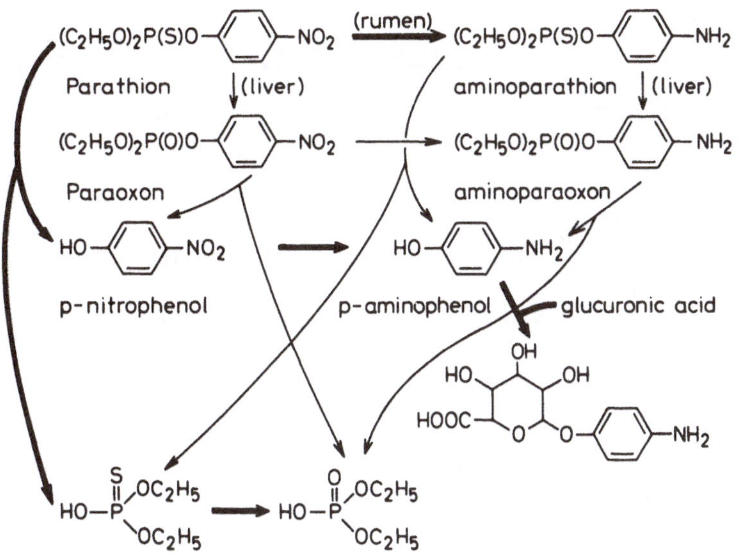

Fig. 19. Metabolic pathway of parathion in cattle (O'Brien 1960, Ahmed *et al.* 1958).

treated with parathion. The liver plays an important role in the transformation of parathion to paraoxon. Under the influence of microsomal enzymes and with paraticipation of NADPH and molecular oxygen, not only the O-analog but also *p*-nitrophenol and diethylthiophosphoric acid are formed (Nagatsugawa *et al.* 1968). For further detailed studies about the effects of liver enzymes, which transform paraoxon mainly to diethylphosphate but also to O-desethylparaoxon, see Kojima and O'Brien (1968). Paraoxon was hydrolyzed by poultry liver tissue to a lesser degree than by mammalian liver (Murphy 1966). Paraoxon was decomposed by an enzyme called E 600-esterase by Aldridge (1953) but which is identical with A-esterase. It was present in the tissues (especially in the serum) of rabbits, but also in rats, sheep, goats, horses, etc. in different amounts. Furthermore, aromatic plasma esterases participated in the hydrolysis process (Mounter and Whittaker 1953). The serum-albumin, or an enzyme which is present in it, cleaved the paraoxon in rabbits > pigs > cattle > horses (Erdös and Boggs 1961).

Isopropyl parathion was metabolized in the mouse in such a way that monoisopropyl parathion and monoisopropyl paraoxon occured in the urine, aside from the substance itself and its O-analog. The only water-soluble metabolite was diisopropyl thiophosphoric acid (Camp *et al.* 1969); they reported the degradation pathway in Figure 20.

The mouse — as a model animal — had a high elimination rate (Wirth 1949) so that daily repeated paraoxon applications did not create toxic symptoms; the elimination rate was 0.1 mg./kg. in two hours.

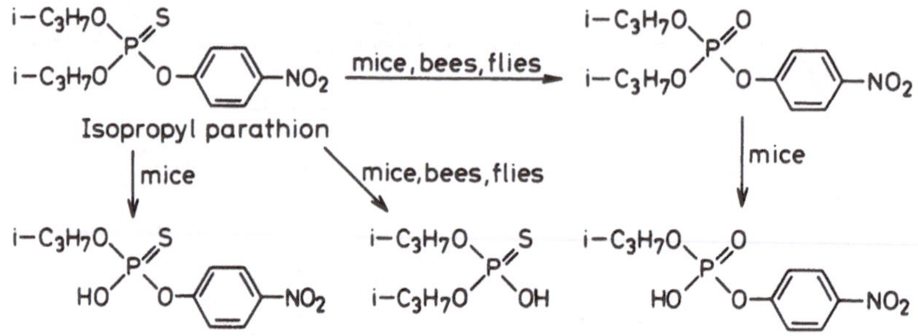

Fig. 20. Metabolic pathway of isopropyl parathion (CAMP *et al.* 1969).

The transformation of parathion and aminoparathion in rats was different from that in cattle. Rats decomposed parathion rapidly and eliminated it. In 24 hours 66 percent parathion and 68 percent aminoparathion were eliminated with the urine after an application each of ten mg./kg. *per os* (AHMED *et al.* 1958). For excretion within two days after parathion treatment, 99.5 percent was present as hydrolysis products including about 0.5 percent aminoparathion; the analogous values after aminoparathion application were 96.3 percent and 3.7 percent. There was a probable trace of acetylaminoparathion.

PLAPP and CASIDA (1958 b) reported the following excretion concentrations in urine of rats after 1.5 μg./g. *per os:* $(RO)_2P(S)OH$ = 78 percent, $(RO)_2P(O)OH$ = 16 percent, RO(ϕO)P(O)OH = two percent, and RO(ϕO)P(S)OH = four percent.

JENSEN and PEARCE (1952) prepared S^{35}-parathion for investigations on rabbits. After cutaneous and *i.v* application it was rapidly excreted with the urine. The S^{35} was present in the metabolites. There was no accumulation in the blood and organs. After dermal treatment with 125 mg./animal, the blood level reached maximum with 0.8 p.p.m. after four days. The concentration in the urine increased in six days to ten p.p.m. and decreased in 14 days to two p.p.m. (JENSEN *et al.* 1952). Rabbits excreted in 24 hours after 0.2, 1.0, and 5.0 mg./kg. *per os* 43, 39, and 57 percent, respectively, of the applied dosage (v. EICKEN 1954).

The major excretion product in the urine of dogs was also *p*-nitrophenol (v. EICKEN 1954), while *p*-aminophenol appeared only in traces (GARDOCKI and HAZLETON 1951).

From the demonstrations of reduction of parathion to the amino derivative in the rumen it is understood that conjugated [26] *p*-aminophenol is excreted with the urine as sulfate or glucuronide, while the other mammals as nonruminants excreted free *p*-nitrophenol (PANKASKI *et al.* 1952, AHMED *et al.* 1958).

[26] For the metabolic behaviour of conjugated glucuronic acid, ethereal sulfates, and diazotized amino groups in rabbits as a model see SMITH and WILLIAMS (1949).

AHMED *et al.* (1958) discussed as possible excretory and other products in cattle aminoparathion, diethylphosphoric acid, diethylthiophosphoric acid, *p*-aminophenylglucuronide, small amounts of parathion, and small amounts of paraoxon. Quantitative recoveries for cattle were described. After application of parathion the maximum concentration of parathion and/or its metabolites was reached in rumen fluid after 1/2 hour, in jugular vein blood after 1.5 hours, in urine after 11 hours, in feces after 29 hours, and in milk after 47 hours (Table CXXXV).

Table CXXXV. *Parathion and metabolites present after oral administration to a cow of P^{32}-parathion* (AHMED *et al.* 1958).

Substrate	Hours after admin. [a]	Parathion equivalents [b] (p.p.m.)				
		Parathion	Amino-parathion	Paraoxon	Amino-paraoxon	Hydrolysis products
Urine	0–24	1.2	170	0.0	8 [c]	239
Blood	0.5	0.18	0.32	0.29	0.12	3.0
	2.0	0.14	0.15	0.14	0.27	4.3
	6.0	0.07	0.04	0.04	0.42	2.7
Rumen fluid	0.5	10.0	7.5	0.0	0.0 [d]	0.28
	2.0	2.7	8.3	0.0	0.0 [d]	0.34
	6.0	0.69	2.6	0.0	0.0 [d]	1.6

[a] 6.7 mg./kg.
[b] P.p.m. as hydrolysis products based on radioactivity not extractable from aqueous phase into chloroform; p.p.m. of other metabolites based on column chromatography with Celite-isooctane-methanol chromatography of chloroform-soluble metabolites.
[c] Extracted for recovery of amino derivatives and yielded aminoparathion with no definite absorption band of P=O at 1,260 cm.$^{-1}$
[d] Up to five percent of a polar metabolite of parathion present; possibly aminoparaoxon, but properties not determined.

For the human being ROAN *et al.* (1969) observed good correlation between the excretion of *p*-nitrophenol in the urine and the pesticide concentration. The excretion of the metabolite *p*-nitrophenol with the urine of people who came into contact with parathion was very rapid and ended after 48 hours (ARTERBERG *et al.* 1961). v. EICKEN (1954) measured the excretion rate for human beings as 70 percent in 22 hours. For further comparative data about excretion in human urine see LIEBEN *et al.* (1953).

BÄR (1964 b) considered the residue question important only in the case of parathion, especially since organic P-compounds in animals can be detected in small quantities only with very sensitive methods.

The autoradiography of P^{32}-parathion in mice after *s.c.* injection showed the radioactive material was only slowly resorbed from the subcutaneous fat depots. For low blood levels there was a slight cumulation in the central nervous system, in the muscles, and in bone marrow. Higher concentrations were present in liver, kidney, fat, digestive channel, thyroid gland, spleen, and lung. The highest radioactivity was in the salivary glands and the brown neck fat [27] (FREDRIKSON and BIGELOW 1961).

HAZLETON and HOLLAND (1950) pointed out that for rats, after several applications of ten to 100 p.p.m. of parathion in the feed, the analyses for parathion in the tissues were negative.

KUBISTOVA (1959) applied P^{32}-labelled parathion to rats and found toxic reactions by oxidation to the O-analog occured in the liver (64 percent), in the lung (13 percent), in the kidney (1.5 percent), and in the intestines (21 percent). No oxidation was detected in heart muscle, spleen, pancreas, brain, and ovary.

The transformation ratio of parathion to paraoxon in rat tissue homogenate was 75 percent in 24 hours (KUBISTOVA 1956); on the other hand, only 4.4 percent of the parathion was oxidized to paraoxon *in vivo* in one hour. The half-life was about 15 hours. Paraoxon apparently has a short residence time.

GIACHETTI *et al.* (1966) found paraoxon in the brain of rats by glc after 18 hours, after *i.p.* application of one mg./kg. body wt.; paraoxon was missing after 48 to 92 hours, but traces of its metabolites were detected.

Parathion and also paraoxon rapidly penetrated through rabbit skin (FREDRIKSON 1962, PERKOW 1956, HAZLETON and HOLLAND 1950). NABB *et al.* (1966) reported the average speed of this resorption as 0.059 and for paraoxon as 0.32 μg./min./cm². JENSEN *et al.* (1952) established less than 0.5 p.p.m. in the tissues five days after cutaneous application of 125 mg. of parathion/animal. On the other hand, the blood contained four p.p.m. after 20 days and the spleen two p.p.m. The concentration in liver at both times was 0.3 p.p.m. It is noteworthy that these values are based on S^{35}-detection

Table CXXXVI. *Parathion equivalents in two rabbits on the fifth and twentieth days after dermal application* [a] (JENSEN *et al.* 1952).

Tissue	Parathion equivalent (p.p.m.) after	
	5 days	20 days
Urine	4.28	0.56
Blood	3.79	0.11
Bile	0.31	0.06
Liver	0.31	0.31
Fat	0.90	0.11
Muscle	0.21	0.11
Brain	0.13	0.13
Heart	0.21	0.10
Spleen	2.02	0.51
Kidney	0.22	trace

[a] 125 mg./animal.

[27] So-called hibernating gland.

so that nothing can be said about the absolute concentration of the active substance. Table CXXXVI shows the individual data.

DANGSCHAT [28] (1965) did not find free parathion in the liver with a biological method which detected one to 100 p.p.m. in tissues, nor when toxic dosages of five or ten mg./kg. body wt. were applied. In freshly killed animals the muscles contained five and ten p.p.m., respectively, and within 15 minutes after killing also five and ten p.p.m.; one hour after killing there was no free alkylphosphate.

After *per os* treatment with a fatal dosage (25 mg./kg. as WP) no parathion is found in the dog immediately after death in gall bladder, liver, kidney, abdominal fat, saliva, or intestines; two to seven p.p.m. appeared in blood, spleen, lungs, brain, and spinal cord. After a fatal *i.v.* dosage parathion was also detected in urine, liver, bile, kidney, spleen, and lung. The 90-day feeding of parathion to dogs resulted in negative analytical findings 24 hours after the last application in serum, blood, brain, liver, and lungs, while traces were found in urine and bladder. After daily application of one mg./kg. body wt., the tissues were free of parathion. With a dosage of three mg./kg. body wt. daily, traces occured in spleen, kidney and intestines, but 13 p.p.m. was detected in the spinal cord (HAZLETON and HOLLAND 1950).

For cattle 43 percent of the applied radioactive dosage was excreted with the urine in five days, and 24 percent with the feces; 70 percent of the urine fraction was aminoparathion (AHMED *et al.* 1958). They also found in the first 24 hours after application 40.7 percent of the radioactive material in the urine was aminoparathion and 1.8 percent aminoparaoxon. Paraoxon was not found in the urine: only very small quantities (approximately one p.p.m.) were excreted as parathion with the urine. The hydrolysis products in cattle urine consisted of seven percent diethylphosphoric acid in from zero to three hours and 26 percent in from 36 to 47 hours. The remainders of 74 and 93 percent, respectively, consisted predominantly of diethylthiophosphoric acid (Table CXXXVII).

Table CXXXVII. *Parathion and metabolites present in cattle fat and urine at various times after oral administration* (AHMED *et al.* 1958).

Hours after administration [a]	Parathion equivalents (p.p.m.)		
	Fat biopsies		Hydrolysis products in urine
	Parathion + paraoxon	Aminoparathion + aminoparaoxon	
2	0.10	0.19	0.48
6	0.08	0.14	0.57
24	0.03	0.02	0.78

[a] 6.7 mg. of P^{32}-parathion/kg.

[28] This author does not report the mode of application.

DAHM *et al.* (1950 a) did not find any parathion with a colorimetric method in jugular blood of cows which had been treated over 81 days with parathion as a 25 percent WP at 0.02 to 0.11 mg./kg. body wt., and finally with 0.88 mg./kg. body wt. PANKASKI *et al.* (1952) fed parathion residue-containing hay to cows. Over 61 days 0.33 mg. of parathion/kg. body wt. daily was tolerated. With weekly increasing dosages, one to 32 mg./kg. body wt. were tolerated; hereby, the amount of diazotizable substances in the urine increased. No parathion, free *p*-nitrophenol, or free *p*-aminophenol were found in blood and urine. However, after acid hydrolysis of a composited sample of urine, after daily application of two mg. of parathion/kg. body wt., five µg./ml. of *p*-aminophenol was detected, and 15 µg./ml. after seven mg./kg. body wt. To the contrary, AHMED *et al.* (1958) pointed out: "Their results do not rule out the possibility that O,O-diethyl O-*p*-aminophenylphosphorothioate (aminoparathion) might be a major excretory metabolite and *p*-aminophenylglucuronide of lesser quantitative importance."

For comparison, findings about tissue concentrations in human beings, established after organophosphoric acid ester fatal poinsonings, may be macabre but still interesting. The relatively numerous pesticide poisoning data are explained by the unwanted increase of suicides, which consequently led to an intense study of the problems. In most of the suicide cases a considerably higher than lethal dosage was taken by the persons in question. NEAVE (1954 and 1955 b) reported the lethal dosage for the adult human

Table CXXXVIII. *Residues in various human organs and tissues, expressed as methyl parathion, from cases of lethal Wolfatox poisoning* (FAZEKAS and RENGEI 1967).

Organ or tissue	Apparent methyl parathion (mg./kg. or mg./l.) in					
	Case 1 [a]	Case 2 [b]	Case 3 [c]	Case 4 [d]	Case 5 [e]	Case 6 [f]
Bridge and extended marrow	0.54	0.24	0.02	—	0.01	0.01
White substance	0.39	0.52	0.02	0.77	0.01	0.01
Grey substance	—	—	0.01	0.91	0.01	0.01
Main ganglion	0.42	—	0.02	—	0.01	0.02
Cerebellum	—	0.42	0.02	0.86	0.01	0.01
Stomach and contents	1,891	1,154	1.35	2.2	0.09	0.02
Spleen	0.51	0.73	0.10	0.71	0.04	0.06
Liver	1.02	0.74	0.32	1.91	0.12	0.21
Heart	0.55	0.58	0.04	0.93	0.03	0.03
Lungs	0.21	0.29	0.01	0.17	0.01	0.01
Small intestines and contents	915	370	0.20	1.34	0.16	0.07
Blood	0.73	0.43	0.13	0.94	0.02	0.01
Kidneys	1.12	0.99	0.46	1.85	0.17	0.27
Urine	—	1.75	—	—	0.09	—

[a] Survived 20 hours.
[b] Survived 24 hours.
[c] Survived 28 hours.
[d] Survived 33 hours.
[e] Survived 65 hours.
[f] Survived 70 hours.

being as 6.13 mg./kg. body wt. For children it was much lower (MARESCH 1957). According to LENDLE (1954), the lethal dosage for the adult human being was about one g./100 kg. body wt. FAZEKAS and RENGEI (1967) determined *p*-nitrophenol from methyl parathion poisoning cases (Table CXXXVIII).

Parathion concentration data reported by PRIBILLA (1954) are of interest for comparison (Table CXXXIX).

In Table CXL further quantitative data of parathion and methyl parathion residues in corpse tissues have been summarized from the literature. Only those data were considered for which the approximate quantity of amount received was known. The data differ considerably in dependence on detection method and time after parathion intake.

Parathion and methyl parathion in food: CUMMINGS (1965) found in the Baltimore area 0.07 p.p.m. of parathion in the total human diet and also 0.07 p.p.m. in meat, fish, and poultry. During a half-hour cooking process parathion was hydrolyzed in vegetables 49 to 64 percent (mashed potatoes), and 91 to 93 percent (cabbage mash). The corresponding hydrolysis rates for methyl parathion were 59 to 62 and 76 to 78 percent, respectively (ASKEW *et al.* 1968).

34. PHORATE. — Phosphorodithioic acid, O,O-diethyl *S*-[(ethylthio)methyl] ester

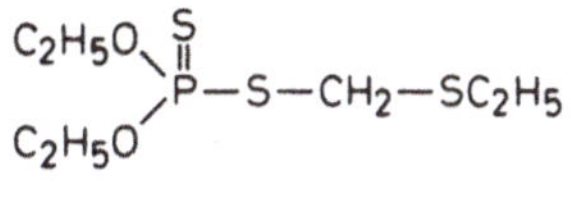

Alternate names: Thimet, ENT 24042, 3911.
Application: Contact insecticide, systematically effective.
Toxicity: See Table CXLI.
Detection: See BUNYAN and TAYLOR (1966), SUTHERLAND *et al.* (1964), MCLEOD *et al.* (1969).
Tolerances and restrictions: In the U.S.A., one-to-three p.p.m. in various plant products (FREAR *et al.* 1969).
Metabolism and residues: Phorate was attacked only slowly by the rumen fluid (AHMED *et al.* 1958). It was oxidized in plants to components which exhibited a higher ChE inhibition than phorate itself.

Investigations on tissue contents have been made for rats, poultry, and cattle. Rats excreted, after a single treatment of 2.0 mg./kg. body wt. P^{32}-phorate, 35 percent of the radioactive material with the urine in 144 hours and 3.5 percent with the feces; after six daily dosages of one mg./kg. body wt., 12 percent appeared in the urine and six percent in the feces in seven days. On the sixth and seventh days the same amounts of phorate metabolites were found in urine and feces. Residue determinations of radioactive metabolites of phorate were difficult (BOWMAN and CASIDA 1958). The natures of nonextractable phorate derivatives in rat tissues are unknown. It is unlikely that phorate is degraded to phosphoric acid, since even after

Table CXXXIX. *Parathion in organs of poisoning cases* (PRIBILLA 1954).

Age (years)	Sex	Dosage and survival time	Parathion (μg./100 g. of tissue) [a] in								
			Stomach and contents	Small intestine and contents	Liver	Lung	Brain	Muscle	Kidney	Urine	Blood [b]
9	♂	10 ml., ~ 10 min. vomiting	5,350	—	traces	—	traces	traces	—	—	$S+S+$
58	♀	1 sip, some min. vomiting	(4.07 g.)	—	n. d.	—	n. d.	n. d.	n. d.	—	$S+S+$
23	♂	? ~ 1/2 hr. vomiting	430	6,020	200	n. d.	n. d.	n. d.	160	—	140
20	♀	2 vials, few. min.	258 [c]	258 [c]	49	95	14	24	64	312	$S+S+$
33	♂	? ~ 1/2 hr.	1,533	—	103	—	29	86	70	—	200
48	♂	1 vial ?	1,734	2,625	13	—	n. d.	36	42	—	n. d.
45	♂	1 sip, 7 hr. vomiting	51	46	88	—	—	16	130	—	$S+S+$
38	♂	1 vial ?	3,450 [c]	3,450 [c]	84	—	—	82	111	—	80
40	♀	? 31.5 hr.	144 [c]	144 [c]	56	—	66	1,240	—	—	n. d.
45	♂	? ~ 60 hr.	133	—	172	182	126	60	660	—	63

[a] n. d. = none detectable.
[b] $S+S$ = reaction according to SCHWERD and SCHMIDT test.
[c] Combined stomach, small intestine, and contents.

Table CXL. *Residues in corpse tissues after parathion and methyl parathion poisoning.*

Dosage absolute a. i. (g.)	Residues (mg.-%) [a]							Reference
	Stomach content		Small intestines	Brain	Liver	Kidney	Spleen	
	mg.-%	ml.						
			Parathion					
0.3 [b]	177	(127)	3.0 (70 g.)	—	—	—	—	Naeve (1954 and 1955 b)
1.8	1.7	(90)	1.1 (70 ml.)	13 µg.-% (200 g.)	5 µg.-% (200 g.)	25 µg.-% (80 g.)	—	Schweitzer (1958)
10	100	(950)	—	—	—	—	3.1	Fretwurst & Naeve (1954 and 1955)
8	715	(250)	—	—	—	—	1.3	
5	955	(100)	—	—	—	—	1.8	
~ 20	200	(150)	—	—	—	—	1.4	
3–4	290	(250)	—	—	—	—	0.9	
1 ml. [b]	—	—	—	—	— [e]	—	22 [e]	Leonhardt (1952 and 1954)
			Methyl parathion [f]					
200 [c]	115	—	0.37	0.04	0.07	0.10	0.07	Fazekas & Bengei (1967)
100 [c]	0.16	—	0.02	0.002	0.03	0.05	0.01	
100–200 [c]	0.22	—	0.13	0.08	0.20	0.19	0.07	

[a] Data in parentheses = absolute content.
[b] 6.13 mg.-%.
[c] E 605 forte.
[d] Wolfatox.
[e] Press juice spleen and liver 17.5.
[f] Compare Table CXXXVIII.

Table CXLI. *Acute toxicities of phorate for rats.*

Mode of application	LD_{50} (mg./kg.)	Reference
per os	2.1	HOLMSTEDT (1959)
per os	3.7	MARTIN (1961)
s. c. [a]	8–10 [b]	BOWMAN & CASIDA (1958)

[a] Male.
[b] Oxidation products are more toxic.

longer intervals it was not possible to find radioactive phosphoric acid in the urine. The direct bonding of phorate to tissue is also improbable, since it is relatively easy to recover phorate which had been applied to tissue. It is possible that radioactive phorate is present in form of phosphorylated protein.

BUNYAN and TAYLOR (1966) found practically no phorate in meat and organs of pheasants after application of 6.2 to 21.7 mg./kg. body wt. In other investigations with pheasants and pigeons BUNYAN *et al.* (1959) also established no residues after prior feeding over 14-, 28-, and 42-day periods with 100 p.p.m. of phorate.

P^{32}-Phorate was given to a cow by BOWMAN and CASIDA (1958) in a highly toxic dosage of 3.04 mg./kg. body wt. *per os*, whereby the acute symptoms that appeared were controlled with atropine injections. The blood level as expression of the resorption rate increased within six to eight hours. Between 18 to 36 hours after application the content of chloroform-soluble metabolites in blood increased slightly. The cow excreted 59 percent of the radioactive material within 72 hours. After separation into chloro-

Table CXLII. *Residues in tissues 96 hours after oral administration* [a] *of* P^{32}*-phorate to a cow* (BOWMAN and CASIDA 1958).

Tissue	Total radio-active equiv. (p.p.m.)	Radioactive equiv. extractable with [b]	
		Chloroform (p.p.m.)	Acetone (p.p.m.)
Liver	10.3	0.50	0.50
Kidney	5.2	0.80	0.50
Lung	1.5	0.20	0.10
Heart	0.64	0.59	0.02
Muscle (loin)	0.29	0.00	0.02
Brain	0.24	0.05	0.02
Fat (mesentery)	0.03	0.00	0.00

[a] 3.04 mg./kg.
[b] Remainder of radioactivity was in acetone-powders of the tissues.

form-soluble and water-soluble fractions, the entire activity was found in the aqueous phase. Therefore, only hydrolysis products appeared in the urine of the cow. In the beginning the O,O-diethyl thiophosporic acid dominated, while later O,O-diethyl phosphoric acid prevailed; excretion of O,O-diethyl dithiophosphoric acid was consistently low over the entire period. Only 0.8 percent of the applied radioactivity appeared in the feces within 96 hours; 20 percent of these products was chloroform-soluble six hours after application and ten percent in 12 hours. The chloroform-soluble products were O,O-diethyl-*S*-(ethylsulfinylmethyl) dithiophosphate and/or O,O-diethyl-*S*-(ethylsulfonylmethyl) dithiophosphate, and at the end non-oxidized phorate was excreted. Residues for the individual tissues are in Tables CXLII and CXLIII. The highest values were for liver and kidney tissues.

Table CXLIII. *Total phorate equivalents in tissues 96 hours after oral administration* [a] *of* P^{32}*-phorate to a cow* (BOWMAN and CASIDA 1958).

Range of phorate equiv. (p.p.m.)	Tissues (in decreasing order)
2.78–1.04	rumen wall, omasum wall, reticulum wall, parotid gland, submaxillary gland, gall bladder, adrenal gland, rib bone, subiliac lymph node
0.89–0.52	submaxillary lymph node, small intestine wall, appendix wall, intestine wall near rectum, abdominal wall, pancreas, spleen, tongue, supramammary lymph node
0.48–0.11	dorsi muscle, urinary bladder, mammary gland, placenta, leg muscle, thyroid gland, back muscle, small intestinal fat, sheath of spinal cord, hide
0.06–0.02	spinal cord, abdominal fat, large intestine wall, large intestine fat, subcutaneous fat, kidney fat

[a] 3.04 mg./kg.

35. PHOSDRIN. — Crotonic acid, 3-hydroxy-, methyl ester, dimethyl phosphate

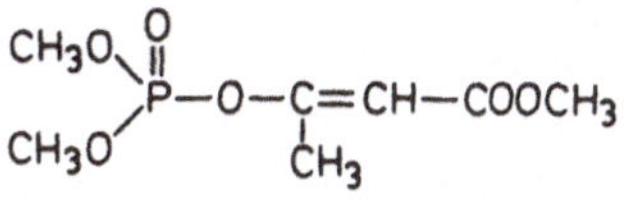

Alternate names: Phosdrin, mevinphos, 2046.
Application: Contact and systemic insecticide against biting and sucking insects, mites, etc. in plant protection; short residual effect (CASIDA *et al.* 1956).

Toxicity: See Table CXLIV. Immediately effective insecticide (as O-compound); atropine responds well in poisoning cases (STOECKEL and MEINICKE 1966).

Table CXLIV. *Acute toxicities of Phosdrin for rodents.*

Animal species	Sex	Mode of application	LD_{50} (range) (mg./kg.)	Reference
Mouse	—	*per os*	8.9	HOLMSTEDT (1959)
Mouse	♂	*per os* [a]	7.8 (6.8–8.9)	KODAMA *et al.* (1954)
Mouse	♀	*per os*	4.3 (2.7–6.9)	KODAMA *et al.* (1954)
Rat	—	*per os*	4.0	COREY *et al.* (1953)
Rat	—	*per os*	4.0–7.0	PONSOLD & BOHN (1965)
Rat	♂	*per os* [a]	6.8 (5.4–8.6)	KODAMA *et al.* (1954)
Rat	♀	*per os*	6.0 (5.2–7.0)	KODAMA *et al.* (1954)
Rat	—	*s. c.*	0.8	KRUEGER & CASIDA (1957)

[a] Technical material.

Two to five p.p.m. of Phosdrin in the feed of rats during long-term feeding slightly decreased the plasma and erythrocyte ChE in 13 weeks, but not the ChE in the brain. Two to five p.p.m. gave a slight inhibition for the dog; clinical symptoms of poisoning appeared after 75 p.p.m. (CLEVELAND and TREON 1961); a slight ChE inhibition existed for rats after application of 12.5 p.p.m. in the feed (KODAMA *et al.* 1953). For data for cumulative toxicity, see MORSE *et al.* (1953).

Tolerances: In the U.S.A., 0.25 to 0.5 p.p.m. in plants and fruit; one p.p.m. in lucerne and clover (FREAR and FRIEDMANN 1968).

Detection: See PORTER *et al.* (1964), BURGER and JANSEN (1965) (qualitative), PONSOLD and BOHN (1965), DUGGAN *et al.* (1967), and FARAGO (1968) (human tissue).

Metabolism and residues: Phosdrin is unstable; fresh rumen fluid attacked Phosdrin in 24 hours (AHMED *et al.* 1958). After *per os* application of P^{32}-Phosdrin the radioactivity in blood reached its maximum in two to four hours; it decreased rapidly within 24 hours. Phosdrin was not cumulated in the tissues. It was rapidly detoxified. Phosdrin was fed one to 20 p.p.m. to cattle over a 12-week period; after 12 weeks the Phosdrin concentration in all organs was <0.03 p.p.m. as assayed by ChE inhibition (CASIDA *et al.* (1958). After extraction of fat, heart, muscle, brain, and spinal cord of a steer which had received *per os* one mg./kg. body wt. of P^{32}-Phosdrin for seven days, the tissues contained too low an amount for a determination of the fractions. After seven days' application of Phosdrin at one mg./kg. body wt. the established radioactivities were predominantly present in the hydrolysis products. The liver contained 1.17 p.p.m. of Phosdrin and metabolites, kidney 0.40 to 0.43 p.p.m., lung, rumen, and ovaries 0.21 to 0.23 p.p.m., tongue, heart, and ribs 0.13 to 0.19 p.p.m., and brain, bone marrow, loin muscles, renal, intestinal, and subcutaneous fat <0.01 p.p.m. After fractionation 0.3 p.p.m. of Phosdrin was in the liver, 0.04 p.p.m. in the kidneys, and less in the other organs. Calculated from the total activity fat contained <0.1 p.p.m. of Phosdrin or <0.03 p.p.m., when measured by ChE inhibition. The rapid excretion agreed with the low residues in the organs, which reached 77 percent in three days, of which more than half was excreted through the kidneys within the first 12 hours (application two mg. per kg. *per os*). The only excretion product was dimethylphosphoric acid (CASIDA *et al.* 1958).

O'BRIEN (1960) postulated a very simple metabolic scheme for Phosdrin, which undergoes a rapid hydrolysis:

$$(CH_3O)_2P(O)O\underset{\substack{|\\ CH_3}}{C}=CHCOOCH_3 \rightarrow (CH_3O)_2P(O)OH$$

It is also possible that there is hydrolysis to Phosdrin-acid at first, followed by a degradation to dimethylphosphate:

$$(CH_3O)_2P(O)O\underset{\substack{|\\ CH_3}}{C}=CHCOOCH_3 \rightarrow (CH_3O)_2P(O)O\underset{\substack{|\\ CH_3}}{C}=CHCOOH$$

Supplement: FARAGÓ (1968) found the following residues in mg.-% in the tissues of human beings after suicide with Phosdrin: stomach 7.08, intestines 0.44, blood 0.20, liver 3.55, kidney 0.39, and urine 0.43.

36. PHOSPHAMIDON.* — Phosphoric acid, dimethyl ester, ester with 2-chloro-*N*,*N*-diethyl-3-hydroxycrotonamide; mixture of α- and β-isomers plus one to two percent side products such as dechlorophosphamidon and γ-chlorophosphamidon.

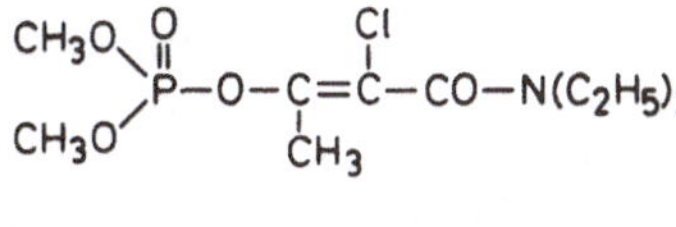

Alternate names: Dimecron.
Application: Systemic insecticide, effective against aphids and mites, with average persistence on or in plants (ANONYMOUS 14); its concentration reached on the average $<$one p.p.m. in four to ten days.
Veterinary application: 0.1 to 0.2 percent a.i. as spray and dip against ticks (ANONYMOUS 14).
Toxicity: See Table CXLV. Phosphamidon was toxic for bees (MARTIN 1961).

Because of the rapid decomposition of the effective substance on forage (pasture grass, lucerne, and others), animals can graze on "normal" treated areas without observing incidents. After feeding of cows with grass which

* Editor's note: See vol. 37 of Residue Reviews which is entirely devoted to phosphamidon.

Table CXLV. *Acute toxicities of phosphamidon for various animals.*

Animal species	Sex	Mode of application	Toxic dos. (mg./kg.)	LD_{50} (mg./kg.)	
Mouse	—	*per os* [a]	—	11.2–13.0	ANONYMOUS 14
Mouse	♂	*i. p.* [b]	—	6	CLEMONS & MENZER (1968)
Rat	♂	*per os* [c]	—	22.5	KLOTZSCHE (1964)
Rat	—	*per os* [a]	—	16.8	KLOTZSCHE & MARTIN (1961)
Rat	—	*per os*	—	20.0	JAQUES & BEIN (1960)
Guinea pig	—	*per os*	50	—	DRUMMOND (1960)
Guinea pig	—	*s. c.*	50	—	DRUMMOND (1960)
Birds	—	*per os*	—	1–5	ANONYMOUS 14

[a] Technical product.
[b] Aqueous solution.
[c] Twenty percent solution.

had been treated with phosphamidon in this way, no sickening effect was observed (ANONYMOUS 14). Applications both as dip and as spray proved to be harmless to treated animals.

Phosphamidon causes only a relatively small ChE inhibition; however, according to BULL *et al.* (1967) the *trans*-isomer is a strong ChE inhibitor. Regeneration was rapid, which is a characteristic of the enol-phosphates. Three mg./kg. inhibit brain ChE 50 percent in 14 days for rats, but not the periphery ChE. In a chronic test the no-effect dosage for dogs, with regard to ChE inhibition, was 0.5 mg./kg./day, and with regard to other criteria such as growth development of dogs and rats, five mg./kg. (ANONYMOUS 14).

Tolerances: The ADI is reported, with the use of the factor 100, as 0.0025 mg./kg.; with the use of the factor ten, which seems to be capable of being substituted after judgment of the ChE inhibition, 0.01 mg./kg. As a comparison the tolerance value for harvested edible fruit is 0.5 to 1.0 p.p.m. (ANONYMOUS 14) in some countries; in the U.S.A, 0.1 to 1.0 p.p.m. (FREAR *et al.* 1969).

Detection: See PACK *et al.* (1964).

Metabolism and residues: Phosphamidon was not cumulated in the tissues (ANONYMOUS 14); it was extremely rapidly decomposed in warm-blooded animals and by isolated tissues (ANLIKER *et al.* 1964), and also when high dosages such as three mg./kg .body wt. are applied (ANONYMOUS 14). BULL *et al.* (1967) conducted model investigations concerning the metabolic fate of the *cis*- and *trans*-isomers of phosphamidon in plants and insects and established a short half-life and a degradation to metabolic products which are formed through oxidation or hydrolysis. CLEMONS and MENZER (1968) followed the oxidative metabolism of labelled phosphamidon (C^{14} and P^{32}) in rats and goats. They found traces of phosphamidon in the urine. Nine organo-soluble metabolites were in the urine of goats and eight organo-soluble metabolites were in the urine of rats. More than 90 percent of the radioactive products in the urine of rats were insoluble in chloroform, meaning they were nontoxic metabolites. Three of these were identified as oxidation products and one as a hydrolysis product.

CLEMONS and MENZER (1968) concluded that the oxidative desethylation of phosphamidon is of great importance for animal metabolism. Aside from traces of phosphamidon, larger amounts of desethylphosphamidon and phosphamidon amide appeared. The major part of the radioactive material was excreted within 24 hours with the urine. The level for rats was higher than for goats. Female rats clearly excreted more P^{32}-labelled substances than male animals. Within 72 hours for male rats, 71.8 percent P^{32}-metabolites and 42.7 percent C^{14}-metabolites appeared in the urine, for female rats 67.2 percent P^{32}- and 44.3 percent C^{14}-products. The percent data related to the total applied dosage of two or four mg./kg. body wt., respectively. In the feces of male rats, 12.6 percent C^{14}-products was found and 10.1 percent C^{14}-products in female rats (CLEMONS and MENZER 1968).[29]

Further reports signify the following: After *per os* application of three mg./kg. C^{14}-phosphamidon to rats, about 95 percent of the applied radioactivity was again found in 72 hours. In these tests about 49 percent was found after 12 hours, and about 86 percent of the radioactivity after 24 hours in the urine, while the smaller residue was established in the feces and the breath. However, according to these reports the metabolites in urine and feces, respectively, are not phosphamidon or desethylphosphamidon (<0.0001 p.p.m.) (ANONYMOUS 13)[30], which appeared as the prevailing metabolite in plant metabolism and the concentration of which was <1.0 p.p.b. according to ANLIKER *et al.* (1964)[30]. After five days' feeding with a ration which contained ten p.p.m. C^{14}-phosphamidon, no significant residues (<0.0001 p.p.m.) could be established in muscles, fat, liver, kidneys, brain, etc. (ANONYMOUS 13).

No active substance could be detected in the tissues of cows which received five and 20 p.p.m. of phosphamidon in the ration (ANONYMOUS 14)[30].

CHAMBERLAIN and STUFF (1960) found, for the milk cow after five days' feeding of a total of 275.94 mg. of C^{14}-phosphamidon, maximum excretion of radioactive substances in the 52-hour urine sample. Within the five-day test period, 62.6 percent of the applied dosage was excreted, and after the last treatment the urine activity decreased to 0.19 μg.-equivalents/mg. Only three percent of the radioactivity appeared in the feces in four days of the five day test.

---

[29] Of the identified metabolites desethylphosphamidon exhibited for male rats an *i. p.* LD_{50} of 7.0 mg./kg., Phosphamidon amide and dechlorophosphamidon an LD_{50} of 2.5 mg. per kg. body wt., while the LD_{50} of phosphamidon was 6.0 mg./kg.

[30] It cannot always be established with certainty whether data of the same authors were possibly used for the individual anonymous literature citations.

In another experiment with oxen (ANONYMOUS 13) receiving 20 p.p.m. of phosphamidon for five days, neither one nor five days after the application could phosphamidon or one of its known metabolites be detected (<0.005 p.p.m.) in muscles, fat, kidney, liver, lung, and brain.

According to CLEMONS and MENZER (1968), the goat excreted in 72 hours 47.1 percent of P^{32}-labelled phosphamidon or 41.7 percent of C^{14}-labelled material with the urine. Only 0.072 percent C^{14}-substances appeared in the feces. The totalled residues which had been obtained from the individual tissue fractions after 72 hours gave 0.451 percent of P^{32}- and 0.138 percent of C^{14}-phosphamidon for the liver and for the kidney correspondingly 0.179 percent and 0.032 percent, respectively, based on the starting dosage of three mg./kg. P^{32}- and C^{14}-phosphamidon for a 44.5 kg. goat.

Special remarks: The cooking process destroys phosphamidon 80 to 100 percent within 15 minutes (ANONYMOUS 14).

37. RUELENE. — Phosphoramidic acid, methyl-(4-*tert*-butyl-2-chlorophenyl) methyl ester

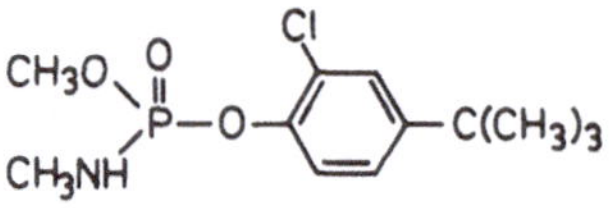

Alternate names: Dowco 132.

Application: See also HERLICH *et al.* 1961. Ruelene is a systemic insecticide of low toxicity (RADELEFF 1964). Furthermore, it has contact insecticidal and anthelmintic effects (ANONYMOUS 1). These effects occured faster than for the corresponding P = S compound [31] (SCHRADER 1963).

For outside application, the pour-on procedure according to ROGOFF and KOHLER (1960) as well as KOHLER and ROGOFF (1962) [32] with 7.2 to 9.6 g./animal (young cattle) was successful against bot-fly attack. SCHARFF (1962) reported that bot-fly attack was controlled with an application of 40 to 70 mg./kg. with a reduction rate of 99 percent (see also HARVEY and BRETHOUR 1961, ROSENBERGER *et al.* 1961, MCGREGOR *et al.* 1959, and others). Also, horn fly attack was controlled with the pour-on technique (ROGOFF and KOHLER 1961).

In a dip for bot-fly control 0.25 percent Ruelene was required (SCHARFF 1962), and likewise a concentration of 0.25 percent for sprays was necessary

[31] The systemic insecticide Narlene (Dowco 109) is closely related to Ruelene:

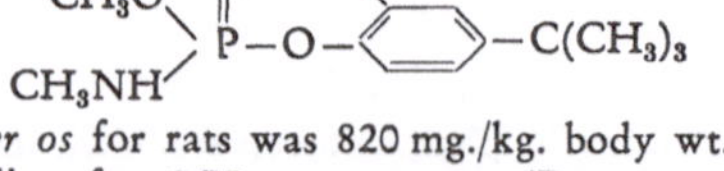

The acute LD_{50} *per os* for rats was 820 mg./kg. body wt. (FREAR 1965). There was good effect against bot-flies after 0.75 percent spray (ROGOFF *et al.* 1960); after oral application with feed (DRUMMOND and MOORE 1960, FRENCH *et al.* 1958) or after injection (DRUMMOND and GRAHAM 1959), it was effective against *Dermatobia* (MCGREGOR *et al.* 1958).

[32] See reports of toxicities for cattle.

(ROGOFF and KOHLER 1960). Bot-fly control was also possible with oral application and with continuous treatment with mineral salt mixtures (KOHLER and ROGOFF 1961). A good effect against lice attack was obtained with a dip of 0.25 percent Ruelene (SCHARFF 1962). For the back-rubber procedure a five percent Ruelene formulation in oil was used (RAUN and FRENCH 1961).

There was good anthelmintic effect with oral application; 30 to 50 mg./kg. body wt. were used for cattle against worm attack in stomach and intestines, and 100 to 150 mg./kg. body wt. for sheep and goats (SCHRADER 1963, ALICATO 1960, BAKER *et al* 1959, DOUGLAS and BAKER 1959, DOUGLAS *et al.* 1959, GALVIN *et al.* 1959, GORDON 1958, HERLICH *et al.* 1961, ROOS and KARR 1960, SHAVER and LANDRAM 1959, and others). The effect on fly larvae in chicken feces after oral intake was poor (SHERMAN and ROSS 1961).

Table CXLVI. *Acute toxicities of Ruelene for various animals after oral treatment.*

Animal species	Toxic dos. (mg./kg.)	LD_{50} (mg./kg.)	Reference
Mouse	—	1,080	METELICA (1967)
Rat	—	950	FREAR (1965)
Rat	—	~ 1,000	MARTIN (1961)
Rat	—	~ 1,000	SCHRADER (1963)
Rat	—	1,030	METELICA (1967)
Rat [a]	—	635	DURHAM (1967)
Rat [b]	—	460	DURHAM (1967)
Pig	15	—	RADELEFF (1964)
	~ 10		ANONYMOUS 1
Goat	max. nontox. 150 min. tox. 200	—	RADELEFF & BUSHLAND (1960)
Sheep	160	—	ANONYMOUS 1
Sheep	200 300	—	RADELEFF (1964)
Sheep	max. nontox. 150 min. tox. 200	—	RADELEFF & BUSHLAND (1960)
Calf	50	—	RADELEFF (1964)
Calf	max. nontox. 25 min. tox. 50	—	RADELEFF & BUSHLAND (1960)
Cattle	100	—	RADELEFF (1969)
Horse	~ 40	—	ANONYMOUS 1
Horse	50	—	RADELEFF (1961)
Horse	max. nontox. 25 min. tox. 50	—	RADELEFF & BUSHLAND (1960)

[a] Male.
[b] Female.

Toxicity: See Table CXLVI. Ruelene belongs to the so-called less toxic organophosphate esters. It was also formed in the animal body from the less toxic S-compounds such as DOWCO 109 (Radeleff 1960).
Detection: By paper chromatography or TLC (Watts 1967); the latter method had a sensitivity of 0.1 ng.
Restrictions and tolerances: Ruelene as a systemic insecticide for cattle, sheep, and goat received an extension until Jan. 1, 1970 in the U.S.A. (Frear *et al.* 1969). Knipling and Westlake (1966) mentioned a 28-day waiting period before slaughtering. Beesley (1966) cited the recommendation of the producers of Ruelene that the meat of treated animals not be used as food for at least four weeks.
Metabolism and residues: Ruelene is partially attacked by the rumen microorganisms (Bauriedel and Swank 1962).

Ruelene is rapidly resorbed and with cattle reached maximum concentration in blood in six hours after *i.m.* injection, and in 12 hours after dermal application. Two hours after *i.m.* injection and four hours after dermal application the blood concentration reached 0.5 and 1.8 p.p.m., respectively (Plapp *et al.* 1960 b). These values corresponded to those of Bauriedel and Swank (1961) for sheep, which reached 24 p.p.m. four hours after 100 mg./kg. *per os.*

Ruelene was completely metabolized (Plapp *et al.* 1960 b). Luschin (1966) reported that part of the compound is decomposed within 24 to 36 hours. The last products, such as phosphoric acid and phosphate, enter the phosphorus metabolism of the animals.

The major part of this insecticide was eliminated mostly with the urine in the form of degradation products. After *i.m.* injection of 11 mg./kg. body wt. the excretion of Ruelene or its metabolites reached maximum in urine after 12 to 18 hours. A total of 35 percent in the urine and 12 percent in the feces of the applied dosage was recovered (Plapp *et al.*, Unpublished data; Plapp *et al.* 1960 b). After dermal application of 40 mg./kg. body wt. 12 percent appeared in the urine with only traces in the feces. Maximum excretion with the urine and feces lay between eight and 12 hours (Gatterdam, Unpublished data; Plapp *et al.* 1960 b). The excretion of Ruelene and its hydrolyzed metabolites was slow on the whole; however, Plapp *et al.* (1960 b) found that within two weeks cattle treated orally or *i.m.* excreted only 35 to 42 percent with the urine or feces. It can be concluded from these findings that certain quantities remained in the organism as residues; however, no unchanged Ruelene was generally found.

Bauriedel and Swank (1962) established for sheep that excretion with the urine was 85 percent of the applied quantity, the larger part of which was found within 24 hours; 75 percent was hydrolysis products.

Buttram and Arthur (1961 b) assumed the degradation of Ruelene in poultry took place by attack at the P – N and P – O – C groups. For sheep Ruelene was decomposed to inorganic phosphate, which was also proved by the P^{32}-content of the bones. Figure 21 contains the possible metabolic routes. According to this scheme, cleavage of the molecule takes place either at the methyl ester bond or at the acidamide bond and the phosphate ester bond so that butylchlorophenol may be formed, also. KEDENBURG (1965) established for cattle no measurable active components in meat or in liver and kidney 21 days after pour-on treatment; butylchlorophenol was not established. No residues were found in meat 21 days after dermal treatment with the common practical dosage, nor in *s.c.* fatty tissue after 28 days (LUSCHIN 1966). BAURIEDEL and SWANK (1962) did not find ChE-inhibiting Ruelene as such in the tissues of sheep seven days after application of 200 mg./kg. body wt. Ruelene did not remain in the fatty tissue of the body. On the other hand, KEDENBURG 1965) reported traces of Ruelene in cattle in the *s.c.* fatty tissue of the back 21 days after a pour-on treatment with 14.3 g. of Ruelene/500 kg. body wt., whereby a concentration of 0.1 p.p.m. fresh wt. was present. In the same tissue 4-*tert.*-butyl-2-chlorophenol at 0.04 to 0.08 p.p.m. was established.

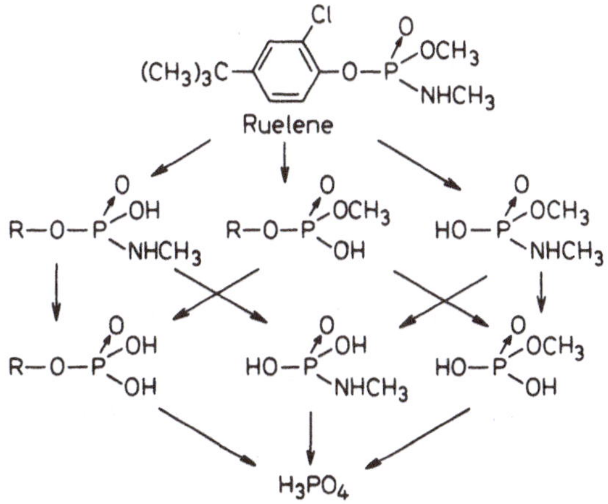

Fig. 21. Possible routes for the hydrolysis of Ruelene to inorganic phosphate (BUTTRAM and ARTHUR 1961 b): *R*=$(CH_3)_3C$– 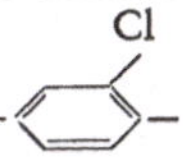 – .

Measurable P^{32}-activities in chloroform extracts of sheep tissue from animals treated with P^{32}-Ruelene are in Table CXLVII, in which the slowed-down decomposition rate in the heart muscle is obvious; there seemed to be mainly phospholipids present here, the same as in pancreas, as concluded from the analogous behaviour after application of inorganic phosphate (BAURIEDEL and SWANK 1962).

BUTTRAM and ARTHUR (1961 b) also investigated residues in tissues of chickens which had received 100 p.p.m. of P^{32}-Ruelene over seven days with the feed. Of the Ruelene consumed, 29 percent was excreted with the feces in 21 days, while 17.5 percent was present after one day and 27 percent after seven days; maximum excretion was on the fourth day. Six metabolites

Table CXLVII. *P^{32}-activity of chloroform extracts of sheep tissue from animals treated with P^{32}-Ruelene* (Bauriedel and Swank 1962).

Tissue	Ruelene equivalent (p.p.m.) after							
	Ruelene dosage 100 mg./kg.				Ruelene dosage 200 mg./kg.			
	3 days	7 days	14 days	21 days	7 days	14 days[a]	14 days[a]	21 days
Blood	0.1	0.3	—	0.0	—	0.0	—	—
Bile	0.1	0.3	—	0.0	—	0.0	—	—
Liver	1.5	1.0	0.1	0.1	0.1	0.0	0.1	0.0
Kidney	0.3	0.3	—	0.1	0.1	0.0	0.0	0.0
Spleen	0.1	0.2	0.0	0.0	0.1	0.1	0.1	0.0
Pancreas	4.5	0.2	0.1	0.1	0.1	0.1	4.4	0.1
Heart muscle	0.7	0.6	0.8	0.7	0.7	1.0	0.8	0.5
Tenderloin	0.1	0.1	0.1	0.2	0.2	0.3	0.2	0.4
Shoulder muscle	0.1	0.1	0.1	0.1	0.2	0.2	0.1	0.2
Rump muscle	0.1	0.1	0.1	0.1	0.2	0.3	0.3	0.3
Omental fat	0.0	0.0	0.0	0.0	0.0	0.0	0.0	0.0
Perirenal fat	0.0	0.1	0.0	0.0	0.0	0.0	0.0	0.0
Subcutaneous fat	0.0	0.0	0.0	0.0	0.1	0.0	0.0	0.0

[a] Averages of two different animals sacrificed at the same time.

out of presumably nine were isolated. Fourteen to 38 percent of the radioactivity present in the acetonitrile fraction and <1.0 percent in the *n*-hexane fraction proved to be Ruelene. Much of the radioactivity in the feces was in the aqueous extract, which also demonstrated rapid decomposition. The highest residues were in liver, kidney, and bones. Radioactivity was persistent in bones for two weeks after going back to normal feed without pesticide; this showed the decomposition of Ruelene as far down as phosphoric acid. No radioactive P^{32} was detected in fat (Table CXLVIII). The absence of acetonitrile-soluble radioactive components (<0.04 p.p.m.) in blood, brain, breast muscle, thigh, upper arm, fat, and skin showed no free Ruelene present. Only in liver, kidney, and stomach were such acetonitrile-soluble substances found, which again decreased three days after discontinuation of Ruelene feeding. Most of the nonextractable substances were acid-soluble (80 to 98 percent); the remainder were phospholipids and RNA (Buttram and Arthur 1961 b).

Remarks for evaluation: After spray treatment of cattle with Ruelene at 0.5 percent (5×) and 0.75 percent (1×) concentrations only in the rib pieces was there slight change in taste, while kidney and liver were not significally different from the control samples (Brogdon and Dawson 1965).

Kedenburg (1965) reported that cooking and frying of Ruelene-containing tissues did not cause appreciable inactivation; heat inactivation at 100° C. was slight. On the contrary, traces of Ruelene in fat were quantitatively destroyed in 15 minutes at the higher temperatures of melting. Under physiological conditions (37° C. and pH 7.0) liver and kidney tissues rapidly decomposed Ruelene. Muscle tissue was less active. This decomposi-

Table CXLVIII. *Residues in tissues of laying hens fed P^{32}-Ruelene* (BUTTRAM and ARTHUR 1961 b).

Tissue	Ruelene equivalent (p.p.m.) [a] after							
	Ruelene feeding period			Normal feed after treatment				
	1 day	3 days	7 days	1 day	3 days	7 days	10 days	14 days
Blood	0.09	0.41	1.05	0.94	0.75	0.34	0.05	< 0.04
Bone	0.10	0.86	1.92	1.42	1.71	1.53	0.66	0.85
Brain	< 0.04	0.12	0.31	0.35	0.23	0.28	0.15	0.16
Breast	< 0.04	0.20	0.56	0.59	0.60	0.53	0.23	0.21
Drumstick	< 0.04	0.30	0.58	0.56	0.38	0.46	0.20	0.08
Fat	< 0.04	< 0.04	< 0.04	< 0.04	< 0.04	< 0.04	< 0.04	< 0.04
Gizzard	0.98 (0.15)	0.52 (0.23)	0.79 (0.20)	0.77 (0.10)	0.43	0.17	0.06	< 0.04
Kidney	1.11	2.42 (0.16)	3.59 (0.16)	2.55 (0.15)	1.64	0.80	0.31	0.23
Liver	1.63 (0.08)	3.27 (0.08)	4.20 (0.06)	2.61	1.42	1.10	0.44	0.21
Skin	0.05	0.16	0.30	0.24	0.17	0.13	< 0.04	< 0.04

[a] Numbers in parentheses indicate the p.p.m. of acetonitrile-soluble residues; all other tissues contained below 0.04 p.p.m. of acetonitrile solubles.

tion in liver and kidney was considerable at +40° C. but very small at −10° C. and stopped completely on the second day of storage.

Furthermore it is doubtful that the antimitotic effect, which can be observed on plants (pea root) after relatively high dosages (NETHERY *et al.* 1965), will show on the mammal directly or after consumption of residue-containing tissue, since such concentrations (e. g., 200 p.p.m.) are rarely reached; furthermore, no mutagenic effect could be obtained with the Müller-Drosophila test.

38. S 125. — Thiophosphoric acid, O,O-diethyl-O-(naphthalimido) ester

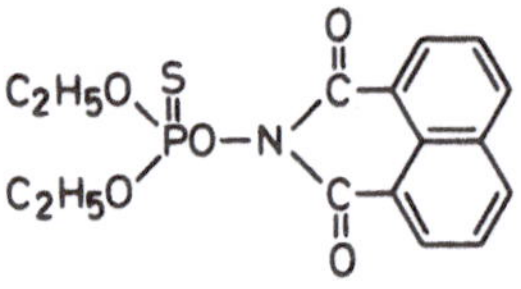

Alternate name: Bayer 22408.
Application: Control of cotton pests; effective against flies, mosquito larvae, and ticks.
Toxicity: See Table CXLIX.

Table CXLIX. *Acute toxicities of S 125 for rats after various application.*

Mode of application	LD_{50} (mg./kg.)	Reference
per os	500	MARTIN (1961)
per os	335	BOYD & ARTHUR (1960)
s.c.	1,000	BOYD & ARTHUR (1960)

Metabolism and residues: S 125 is the thiophosphate of naphthalophos (q. v.). Although it is not available as a trade product on the market, it has been remarkably well investigated. Aside from the use of P^{32}-labelled substances the fluorometric method of GIANG (1961) offers a good means of detection.

Excretion in the urine of rats after *per os* treatment with P^{32}-labelled material was three times higher than after *s.c.* injection and approximately four times higher than after dermal treatment (BOYD and ARTHUR 1960). Furthermore, these authors established only small differences in excretion with feces with respect to application methods. The excretion fractions with the feces after dermal and *s.c.* applications were greater than those in the urine for these application modes. Eliminated products were mainly hydrolyzed S 125, with the larger part in the urine. However, after dermal application, more nonhydrolyzed substance or nonhydrolyzed metabolites were in the feces than after *s.c.* or *per os* treatment. Radioactivity in blood, urine, fat, and heart three days after treatment derived from hydrolysis products. Liver and kidney contained larger quantities, but only a small part was soluble in chloroform. Residues which were considered toxic were found among the chloroform-soluble radioactive materials. There were differences in the amounts of residues dependent on the mode of application. The residues are in Table CL.

Table CL. *S 125 equivalents in tissues of rats treated with P^{32}–S 125* (BOYD and ARTHUR 1960).

Tissue [a]	S 125 equivalent [b] (p.p.m.) after					
	100 mg./kg. (oral)		500 mg./kg. (*s.c.*)		1,000 mg./kg. (dermal)	
	3 days	7 days	3 days	7 days	3 days	7 days
Kidney	0.31	< 0.01	1.10	0.35	< 0.01	< 0.01
Liver	0.94	< 0.01	1.05	0.32	2.22	1.44
Muscle	< 0.01	< 0.01	0.56	0.31	< 0.01	< 0.01
Skin	< 0.01	< 0.01	29	17	270	40

[a] Blood, brain, fat, and heart contained < 0.01 p.p.m. at the three- and seven-day intervals for all routes of administration.
[b] Chloroform-soluble materials.

After dermal application of P^{32}-S 125 in 0.5 percent Triton X100 xylene emulsion to cows, these the same authors found the pesticide content decreased from 18,000 p.p.m. immediately after treatment to 3,500 p.p.m. after 17 days, which meant there was a considerable residual effect which could give rise to later resorption. Expressive of this resorption was the appearance of P^{32}-substances in the feces, which reached maximum five to seven days after treatment (19 to 28 p.p.m. equiv.); in 22 days 32 to 40 percent was excreted. The P^{32}-residues in the feces were fractionated into an acetonitrile phase, a hexane phase, an aqueous phase, and a nonextractable phase, but not characterized.

GATTERDAM *et al.* (1962) refered to a personal communication of CLABORN according to which residues were found in the meat of bulls after a spray with P^{32}-S 125. GATTERDAM also treated bulls with labelled S 125. In the blood of a *per os* treated bull, there was an increase of radioactivity in 24 hours which, with 0.953 µg.-equivalents after oral application, was about 35 times higher than after dermal. No organosoluble radioactivity could be established in the blood of the dermally treated animal; after *per os* treatment only traces could be found. It was established that only 3.2 percent radioactivity of the 24-hour blood sample behaved like S 125 or its O-analog. Four days after dermal application, no radioactivity could be detected in blood any more, while it was still 0.196 µg.-equivalent seven days after *per os* application.

Excretion in urine and feces after dermal application was low. In seven days it was 2.1 percent of the total activity in the urine. After oral treatment the values were considerably higher. Here, within seven days 41 percent of the total activity was excreted with the urine and 49 percent with the feces, whereby the maximum was reached after 24 hours with 268 μg.-equivalents. Excretion for both application modes was more than half the radioactivity in 48 hours. The main excretion products for bulls were diethylphosphoric acid and diethylthiophosphoric acid. After oral intake diethylphosphoric acid increased from 2.0 percent after three hours to 59 percent after 24 hours, while diethylthiophosphoric acid decreased from 88 percent after three hours to 29.5 percent after 24 hours. After dermal application the diethylphosphoric acid increased in the urine from 30.8 percent in six hours to 59.4 percent in 24 hours, while diethylthiophosphoric acid decreased from 61.1 percent after six hours to 32.1 percent after 24 hours. Five to ten percent of the radioactivity was present in the form of two unknown metabolites.

Twelve hours after *per os*, application, 80 percent S 125 and 20 percent O-analog were in the feces; 36 hours after this treatment 65 percent of the activity was diethylthiophosphoric acid and 35 percent was diethylphosphoric acid (GATTERDAM *et al.* 1962). The acetonitrile-soluble components were unchanged S 125, its O-analog, and a methanol fraction. These components of the methanol fraction of the feces exhibited a higher anti-ChE effect than the corresponding fraction in milk. Diethylphosphoric acid and diethylthiophosphoric acid appeared in the water-soluble phase as hydrolysis products. Chloroform-soluble components of the urine were 14 percent unchanged substance and 86 percent O-analog. The water-soluble fraction contained 63 percent diethylthiophosphoric acid and 37 percent diethylphosphoric acid (BUTTRAM and ARTHUR 1961 a).

It can be concluded from the numbers mentioned above that only small residues remained in the tissues. GATTERDAM *et al.* (1962) estimated them to be <0.05 p.p.m. S 125 or its metabolites.

39. SARIN. — Isopropoxymethylphosphorylfluoride

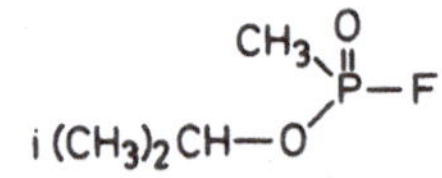

Application: No common practical application; extremely toxic substance.
Toxicity: See Table CLI.
Metabolism and residues: Sarin is a strong ChE inhibitor, which *in vitro* has a strong bond to plasma protein. The bond rate was 35 percent in rat plasma, seven percent in human plasma, and 11 percent in guinea pig

Table CLI. *Acute toxicities of sarin for mice.*

Mode of application	LD_{50} (μg./kg.)	Reference
i.p.	420	HOLMSTEDT (1959)
i.p.	283	VAN METER & KARCZMAN (1968)
s.c.	271	VAN METER & KARCZMAN (1968)

plasma (COHEN *et al.* 1961). Rat plasma contained (like other species) sarinase (CHRISTEN and VAN DEN MUYSENBERG 1965). In plasma of human beings, rats, and mice there is, therefore, a rapid enzymatic hydrolysis of sarin to the nontoxic isopropyl-hydrogen-methylphosphonate (CHRISTEN and COHEN 1963, COHEN *et al.* 1961).

Specific data about tissue residues are not available.

40. SULFOTEPP. — Tetraethyl dithiopyrophosphate

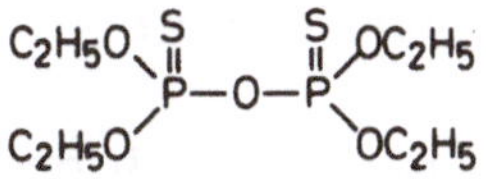

Alternate names: Bayer E-393, Bladafum, ASP-47.
Application: No veterinary application; highly effective contact insecticide in plant protection, fumigant in green houses.
Toxicity: See Table CLII.

Table CLII. *Acute toxicity of sulfotepp for mice after s.c. injection.*

LD_{50} (mg./kg.)	Reference
8	HOLMSTEDT (1959)
5.0	KLIMMER (1964)

Metabolism and residues: Sulfotepp was attacked by the rumen fluid but more slowly than TEPP (q. v.) (AHMED *et al.* 1958). No literature reports are available for tissue residues.

41. TABUN. — Dimethylamidoethoxy phosphorylcyanide

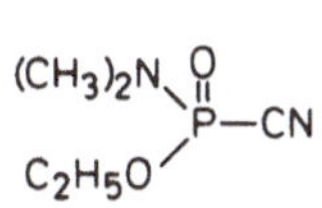

Toxicity: LD_{50} for mice *i.p.* 0.6 mg./kg. (HOLMSTEDT 1959).
Detection: With the help of chemiluminescence of luzigenin (WEBER and MATKOVIĆ 1965).
Metabolism and residues: HEILBRONN *et al.* (1964) investigated its fate in rats and mice which had received atropine and N-methylpyridine-2-aldoxime methansulfonate or N,N-trimethylene-bis(pyridinium-4-aldoxime) dibromide before the *i.v.* application of 0.08 mg./kg. of P^{32}-tabun. In the urine, as the major route of excretion, mainly dimethylaminoethoxyphosphine oxide and traces of ethoxydihydroxyphosphine oxide were found as metabolites, but no intact tabun. There was only slight activity present in the feces. Excretion with the urine was 15 percent of the radioactivity in 24 hours and 32 percent in six days; there were 0.9 and 0.3 percent in the

feces and bile. Lung, kidney, liver, and bones contained the largest quantities in the first 24 hours after injection; smaller quantities were present in brain, heart, and muscles. Maximum radioactivity existed in the kidneys after 20 minutes; values in the liver increased during the first four hours. A diaplacental transfer in the fetus tissue also took place. Tissues with high ChE content, such as muscles, retained only a little P^{32}, while liver and kidney bound much of it. After six days the radioactivity in all tissues except brain and bones decreased considerably.

42. TEPP. — Tetraethylpyrophosphate

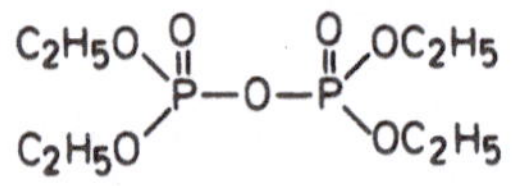

Alternate names: Bladan, Nifos-T, Vapotone.
Application: Pesticide with acaricidal effect in plant protection, dangerous insecticide (FREAR and FRIEDMANN 1968).
Toxicity: See Table CLIII.

Table CLIII. *Acute toxicities of TEPP for mouse and rat.*

Animal species	Mode of application	Toxic dos. (mg./kg.)	LD_{50} (mg./kg.)	Reference
Mouse	*i.p.*	—	0.7	HOLMSTEDT (1959)
Mouse	*per os*	—	7.0	SCHRADER (1963)
Mouse	*s.c.*	1	—	HOLMSTEDT (1959)
Mouse	*per os*	2	—	HOLMSTEDT (1959)
Rat	*per os* [a]	—	2.0	FRAWLEY & FUYAT (1957)
	per os [b]	—	1.2	
Rat	*per os*	0.002 [c]	—	DEICHMANN & WITHERUP (1947)

[a] Male.
[b] Female.
[c] Acute dosage, ml. of a 0.1 percent aqueous solution.

Tolerances: In the U.S.A., "zero-tolerance" is required in plant protection (FREAR and FRIEDMANN 1968).
Metabolism and residues: TEPP was unstable in "moisture" (HAZLETON 1955), and poorly stable in aqueous solution (DEICHMANN and WITHERUP 1947); it was, therefore, rapidly decomposed in the rumen fluid (AHMED *et al.* 1958). It is a strong ChE inhibitor. The enzymatic cleavage of TEPP led to dimethylphosphoric acid, which was not toxic for mammals (CASIDA 1956, FLEISCHER and JANDORF 1952).

Quantitative data about residues in tissues of edible domestic animals do not exist.

43. TRICHLORFON. — Phosphonic acid, (2,2,2-trichloro-1-hydroxy-ethyl)-, dimethyl ester

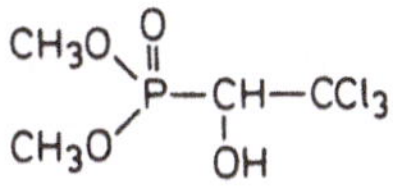

Alternate names: Tugon, Neguvon, Dipterex, Bayer L 13/59, Dylox, Wotexit, chlorophos, chlorofos, trichlorphon.
Application: Insecticide with systemic and antiparasitic effect for outside and inside applications. It was effective against bot-flies, *Dermatobia*, lice, fleas, mites, and *Gastrophilus* spp. (BOLLE 1956, MCGREGOR *et al.* 1954), as well as against filariasis, ascariasis, and intestinal nematodes of ruminants (BEHRENZ *et al.* 1959, GALVIN *et al.* 1959, DIRKSEN and RADEMACHER 1960). Outside application was with a 0.15 to two percent aqueous solution as a wash, with 0.5 to three 1. as a spray, as well as in special formulations with pour-on and spot-on methods. Internal medication was applied with 35 mg./kg. for horses, 30 to 50 mg./kg. for pigs, and 75 to 80 mg./kg. for cattle and sheep. LYONS *et al.* (1967) injected sheep with 70 mg./kg. in order to get an anthelmintic effect (cf. RIEK *et al.* 1958).
Toxicity: See Table CLIV. [33] With regard to the species compatibility of trichlorfon, there were deviations (KAEMMERER 1963). The property of being rapidly decomposed by plasma esterases explained the relatively low toxicity for mammals (ARTHUR and CASIDA 1957).
Restrictions and tolerances: In the U.S.A., 0.2 p.p.m. in vegetables, bananas, and others (FREAR *et al.* 1969). BÄR (1964 a) pointed to the necessity for cooking contaminated meat for one hour ,if slaughtering was done less than six hours after treatment.
Detection: See DUGGAN *et al.* (1967), MCDOUGALL (1964), and DEDEK (1966). Trichlorfon is a widely used insecticide in the area of veterinary medicine so that extensive investigations of it were made. The analytical methods comprised biological, chemical, and radiochemical procedures. Investigations using biological testing methods achieved considerable sensitivity and permitted statements about the remaining insecticidal effect. Specific methodology includes biological with mosquito larvae (BEHRENZ 1959 and 1961); enzyme inhibition test (DU BOIS and COTTER 1955); enzyme inhibition and colorimetric determination of the thiocholine used with bis(*p*-nitrophenyl)-disulfide (KEDENBURG 1965); enzyme-chemical determination with an agar diffusion method in which the enzyme inhibitor penetrated into the enzyme-containing agar (SANDI 1962, FÜHRER *et al.* 1967); colorimetric determination after chromatographic cleanup and oxi-

[33] There are a number of trade products with certain additives (PAM or atropine), which increase the compatibility of trichlorfon: Bubulin (DDR), LD_{50} for rats *s.c.* 2,480 mg./kg. (RAHN 1963); for sheep and goat see SCHULZ and WUJANZ (1961). Addition products of chloral and formamide such as Emittol (Delitia) also improve the toxicity: oral LD_{50} for rat 1,050 to 1,200 mg./kg. (RAHN 1963).

Table CLIV. *Acute toxicities of trichlorfon for various animals.*

Animal species	Mode of application	Toxic dos. (mg./kg.)	LD_{50} (mg./kg.)	Reference
Mouse	*i.p.*	—	500	DU BOIS & COTTER (1955)
Rat	*per os*	—	950–1,100	KLOTZSCHE (1955)
Rat	*per os*	—	450	HOLMSTEDT (1959)
Rat	*per os*	—	625	BOLLE (1956)
Rat [a]	*per os*	—	630	GAINES (1960)
Rat [b]	*per os*	—	560	GAINES (1960)
Rat	*s.c.*	—	400	KRUEGER & CASIDA (1957)
Rat	*i.p.*	—	400	ARTHUR & CASIDA (1957)
Rat	*i.p.*	—	450	DU BOIS & COTTER (1955)
Chicken [c]	*per os*	—	65	SHERMAN & ROSS (1959)
Sheep	*per os*	max. nontox. 200	—	RADELEFF & BUSHLAND (1960)
Cattle	*per os*	max. nontox. 50 min. tox. 75	—	RADELEFF & BUSHLAND (1960)
Calf	*per os*	max. nontox. 5 min. tox. 10	—	RADELEFF & BUSHLAND (1960)
Human	*per os* [d]	7.5 tolerated	—	LEBRUN & CERF (1960)

[a] Male.
[b] Female.
[c] One week old.
[d] Dosed several times.

dation of the insecticide to inorganic phosphorus (LEAHY 1964); TLC (KOLJAKOVA 1968); isotope method with P^{32} (ROBBINS *et al.* 1956); and sensitive detection (0.1 p.p.m.) with glc (ANDERSON *et al.* 1966 a).

Metabolism and residues: Trichlorfon was rapidly resorbed, decomposed, and excreted by the body (BEHRENZ 1961). Because of the low persistence, the residual effect for external application was also very low (BEHRENZ *et al.* 1959). The extremely fast recovery of animals after sublethal dosages also pointed to the very high detoxification rate (DU BOIS and COTTER 1955).

GOOD and CANTOR (1965) pointed out that, although no more trichlorfon as such was found in the tissues (systemic) several hours after treatment, toxic effects could be possible because more toxic, unidentified metabolites could be formed which are able to interfere with the animal enzyme systems and could lead to lethal syntheses. This statement was made as a supposition and may be a remainder of older opinions by THAMM (1960), which also have not been proved as yet. Findings of HASSAN *et al.* (1965 a) will be mentioned here as a model for the formed metabolites. These authors studied the metabolism of P^{32}-trichlorfon in rat brain tissue homogenates. They found four metabolites, three of which were established as being acidic and one as being not acidic. The fraction of total metabolites amounted to 37 percent for monodesmethyltrichlorfon, seven percent for monomethylphosphate, and 16 percent of a metabolite which presumably was 2,2,2-trichloro-1-hydroxyethylphosphoric acid. The nonacidic components remain unidentified.

However, monodesmethyltrichlorfon in brain homogenate did not form during reaction of trichlorfon *in vivo* (HASSAN and ZAYED 1965). It was possibly very rapidly decomposed by serum esterase. The scheme in Figure 22 shows the two possible detoxication routes.

Enzymatic decomposition in the mammal by phosphatases proceded by way of more or less toxic metabolites to inorganic phosphates (DEDEK and SCHWARZ 1966 b). These were unstable *in vivo* and were transformed by phosphorylases to the high-energy carbohydrate-phosphoric acid esters as

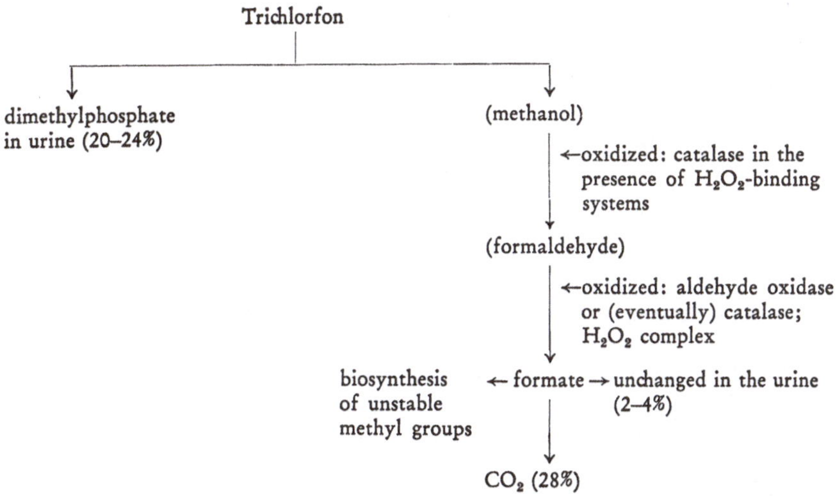

Fig. 22. Possible detoxication pathways for trichlorfon (HASSAN and ZAYED 1965).

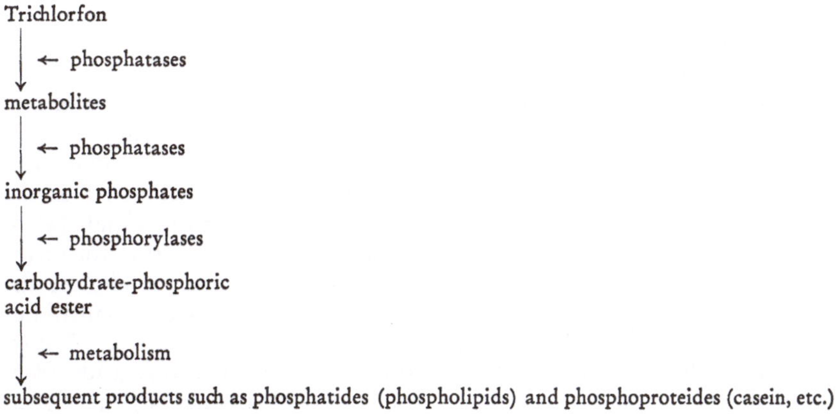

Fig. 23. Generalized metabolism of trichlorfon and other organophosphates (DEDEK and SCHWARZ 1966 b).

intermediate products of the cell metabolism so that the general scheme in Figure 23 was derived.

Trichlorfon is not very stable, especially in aqueous solution, and is cleaved in dependency on the pH value. In an acid environment the attack occured directly on the phosphone-bond (Fig. 24).

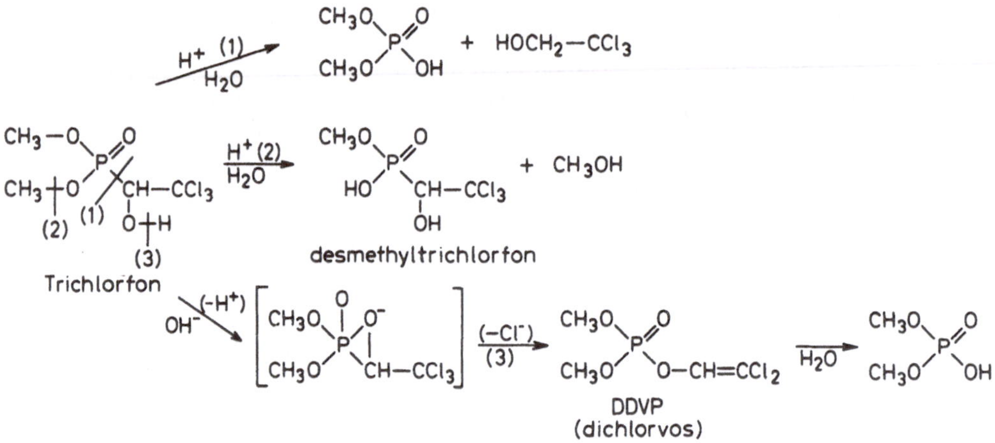

Fig 24. Cleavage of trichlorfon in aqueous medium at bonds (1), (2), or (3) (DEDEK and SCHWARZ 1966 a, DEDEK 1966).

Trichloroethyl alcohol was formed after acid hydrolysis of trichlorfon (MÜHLMANN and SCHRADER 1957); it has a hypnotizing effect. However, trichloroethyl alcohol was conjugated with glucuronic acid and was excreted as urochloralic acid (ARTHUR cited by CASIDA 1956).

During trichlorfon decomposition in neutral and slightly alkaline solution one mole of HCl and one mole of DDVP were formed, which were transformed to dimethylphosphoric acid and dichlorovinyl alcohol; the cleavage product was dichloroacetaldehyde (LORENZ *et al.* 1955).

The major degradation products of trichlorfon which occured *in vivo* were the nontoxic dimethylphosphate and the biologically ineffective but persistent desmethyltrichlorfon (DEDEK and SCHWARZ 1966 a). According to ARTHUR and CASIDA (1958), the first step of trichlorfon decomposition in the liver occured at the C–P bond; major metabolites were dimethylphosphate and monomethylphosphate. At first, a hydrolytic attack at the methyl ester bond(s) seemed to occur in nerve tissue (HASSAN and ZAYED 1965, HASSAN *et al.* 1965 a). ROBBINS *et al.* (1956) believed that for metabolism in cattle rather the cleavage of the O-methyl ester bond(s) or the transformation of the chloral part in the trichlorfon molecule prevailed, but not the decomposition of the C–P bond. According to HASSAN and ZAYED (1965), another equivalent detoxification mechanism occured, aside from the hydrolysis process at the C–P bond, through the already-mentioned attack at the P–OCH_3 bond, which was possibly a phosphatase effect. Small amounts of dichlorvos were found *in vivo*, aside from trichlorfon and chloroform-soluble intermediate products such as phosphorus-containing lipoids (glycerine phosphatides) (SCHWARZ and DEDEK 1966 a).

However, SCHENK (1967) considered the transformation into dichlorvos as being necessary for the biological effect of trichlorfon, a process that occurs in the liver. This metabolite presents no residues problem.

Quantitative data with regard to the P – C hydrolysis are found in Table CLV.

Table CLV. *Metabolism of trichlorfon in two biological systems* (ARTHUR and CASIDA 1958).

Biological system [a]	Percent present as		
	Butonate [b]	Trichlorfon	Hydrolyzed (P–C)
Rat liver homogenates 1 hr.	0.0	86.6	13.4
Rat kidney homogenates 4 hr.	0.0	81.5	18.5

[a] 20 percent homogenates in saline (pH 7.2) containing 1,000 p.p.m. insecticide.
[b] Butyryl ester of trichlorfon.

However, according to DEDEK and SCHWARZ (1966 a), the P – C bond in dichlorvos was attacked more easily by enzymes than the bonds of trichlorfon. The cleavage reactions of trichlorfon and dichlorvos were strongly accelerated by the presence of phosphate-cleaving enzymes (DEDEK 1966), whereby the influence on the reaction was type-specific (Table CLVI).

The cleavage product dichlorvos, formed at pH values of >6.0, is more toxic than trichlorfon. It is possible, as mentioned above, that a large part of the trichlorfon effect is caused by dichlorvos, which is present in equilibrium (DEDEK and SCHWARZ 1966 b), although it occurs in the mam-

Table CLVI. *Half-lives of cleavage of trichlorfon and dichlorvos in vitro* (DEDEK 1966).

Medium [a] (37.5° C.)	Half-lives of P–C bonds	
	Trichlorfon (minutes)	Dichlorvos (hours)
Buffer pH 8.0	53	13.5
Buffer pH 7.0	390	22.5
Buffer pH 7.2	265	17.4
Cattle blood, stabilized with oxalate	62	38/60
Cattle serum, without oxalate addition	32	28/60
Pig serum, without oxalate addition	23	17/60

[a] 100 µg./ml.

mal organism only as a short-lived intermediate product [34] and is cleaved by enzymes more rapidly in mammals than in insects. Dichlorvos contributes only a small part of the trichlorfon. KÜHNERT *et al.* (1963) were able to detect it in cattle. It is also present in pigs; however, 3.5 hours after an *s.c.* injection of 25 mg./kg. it no longer was detected in blood, while it still occurred in the intestines after three hours (SCHWARZ and DEDEK 1965 a). Dimethylphosphate and desmethyltrichlorfon were formed from trichlorfon as further cleavage products, identified by DEDEK and SCHWARZ (1966 b) as long-lived, enzyme-persistent products of low toxicity.

The scheme in Figure 25 is an example of the hydrolytic cleavage in the buffered system of cattle blood with a pH range of 7.1 to 7.3.

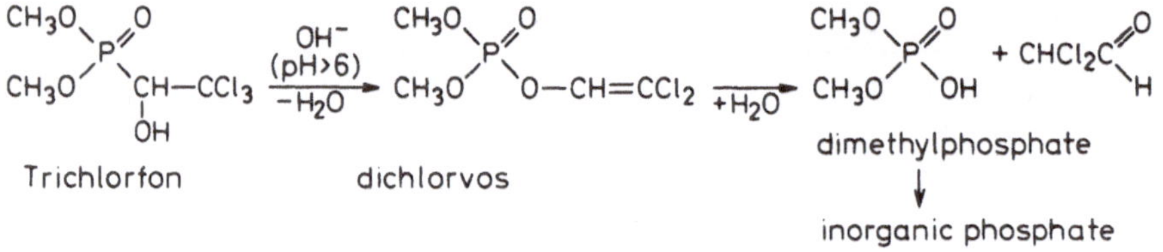

Fig. 25. Hydrolytic cleavage of trichlorfon in beef blood (KÜHNERT *et al.* 1963).

According to SCHENK (1967) and SCHENK and SCHREIBER (1969), the metabolic scheme in Figure 26 for trichlorfon may summarize and explain once more the metabolisms of this material.

DU BOIS and COTTER (1955) proved very early with the use of enzyme inhibition that after an *i.p.* injection of 75 mg. of trichlorfon/kg. body wt. the highest serum concentrations were reached in five minutes, with theoretical concentrations of 75 to 150 µg./ml. but 56 to 115 µg./ml. were actually measured. The decrease in the serum was dependent on the dosage and occurred after 75 mg./kg. in 15 minutes and after 150 mg./kg. in 60 minutes. After application of 150 mg./kg., the serum was free of substance after 60 minutes (BOLLE 1956).

The excretion of trichlorfon in the urine of rats was investigated by DU BOIS and COTTER (1955). They established that from one-to-three percent of an *i.p.* dosage was excreted unchanged with the urine within 24 hours; the values of the following 24 hours could not be measured any more, which means the excretion products were inactive metabolites.

HASSAN *et al.* (1965 b) labelled the two methyl groups of trichlorfon with C^{14}. They found for rats 28 percent of the dosage as $C^{14}O_2$ in the urine. C^{14}-formate and C^{14}-dimethylphosphate were also present at two and 22 percent, respectively. After an *i.p.* injection of 100 mg./kg. of P^{32}-trichlorfon, they found within 48 hours 75 to 85 percent of the total applied dosage of radioactive material in the urine. Three metabolites were recognized with chromatography: mono- and dimethylphosphate (20 to 30 per-

[34] Dichlorvos detection one-to-four minutes after an *i.v.* injection (KÜHNERT *et al.* 1963).

cent and 60 to 70 percent, respectively), as well as an unidentified metabolite (ten percent) which could be neither orthophosphate nor monodesmethylated trichlorfon. The end-product after acid hydrolysis of all P^{32}-trichlorfon metabolites was mono- or dimethylphosphate. HASSAN and ZAYED (1965) also report an excretion rate of >60 percent in 24 hours with the breath and urine of rats, when trichlorfon with C^{14}-labelled methyl groups was applied *i.p.* It was present in the urine as formic acid and dimethylphosphate. BULL and RIDGWAY (1969) after *i.p.* application of P^{32}-trichlorfon or dichlorvos or O-desmethyldichlorvos found only traces of trichlorfon in the urine of rats, but no dichlorvos; however, this was a 16-hour sample of urine. Dimethylphosphate was the highest percentage metabolic product present after injection of trichlorfon and dichlorvos (Table CLVII).

Table CLVII. *Radioactive compounds obtained from the urine of rats treated i.p. with P^{32}-labelled trichlorfon, dichlorvos, or O-desmethyl dichlorvos* (BULL and RIDGWAY 1969).

Compound	Percent of dose, 16 hours after treatment		
	Trichlorfon (dose 5 mg.)	Dichlorvos (dose 0.5 mg.)	O-Desmethyl-dichlorvos (dose 1.7 mg.)
H_3PO_4+ methylphosphate	0.8	9.2	43.6
Unknown E	18.4	0.0	11.2
Dimethylphosphate	37.5	64.1	—
Unknown B	11.1	0.0	0.0
O-Desmethyltrichlorfon	1.4	—	
O-Desmethyldichlorvos	0.8	1.7	21.2
Trichlorfon	0.7	—	—

After 75 mg./kg. *i.p.* no detectable trichlorfon was found in the livers of rats after 15 minutes (DU BOIS and COTTER 1955). After a three-fold LD_{50} treatment of trichlorfon, SCHENK (1967) found residues in the muscles of the fore-limbs, back limbs, and trunks of rats, ten to 25 minutes after death had occurred. The residues were 400 p.p.m. Decontamination was accomplished by cooking for one-and-a-half hours.

ARTHUR and CASIDA (1957) injected 150 mg. of P^{32}-trichlorfon/kg. *i.v.* into a 9.2 kg. dog. Ten minutes after the injection the blood contained only one part trichlorfon and two parts hydrolysis products. After six hours the portion of uncleaved phosphonate was only 0.4 percent and the portion of cleavage products was four times higher. During the first hours after the injection, urine, feces, and saliva contained a high radioactivity. The dog excreted in two days <1 percent of trichlorfon in unchanged form. A sodium salt with organically-bound chlorine occurred as a metabolite, which made up 67 percent of the applied dosage, but did not represent trichlorfon, chloral, trichloroethanol, or inorganic chlorides. After a four-hour hydrolysis with HCl the trichloroethanol formed was 63 percent of the

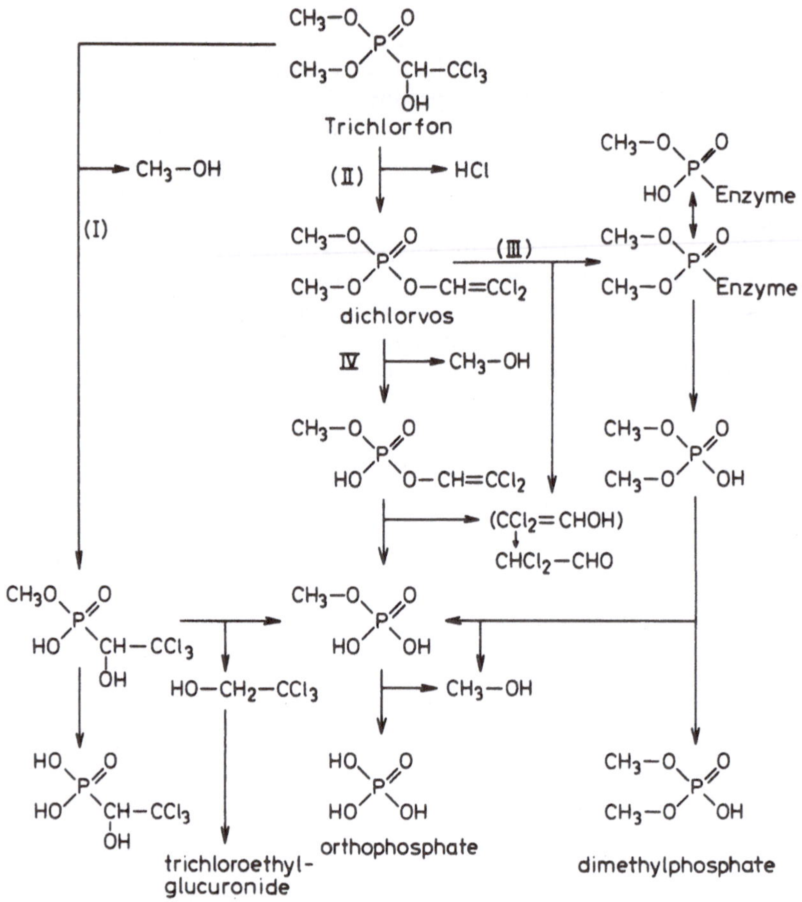

Fig. 26. Metabolism of trichlorfon and dichlorvos in the animal organism (Schenk and Schreiber 1969):

(I) 1. In the acid range water addition leads to cleavage of CH_3 and thus to the non-toxic desmethyltrichlorfon.
2. The methyl group of desmethyltrichlorfon can be cleaved off so that non-methylated trichlorfon is eliminated.
3. The P—C bond in desmethyltrichlorfon is attacked and trichloroethanol results.
4. Trichloroethanol is eliminated as trichloroethyl glucuronide.
5. Monomethylphosphoric acid is formed from desmethyltrichlorfon as a second cleavage product; it can be eliminated as such.
6. The separation of the methyl group from monomethylphosphoric acid is possible so that elimination of orthophosphate occurs.
7. Orthophosphate enters the phosphate pool of the body.

(II) 1. In the pH range of the body dichlorovos is formed from trichlorfon by splitting off HCl.
2. Dichlorvos is demethylated to desmethyldichlorvos.
3. Desmethyldichlorvos decomposes to monomethylphosphoric acid and follows the elimination pathway under I, 5 and 6 above.
4. Furthermore, desmethyldichlorvos can be transformed to dichloroacetaldehyde.

applied dosage and was conjugated with glucuronic acid and excreted with the urine.

The total P^{32}-activity decreased in blood of pigs within a few hours; six to eight minutes after *i.v.* application half of the activity was no longer extractable and after one hour 95 percent of the substance was decomposed. After *i.m.* treatment the substance was detected in blood up to six hours because of continuing resorption; however, no dichlorvos was found after this mode of application (ARTHUR and CASIDA 1957). SCHWARZ *et al.* (1965 a), after an *s.c.* injection of 50 mg./kg. body wt. P^{32}-Bubulin (approx. 25 mg./kg. trichlorfon) into pigs, found ten to 11 p.p.m. in blood after 15 to 60 minutes, and approximately one p.p.m. after five to seven hours. Here, the portion of trichlorfon was 90 percent of the total activity in the beginning and only 25 percent after six hours. The half-lives of trichlorfon and dichlorvos are estimated by DEDEK and SCHWARZ (1966 a) in pig serum without oxalate addition as 23 and 17 minutes, respectively, and that of trichlorfon in the intestinal contents of the pig as two hours (SCHWARZ and DEDEK 1965 a and 1966 a). After *s.c.* injection, radioactive material was also excreted into the intestines of pigs with an increasing count — there must be phosphorus-containing degradation products among them, for the trichlorfon portion of the total radioactivity present in the intestines was 90 percent in the beginning, 80 percent after two hours, and ten percent after six hours. The absolute values in the intestines were: four to five p.p.m. after 20 minutes until about 2.5 hours with one p.p.m. after five-to-seven hours (SCHWARZ *et al.* 1965 a). DEDEK and SCHWARZ (1966 a) were able to detect dichlorvos in chloroform extracts of the intestines. They also established, after *s.c.* application of 25 mg./kg. body wt. of P^{32}-trichlorfon, a slower decrease in concentration in the intestinal contents than in blood because of the lower activity of phosphate-cleaving enzymes.

The half-life of trichlorfon in meat of pigs is approximately two hours (SCHWARZ and DEDEK 1966 a); it was influenced *in vitro* by the acidifying capacity per time unit and the values *in vivo* were dependent on a possible after-resorption, which varied with the mode of application. The concentration decreased in six to seven hours one power of ten. In the back meat 5.0, 1.0, and 0.5 p.p.m. of trichlorfon activity after two, seven, and nine hours,

---

(III) a. Dichlorvos undergoes enzymatic reactions; enzyme-phosphate esters are formed.

b. 1. During reactions with B-esterases (for instance, acteylcholine esterases) relative stable products are formed, which lead to the well-known toxic symptoms.

2. In these cases the hydrolysis is slow; the hydrolysis product is dimethylphosphoric acid.

3. Dimethylphosphoric acid is excreted as such.

4. Dimethylphosphoric acid can also be demethylated and be excreted afterwards as monomethylphosphoric acid and orthophosphate.

c. Reaction products of dichlorvos with A-esterases are immediately cleaved by hydrolysis; one part is transformed to dimethylphosphoric acid.

d. During acyl residue transfer to the enzyme, the rest of the dichlorvos molecule is cleaved off as dichlorovinyl alcohol and is transformed into dichloroacetaldehyde.

respectively, were found. Extrapolated values for 13 to 14, 19 to 21, and 25 to 28 hours were 0.1, 0.01, and 0.001 p.p.m., respectively.

After application by the pour-on method the cutaneous resorption led also to detectable blood levels; however, the carrier solvents were of considerable importance (Dedek and Schwarz 1966 a). The highest blood level of approximately 3.1 p.p.m. was reached with the use of two percent mineral oil formulations (70 mg./100 kg.) after one to two hours. After three hours the level was again under 0.5 p.p.m. After application of 500 mg. of a two percent aqueous trichlorfon solution (20 to 30 mg./kg. body wt.) along the back line, a maximum value of 0.2 p.p.m. of trichlorfon in the blood of milk cows was reached after one to four hours, while the total activity with 0.6 to 0.9 p.p.m. was clearly higher (Schwarz and Dedek 1966 b). The resorption rate was lower from an aqueous solution than from a pour-on formulation. Both 100- and 300 ml. pour-on applications of a 5.7 percent P^{32}-trichlorfon solution led to a time-independent trichlorfon level in blood. The total activity was higher and contained degradation products which were rapidly excreted with the urine. Maximum residues in blood were between ten and 16 hours and reached averages of 0.46 and 0.11 p.p.m., respectively. Concentrations after 60 hours were still 0.1 and <0.02 p.p.m., respectively (milk 14 to 18 hours, 0.5 p.p.m.) (Schwarz and Dedek 1965 b). These tests reflected the importance of the vehicle, the mode of application, and the area wetted.

Behrenz (1959) determined trichlorfon residues in the meat of sheep and cattle, after *per os* application, biologically with 1.5-day old *Chrysomia chlorophyga* or *Lucilia sericata* larvae; concentrations of 0.00001 percent were detectable with this method. One hour after *per os* treatment of sheep with 120 mg./kg., and cattle with 100 mg./kg., of trichlorfon a maximum ten-p.p.m. residue was reached in muscle tissue. Kidneys contained the largest quantity of up to 100 p.p.m. after one hour. Four-to-six hours after treatment residues could no longer be detected (<0.1 p.p.m.). These values are in Table CLVIII.

Möllhof (1967) gave the calculated absolute values according to the data by Behrenz (1959) as in Table CLIX.

Trichlorfon was extensively decomposed in the mammal organism and excreted (Bolle 1956). Dedek and Schwarz (1966 a) reported the half-life

Table CLVIII. *Biologically active trichlorfon residues in sheep and cattle after per os treatment* (Behrenz 1959).

Hours after treatment	Residue (%)	
	Sheep muscle (120 mg./kg.)	Cattle liver (100 mg./kg.)
1	0.001–0.0001	0
2	0.00001	0
4	—	—
6	$<$ 0.00001	0

of cleavage in serum for trichlorfon and dichlorvos, as follows[35]: cattle blood stabilized with oxalate, 62 and 38 minutes, respectively, and cattle serum without oxalate addition, 32 and 28 minutes, respectively. The half-life *in vivo* in cattle blood was six to eight minutes.

Table CLIX. *Trichlorfon residues in tissues after oral treatment* [a] *of sheep with Neguvon tablets* (MÖLLHOFF 1967).

Tissue	Residues (p.p.m.) after		
	1 hr. [b, c] (4 animals)	2 hr. [b, c] (1 animal)	6 hr. [b, c] (2 animals)
Upper thigh			
Right	1–10	~ 0.1	n.d.
Left	1–10	~ 0.1	
Back			
Inside	1–10	< 0.1	n.d.– < 0.1
Outside	1–10	0.1	n.d.– < 0.1
Kidney			
Right	10–100	0.1–1.0	n.d.– < 0.1
Left	10–100	< 0.1	n.d.–< 0.1
Liver	n. d.	n. d.	n. d.

[a] 1.5 times normal dosage, or 120 mg./kg. body wt.
[b] Time between treatment and slaughter.
[c] n. d. = none detectable.

After *per os* application of P^{32}-trichlorfon to cattle at 40 mg./kg., 32.6 mg./kg. (0.13 percent) was found in blood after three hours, 6.5 mg./kg. (0.03 percent) after 12 hours, and 0.7 mg./kg. (0.003 percent) after 45 hours (BOLLE 1956). Investigations of metabolism by ROBBINS *et al.* (1956) with 25 mg./kg. of P^{32}-trichlorfon in *per os* treatment of cattle resulted in maximum radioactivity in blood of 15.1 μg.-equiv./ml. after two hours. After 24 hours, the radioactivity decreased to 0.55 μg.-equiv./ml. Only a small part of the radioactivity originated from unchanged effective substance (1.1 μg. trichlorfon/ml. after two hours). Dichlorvos was not found after *per os* treatment. These tests by ROBBINS *et al.* (1956) were questioned by KÜHNERT *et al.* (1963) because no statement was possible for the whereabouts of more than 30 percent of the P^{32}-trichlorfon. Therefore, P^{32}-Bubulin (a combination product which, aside from 500 g. of trichlorfon also contains five g. of PAM and 1.5 g. of atropine sulfate/liter to increase compatibility) was applied by KÜHNERT *et al.* (1963) to cattle in quantities of 20 mg./kg. *i.v.* and 25 mg./kg. *i.m.* Maximum concentration in blood was reached after two minutes for *i.v.* application, and after one hour for *i.m.* application. Degradation after *i.v.* treatment was rapid: after six to eight minutes half the activity could no longer be extracted; 95 percent of the trichlorfon was decomposed after one hour. Very little dichlorvos occurred

[35] Compare also data in Table CLVI according to DEDEK (1966).

for one to four minutes during the degradation. The decomposition went to phosphate and, eventually, to dimethylphosphate. After *i.m.* injection trichlorfon was detectable in blood for four to six hours; however, it was not possible to detect dichlorvos.

Also after *per os* application of 40 mg./kg. to cattle, P^{32}-trichlorfon left the body, mainly with the urine. Three hours after application, 28 percent of the applied total activity was eliminated through this pathway (Bolle 1956). Only 0.28 percent of the starting activity was detected after 45 hours. According to Robbins *et al.* (1956), the excretion of P^{32}-trichlorfon with the urine of cattle reached its maximum after 2.5 hours; 44 percent of the dosage applied was in the urine after 5.5 hours, and 66 percent after 24 hours, less than 0.5 percent of which was unchanged trichlorfon during the first 12 hours. Of the radioactive products in the 12-hour urine, 77 percent was an unknown metabolite and 16.8 percent was dimethylphosphate and/or dimethylphosphite. Excretion with the feces remained low with three percent of the total activity.

Actual residues in tissues were low, which can easily be understood from the unstable metabolic behaviour of trichlorfon. Thus, Behrenz (1959) established with a biological method that, after an oral application of 100 mg. of trichlorfon/kg. body wt., the highest concentration of active substance in the muscle meat of cattle was reached after one hour and was 0.01 to 0.001 percent. Table CLX contains calculations of concentrations established by Behrenz (1959).

Table CLX. *Trichlorfon residues in muscle meat of cattle after oral treatment* [a] (Möllhoff 1967).

Residue (p.p.m.) after			
1 hr. [b]	2 hr. [b]	4 hr. [b]	6 hr. [b]
10–100	1–10	⩽ 0.1	n. d. [c]

[a] 100 mg./kg. body weight.
[b] Time between treatment and sampling.
[c] n. d. = none detectable.

After *per os* application of 40 mg. of trichlorfon/kg. body wt., 25.6 mg./kg. of skin (0.1 percent) existed after three hours in the skin of cattle (Bolle 1956).

Kedenburg (1965) treated "Höhenfleckvieh" cows with 210 ml. of a six percent trichlorfon pour-on formulation in white oil at 12.6 g./animal. The residues were below the limit of detection 21 days after treatment in liver, kidney, muscle, kidney fat, and *s.c.* fatty tissue. Residue data after dermal resorption were investigated by Adkins (1966). Twenty-four hours after application of a three percent aqueous solution, or an eight percent oily or aqueous pour-on formulation, the residues were low in muscle samples of cattle. Kidney, fat, and liver contained no detectable residues (<0.1 p.p.m.).

Omental fat reached a maximum for two animals of 3.8 to 9.2 p.p.m. and the back fat 0.2 p.p.m. All organ samples were free of residues seven to 14 days after treatment (Table CLXI).

The following can be said for trichlorfon from the various experimental data as a summarization. The inactivation to noninsecticidal substances occurs within four to six hours for cattle and sheep. The maximum concentration in meat is reached about one hour after treatment; it decreases in four to six hours to <0.1 p.p.m., demonstrating that meat is practically free of effective substance six hours after treatment.

Table CLXI. *Residues in cattle tissues after trichlorfon treatment with pour-on applications* (ADKINS 1966).

Tissue	Residue (p.p.m.) [a] after					
	8% aqueous		Oily		3% aqueous	
	1 day	3 days	1 day	3 days	1 day	3 days
Liver	—	—	< 0.1	< 0.1	< 0.1	< 0.1
Kidney	< 0.1	< 0.1	< 0.1	0.2, < 0.1	—	—
Brain	—	—	0.1, 0.2	0.1, < 0.1	—	—
Heart	—	—	0.2	< 0.1	—	—
Leg muscle	< 0.1	< 0.1	0.2, 0.1	< 0.1	< 0.1	< 0.1
Rump muscle	—	—	0.2, 0.1	0.2, 0.1	0.2	0.2, < 0.1
Filet muscle	—	—	< 0.3, < 0.1	0.1, < 0.1	< 0.1	< 0.1
Omental fat	3.2, 9.2	< 0.1, 0.4	0.6, < 0.1	2.3, < 0.1	3.8, 0.1	0.4, < 0.1
Renal fat	< 0.1	< 0.1	< 0.1	< 0.1	< 0.1	< 0.1
Back fat	0.2, < 0.1	< 0.1	< 0.1	0.1, < 0.1	0.1, 0.1	0.2, < 0.1

[a] Duplicate numbers from separate animals.

Remarks for evaluation: Residue quantities after application of trichlorfon are small; they decrease extraordinarily rapidly depending on the time after application. For animals which had been slaughtered very shortly after a therapeutical treatment, the cooking process destroyed the substance, even if it was present in 100- to 1,000-fold quantity. After a one-hour cooking period the trichlorfon content decreased to values which could no longer be measured biologically (BEHRENZ 1959). SCHENK (1967) also succeded in obtaining residue-free meat by cooking 1.5 hours, even when extremely high concentrations of, for instance, 400 p.p.m. were present. Also, no deviations in taste could be established in cooked or fried meat (BEHRENZ 1959). The influence of trichlorfon on the digestive systems of mice, described by RENG and LIEM (1966), should be groundless because of their selection of very high but sublethal dosage for their discussion of the importance of tissue residues.

44. TRICHLORFON, BUTYRIC ACID ESTER (BUTONATE). — The *n*-butyric acid ester of trichlorfon, or butonate [butyric acid, ester with dimethyl-(2,2,2-trichloro-1-hydroxyethyl) phosphonate], exhibited a lower toxicity for warm-blooded animals (oral LD_{50} 1,000 to 2,000 mg./kg., rat) but the same insecticidal effect. Butonate had a half-life in cattle serum of only nine minutes *in vitro* and three to four minutes *in vivo* (DEDEK and SCHWARZ 1967). After *i.m.* application of 50 mg. of butonate/kg. body wt., maximum values in cattle blood reached only 0.1 p.p.m. which is connected with the low water-solubility and the consequently reduced resorption, and also with rapid decomposition (DEDEK and SCHWARZ 1967).

After pour-on application (300 ml. of a five percent solution = 40 mg./kg. body wt.) of a special P^{32}-butonate formulation, there was good resorption. Total radioactivity measured in the blood was ten percent in the beginning and only two percent unchanged butonate after six hours. Extractable toxic fractions were established by DEDEK and SCHWARZ (1967) with 30 percent in the beginning and ten percent later on. The persisting larger residue consisted of nonextractable, nontoxic degradation products. Maximum concentrations for butonate were 0.40 to 0.45 p.p.m. in one to three hours, and for the toxic metabolites 1.2 to 1.3 p.p.m. in two to four hours. DEDEK and SCHWARZ (1967) reported the degradation of butonate to yield dimethylphosphate (nontoxic and major amount of the nonextractable metabolites), trichlorfon, and desmethylbutonate (almost nontoxic, small amount).

Butonate is deacylated *in vitro* and *in vivo* at the α-C atom to form trichlorfon (ARTHUR and CASIDA 1958). Quantitative metabolic reports are in Table CLXII.

45. V-C 13 NEMACIDE. — Phosphorothioic acid, O-2,4-dichlorophenyl-O,O-diethyl ester

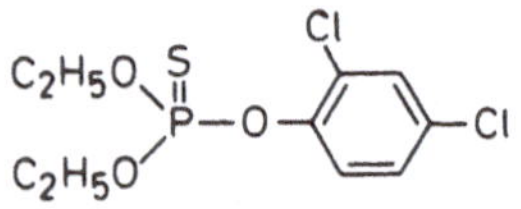

Alternate names: Nemacide.
Application: As spray against screw worm attack on animals; larvicide.
Toxicity: LD_{50} *per os* rat: 270 mg./kg. (MARTIN 1961). Nemacide is activated *in vivo* to a ChE inhibitor.
Detection: See CLABORN and IVEY (1964).
Metabolism and residues: IVEY *et al.* (1964) found in omental fatty tissues an average maximum for cattle after seven days of 5.5 p.p.m., 10.7 p.p.m. for sheep, and 16.3 p.p.m. for goats; corresponding values after two weeks were 2.7 p.p.m., 7.6 p.p.m., and 10.9 p.p.m. The residues were eliminated from the fat in six weeks for cattle and in eight weeks for other animals. No Nemacide residues were found after 57 days in the other tissues. After 27 days muscle meat of cattle contained no residues, but that of goats and sheep still contained 0.11 p.p.m. After 27 days renal fat of cattle contained 1.1 p.p.m. and of sheep and goats 3.6 and 1.2 p.p.m., respectively. Only on the second day after slaughtering were there significant detectable amounts in all organs of sheep; they were 18.7 p.p.m. in renal fat, 2.2 p.p.m. in muscle, 2.8 p.p.m. in heart, 0.1 p.p.m. in liver, 1.0 p.p.m. in kidney, and 1.1 p.p.m. in the brain.

Table CLXII. *Metabolic products from of P^{32}-butonate administered* [a] *to rats and in several biological systems* (ARTHUR and CASIDA 1958 b).

Biological system	Residue (%) present as		
	Butonate	Dichlorvos	Hydrolyzed (P–C)
Rat *in vivo*			
Fat	17.9	44 6	37.5
Liver	2.1	3.6	94.3
Rat *in vitro* [b]			
Liver homogenates, 1 hr.	54.1	28.2	17.7
Liver homogenates, 4 hr.	43.4	33.8	22.8
Kidney homogenates, 1 hr.	51.6	28.1	20.3
Kidney homogenates, 4 hr.	50.5	22.6	26.9
Human blood plasma [c]	65.1	0.9	34.0

[a] Female white rats treated orally with 2,000 mg./kg.; assayed four hours later.
[b] Twenty percent liver and kidney homogenates in saline solution (pH 7.2) containing 1,000 p.p.m. of insecticide.
[c] Human blood plasma (pH 7.2) containing 400 p.p.m. of butonate incubated one hour at room temperature.

Residues of the hydrolysis product 2,4-dichlorophenol were not established seven and 14 days after slaughtering; on the contrary, two days after slaughtering contents of this phenol in sheep heart, liver, and kidney were 0.3, 0.08, and 0.25 p.p.m., respectively.

Summary *

Out of a wide range of synthetically produced organic phosphorus esters it was possible to extract only a few from the literature regarding information on their residues in the tissue of domestic animals. The manner of application or of contamination stipulates the incorporation of variable quantities of active substance in the animal.

The therapeutics used in veterinary medicine involve as a result of their directness on the one hand, and because of the quantity applied on the other hand, the potentially higher estimated "danger". Primarily, the scale for such a danger is the animal itself, which would at first react with toxic symptoms. In any case, the active substance — being directly passed to the animal or taken up secondarily as a residue via plants — will be submitted to the attempts of the animal organism to detoxify it. In that way, for the human being as a meat consumer, "the risk of residues" is considerably diminished. The examples of the casuistic selection demonstrate that processes of hydrolysis and oxidation, and attempts at excretion by the body generally lead relatively rapidly to the destruction or elimination of the

* Translated by the authors.

active substances and/or their metabolites. The metabolites, for the most part, are of a lower toxicity than the original molecules of the active substance.

The primary compatibility of the active substance shown in the animal is an indication that in principle only lesser quantities can be passed on to the human being, and that thereby the danger of a possible secondary toxicity is diminished. First, the animal will react to the active substance and metabolites. A valuation of the danger caused by the absolute amount of active substance (or metabolite) being taken up in the meat inevitably differs from component to component. It depends as much on the metabolic processes (stability to hydrolysis) as on the habitudes and quantity of consumption which must be seen in relation to the absolute toxicity. Therefore, for the estimation of answers to these questions, details on toxicity and indications of metabolism have been taken up in this work as well.

Due to a lack of other standards, one should for the time being make use of the regulative for the so-called tolerance formula, as is commonly done in the field of plant protection. There is one restriction, however, and that is the tolerance figures are given in such a way as though the confrontation were only to take place with one active substance alone. So far, the questions dealing with the concurrence of several active substances ranging from medicines to food-preserving mixtures are completely obscure. These are the things that ought to be given far closer attention in the future.

Résumé *

Le problème des résidus dans la viande après application ou prise d'esters organophosphorés

Malgré le grand nombre d'esters organophosphorés de synthèse produits, la littérature ne donne des informations sur leurs résidus dans les tissus des animaux domestiques que pour très peu d'entre eux.

La voie d'application ou de contamination stipule l'incorporation de quantités variables de substances actives dans l'animal. Les thérapeutiques utilisées en médecine vétérinaire impliquent comme conséquence de leur spécificité d'une part et à cause des quantités appliquées d'autre part, un plus grand danger potentiel. Le danger est en premier lieu pour l'animal lui même, qui réagirait d'abord avec des symtomes toxiques. En tous cas, la substance active — appliquée directement à l'animal, ou prise secondairement comme résidu à partir des plantes — sera soumise aux effets de l'organisme pour la détoxifier. De cette manière, le risque de résidus est considérablement diminué pour les consommateurs de viande. Les exemples de la sélection casuistique démontrent que les processus d'hydrolyse et d'oxyda-

* Traduit par R. Mestres.

tion et les essais de rejet du corps conduisent généralement à une destruction ou une élimination relativement rapide des substances actives seules ou accompagnées de leurs métabolites. Les métabolites, pour la plus grande part, ont une toxicité plus faible que la molécule originale de la substance active.

La compatibilité primaire de la substance active avec l'animal indique en principe que de moindres quantités peuvent être transmises à l'homme et que le danger d'une possible toxicité secondaire est faible. En premier lieu, l'animal réagira avec la substance active et les métabolites. Une évaluation du danger causé par la quantité absolue de substance active (ou de métabolite) retenue par la viande diffère inévitablement d'un composé à un autre. Elle dépend autant du processus métabolique (stabilité à l'hydrolyse), que des habitudes et des quantités consommées qui peuvent être en relation avec la toxicité absolue. Ainsi, pour répondre à ces questions, des détails sur la toxicité et des indications de métabolismes ont été considérés dans ce travail.

En raison du manque d'autres normes, les règles pour l'établissement des soi-disant tolérances devraient être utilisées pour l'instant comme on le fait généralement dans le domaine de la protection des plantes. Il existe cependant une restriction puisque les chiffres des tolérances sont donnés sur considération des effets d'une seule substance active. Ainsi, les questions relatives à l'interaction de plusieurs substances actives allant des médicaments aux mélanges d'additifs alimentaires, sont totalement ignorées. Il conviendrait, dans l'avenir, de préter plus d'attention à ces questions.

Zusammenfassung *

Problematik der Rückstände im Fleisch schlachtbarer Haustiere nach Anwendung bzw. Aufnahme organischer Phosphorsäureester

Aus der großen Fülle synthetisch hergestellter organischer Phosphorsäureester konnten nur einige aus dem Schrifttum hinsichtlich der Angaben von Rückstandswerten im Gewebe der Haustiere herausgestellt werden. Die Art der Anwendung oder der Kontamination bedingt das Inkorporieren unterschiedlicher Wirkstoffmengen in die Tiere.

Die als veterinärmedizinische Therapeutika eingesetzten Produkte bringen durch ihre Unmittelbarkeit einerseits und infolge der Applikationsmenge andererseits die potentiell höher zu veranschlagende „Gefahr" mit sich. Maßstab einer solchen Gefahr ist primär das Tier selbst, das zuerst mit toxischen Erscheinungen antworten würde. In jedem Falle wird der Wirkstoff — direkt in das Tier verbracht oder sekundär über die Pflanze als Rückstand aufgenommen — dem Abbaubestreben des tierischen Organismus

* Original von den Autoren.

unterworfen. Das „Restrisiko" für den Menschen als Fleischkonsumenten ist dadurch stark verringert. Die Beispiele der kasuistischen Sammlung lassen erkennen, daß Hydrolysevorgänge, Oxydationsprozesse und Ausscheidungsbestrebungen des Körpers im allgemeinen relativ schnell zur Zerstörung bzw. Elimination der Wirkstoffe und/oder ihrer Metaboliten führen. Die Metaboliten sind zumeist von minderer Toxizität als die ursprünglichen Wirkstoffmoleküle.

Die primäre Verträglichkeit des Wirkstoffes am Tier gibt einen Hinweis darauf, daß auf den Menschen grundsätzlich nur geringere Quantitäten überkommen können, und daß sich damit die Gefahr einer (sekundären) Intoxikationsmöglichkeit verringert. Das Tier setzt sich zuvor mit Wirkstoff und Metaboliten auseinander. Eine Beurteilung der Gefahr durch die absolut aufgenommenen Wirkstoff-/Metaboliten-Menge mit dem Fleisch differiert zwangsläufig von Stoff zu Stoff. Sie hängt von den metabolischen Vorgängen (Hydrolysebeständigkeit) genauso ab wie von den Verzehrsgewohnheiten und Verzehrsmengen, die in Bezug zur absoluten Giftigkeit zu stellen sind. Zur Beurteilung dieser Fragenkomplexe wurden daher Toxizitätsangaben und Stoffwechselhinweise in die Arbeit mit aufgenommen. Infolge Fehlens anderer Maßstäbe sollte man sich zur Zeit der Regulative der sog. Toleranzformeln — wie im Pflanzenschutzbereich üblich — bedienen.

Jedoch besteht dabei die Einschränkung, daß die Bezugswerte sich so ausrichten, als ob die Konfrontation nur mit einem Wirkstoff erfolge. Völlig ungeklärt sind bisher die Fragen, die sich um das Zusammentreffen von mehreren Wirkstoffen (Wirkstoffrendezvous) ranken und vom Arzneimittel bis zum Lebensmittelkonservierungszusatz reichen. Hierauf müßte das Augenmerk künftig viel stärker gerichtet werden.

References

ACKERMANN, H.: Studien zur Analytik biologisch aktiver Phosphor-, Thiophosphor- und Phosphonsäureester mit Hilfe eines kombinierten dünnschichtchromatographisch-enzymatischen Verfahrens unter besonderer Berücksichtigung toxikologischer Aspekte. Habil. Schr. Humboldt-Universität Berlin (1967).

—, and R. ENGST: Vorkommen von phosphororganischen Insektiziden im Fetus. Arch. Toxicol. **26**, 17 (1970).

—, B. LEXOW, and E. PLEWKA: Nachweis und Identifizierung von Insektiziden Phosphor-, Thiophosphor-, Phosphon- und Carbaminsäureestern in biologischem Material. Arch. Toxicol. **24**, 316 (1969).

ADAMS, J. M., and C. A. ANDERSON: Spectrophotofluorometric method for Guthion residues in milk and animal tissues. J. Agr. Food Chem. **14**, 53 (1966).

ADKINS, T. R., Jr.: Residues in cattle tissues following back-line and spray application of Trichlorfon. J. Econ. Entomol. **59**, 1423 (1966).

—, D. H. KROPF, and S. G. WOODS: Residue deposition of Co-Ral in the tissues of back-line-treated cattle. J. Econ. Entomol. **56**, 759 (1963).

AHMED, M. K., J. E. CASIDA, and R. E. NICHOLS: Bovine metabolism of organophosphorus insecticides significance of rumen fluid with particular reference to parathion. J. Agr. Food Chem. **6**, 740 (1958).

AKINTONWA, D. A. A., and D. H. HUTSON: Metabolism of 2-chloro-1-(2,4,5-trichlorphenyl)vinyl dimethylphosphate in the dog and rat. J. Agr. Food Chem. **15**, 632 (1967).
ALDRIDGE, W. N.: Some properties of specific cholinesterase with particular reference to the mechanism of inhibition of diethyl *p*-nitrophenyl thiophosphate (E 605) and analogues. Biochem. J. **46**, 451 (1950).
— Serum esterasis. An enzyme hydrolysing diethyl *p*-nitrophenol phosphate (E 600) and its identity with the A-esterase of mammalian sera. 2. Communication. Biochem. J. **53**, 117 (1953).
—, and J. M. BARNES: Some problems in assessing the toxicity of the organophosphorus insecticides towards mammals. Nature **169**, 345 (1952).
ALICATO, J. E.: Incidence of parasites in calves in Hawaii and the treatment of *Cooperia punctata* with special reference to the efficacy of Ruelene. Amer. J. Vet. Research **21**, 440 (1960).
ALLEN, A. D.: Selbstbehandlung zur Kontrolle der kleinen Stech- oder Hornfliege an Rindern. Vet. Med. Nachr. **3**, 210 (1966).
ANDERSON, C. A., J. M. ADAMS, and D. MCDOUGALL: Photofluorometric method for determination of Co-Ral residues in animal tissues. J. Agr. Food Chem. **7**, 256 (1959).
ANDERSON, R. J.: The responsibilities of veterinary practitioners as to the use of pesticides. J. Amer. Vet. Assoc. **147**, 1584 (1965).
—, C. A. ANDERSON, and T. J. OLSON: A gas-liquid chromatographic method for the determination of Trichlorfon in plant and animal tissues. J. Agr. Food Chem. **14**, 508 (1966 a).
— —, and M. L. YAGELOWICH: A photofluorometric method for the determination of Maretin (N-hydroxy-naphthalimide diethylphosphate) residues in animal tissues. J. Agr. Food Chem. **14**, 43 (1966 b).
—, J. S. THORNTON, C. A. ANDERSON, and D. B. KATAGUE: Determination of Fenthion residues in plant and animal tissues by electron-capture gas chromatography. J. Agr. Food Chem. **14**, 619 (1966 c).
ANLIKER, R., K. SCHMID, and R. BLATTNER-GESELL: Metabolism of phosphamidon by rat-liver homogenates. Ciba-Schrift CCI No. 0850 (1964).
ANONYMOUS 1: Ruelene. In: The Merck veterinary manual, 3ed., p. 1045. Rahway, N. J.: Merck & Co. (1967).
— 2: Chemikalien in unserer Umwelt. Nachr. Chemie Techn. **16**, 44 (1968).
— 3: Fleischverbrauch wird weiter steigen. Kraftfutter **51**, 198 (1968).
— 4: Residue problems compounded by big feedlots. J. Amer. Vet. Med. Assoc. **151**, 741 (1967).
— 5: Study on pesticide residues in food. J. Amer. Vet. Med. Assoc. **147**, 468 (1965).
— 6: Feed additive compendium, 1967. p. 332. Minneapolis: Miller Publishing Co. (1966).
— 7: Asuntol 50%iges Netzpulver. "Bayer" Leverkusen D. 4–636/30031, wissensch. Prospekt.
— 8: Maretin. "Bayer" Leverkusen D. 1–627/30758, wissensch. Prospekt.
— 9: Tiguvon. "Bayer" Leverkusen D. 1–6106/30638, wissensch. Prospekt.
— 10: Bromophos. "Cela" Ingelheim, Ausg. Nov. 1965, wissensch. Dokumentation.
— 11: Co-Ral 25% wettable powder. "Chemagro Corporation" CO 3–658, wissensch. Prospekt.
— 12: Guthion (Bayer 17147). "Chemagro Corp.", wissensch. Prospekt.
— 13: Investigation on the excretion of phosphamidon by rats and cattle given single doses or diets containing C^{14}-labelled phosphamidon. "CIBA" AG Basel 0055, wissensch. Dokumentation.
— 14: Dimecron. "CIBA" AG Basel, 1967, wissensch. Dokumentation.
— 15: Kommission für Pflanzenschutz-, Pflanzenbehandlungs- und Vorratsschutzmittel. II. Mittlg. Deutsche Forschungsgemeinschaft, Bad Godesberg, März (1962).
— 16: Kommission für Pflanzenschutz-, Pflanzenbehandlungs- und Vorratsschutzmittel. IV. Mittlg. Deutsche Forschungsgemeinschaft, Bad Godesberg, April (1965).
— 17: Kommission für Pflanzenschutz-, Pflanzenbehandlungs- und Vorratsschutzmittel. III. Mittlg. Deutsche Forschungsgemeinschaft, Bad Godesberg, April (1965).

ANONYMOUS 18: EPN technical data sheet. "Du Pont de Nemours & Co.", Wilmington, Del., wissensch. Dokumentation, Feb. (1967).
— 19: FDA proposes policy statement on negligible pesticide residues. Feedstuffs **40** (9), 8 (1968).
— 20: FAO-agricultural studies No. 73, "Pesticide Residues in Food." WHO-Tech. Rept. Series No. 370, Rome (1967).
— 21: What's New in Food and Drug Research No. 50, p. 4 (1967).
— 22: More on negligible residues. What's New in Food and Drug Research, p. 4, Oct. (1967).
— 23: Monitoring pesticides for safety. What's New in Food and Drug Research, p. 4, June (1967).
— 24: Pesticide residues no cause for alarm. What's New in Food and Drug Research, p. 3, Oct. (1968).
— 25: Diazinon zur Bekämpfung von Ektoparasiten an Haustieren, Stand 1962/63. Information aus der Abt. für Schädlingsbekämpfung "J. R. Geigy AG", Basel.
— 26: Diazinon formulations. Tech. Bull. No. 65–1, GAC 100–265. "Geigy Agricultural Chemicals", Ardsley, N. Y.
— 27: Schriftliche Mitteilung. "Geigy AG", Basel, 8–59.
— 28: Results of tests on the amount of residue remaining including a description of the analytical method used. "Hercules Powder Co.", Section D, Kerrville/Tex.-Corvallis/Ore.
— 29: Warbex. "Lederle", München, 17/6095/3000, wissensch. Prospekt.
— 30: Federal Register, part 120, p. 8758, Sept. (1962).
— 31: Ungarische Höchstmengenverordnung. Mezögazdasági és Elelmezésügyi Ertesitö (Gesetzblatt), Sept. 2 (1970).
— 32: Ronnel petition filed. Feedstuffs **37** (13), 2 (1965).
— 33: WHO Tech. Rept. Series, No. 227. "Toxic Hazards of Pesticides to Man." Geneva (1962).
— 34: WHO Tech. Rept. Series, No. 240. "Principles Governing Consumer Safety in Relation to Pesticide Residues." Geneva (1962).
— 35: WHO Tech. Rept. Series, No. 144. "Procedures for the Testing of International Food Additives to Establish their Safety for Use." Geneva (1958).
— 36: Verordnung über Pflanzenschutz-, Schädlingsbekämpfungs- und Vorratsschutzmittel in oder auf Lebensmitteln pflanzlicher Herkunft (Höchstmenge – VO – Pflanzenschutz-). Nov. 30 (1966); Bundesgesetzblatt – Teil I (Nr. 53), S. 667, Dez. 10 (1966).
APPLEGATE, H. G., and G. CHITTWOOD: Automation of pesticide analysis. Bull. Environ. Contam. Toxicol. **3**, 211 (1968).
ARTERBERRY, J. D., W. F. DURHAM, J. W. ELLIOT, and H. R. WOLFE: Exposure to parathion. Arch. Environ. Health. **3**, 476 (1961).
ARTHUR, B. W., and J. E. CASIDA: Metabolism and selectivity of O,O-dimethyl 2,2,2-trichloro-1-hydroxyethyl phosponate and its acteyl and vinyl derivates. J. Agr. Food Chem. **5**, 186 (1957).
— — Biological and chemical oxidation of tetramethyl phosphorodiamidic fluoride (Dimefox). J. Econ. Entomol. **51**, 49 (1958 a).
— — Bilogical activity of several O,O-dialkyl *alpha*-acyloxyethyl phosphonates. J. Agr. Food Chem. **6**, 360 (1958 b).
— — Biological activity and metabolism of Hercules AC-528 components in rats and cockroaches. J. Econ. Entomol. **52**, 20 (1959).
ASKEW, J., and T. H. MITCHELL: The gas chromatographic examination of organophosphorus pesticides. V. The effect of cooking on organophosphorus pesticides residues. J. Chromatog. **32**, 417 (1968).
AVERELL, P. R., and M. V. NORRIS: Estimation of small amounts of O,O-diethyl O-*p*-nitrophenyl thiophosphate. Anal. Chem. **20**, 753 (1948).
BABAD, H., and T. N. TAYLOR: Nuclear magnetic resonance studies of the phosphorus pesticides. V, part II. A rapid determination of the isomer ratio of Systox. Anal. Chim. Acta **40**, 387 (1968).

Bär, F.: Tierarzneimittel und Aufzuchtmittel in der landwirtschaftlichen Praxis. Schriftenreihe Medizin und Ernährung 4. München: Pallas Verlag Dr. Edmund Gans (1964 a).

— Der Nachweis von Insektiziden in Nahrungsmitteln und die Bedeutung für die Gesundheit. Dtsch. Med. J. 15, 672 (1964 b).

Baker, N. F., and A. P. Douglas: Trial with a new organic phosphate as an anthelmintic in cattle. Amer. J. Vet. Research 20, 278 (1959).

Barnes, J. M., and F. A. Denz: Experimental demyelination with organophosphorus compounds. J. Pathol. Bacteriol. 65, 598 (1953).

Batchelder, G. H., G, G. Patchett, and J. J. Menn: Methyl Trithion. In G. Zweig (ed.): Analytical methods for pesticides, plant growth regulators, and food additives, Vol. II. New York-London: Academic Press (1964).

Batte, E. G., D. J. Moncol, A. C. Todd, and R. S. Isenstein: Critical evaluation of an anthelmintic for swine. Vet. Med. 60, 539 (1965).

Bäumler, J., and S. Rippstein: Gaschromatographische Bestimmung von Insektiziden im Blut mit dem Halogen-Phosphor-Detektor. Arch. Toxicol. 25, 57 (1969).

Bauriedel, W. R., and M. O. Swank: Residue and metabolism of radioactive 4-tert.-butyl-2-chlorophenylmethyl methylphosphoramidate administered as a single oral dose to sheep. J. Agr. Food Chem. 10, 150 (1962).

Beck, J., and M. Sherman: Detection by thin-layer chromatography of organophosphorus insecticides in acutely poisoned rats and chickens. Acta Pharmacol. 26, 35 (1968).

Beck, W., J. Gebeshuber, D. Gesswagner, E. Glofke, E. Kahl, K. Lebeda, and E. Stastny: Beitrag zur Kenntnis der möglichen Beeinflussung von Wild durch Pflanzenschutzmittel. Pflanzensch.-Ber. 5/6/7, 69 (1968).

Beesley, W. N.: Die Anwendung systemisch wirkender Insektizide zur Dasselbekämpfung in England. Vet. Med. Nachr. 1, 28 (1966).

Behrenz, W.: Biologische Bestimmung des Wirkstoffgehaltes im Fleisch von Schafen und Rindern zu verschiedenen Zeiten nach peroraler Behandlung mit Neguvon. Arch. Lebensmittelhygiene 10, 64 (1959).

— Über die Ausscheidung von Neguvon in der Milch nach einmaliger oraler und perkutaner Anwendung des Präparates bei Milchkühen. Vet. Med. Nachr. 3, 133 (1961).

— Experimentelle Arbeiten mit Ektoparasiten der Schafe. Lujet, ein neues Präparat zur Ektoparasitenbekämpfung bei Schafen. Vet. Med. Nachr. 3, 34 (1962).

— Entwicklung systemisch wirkender Insektizide und Acarizide für die Veterinärmedizin. Medizin u. Chemie VII, 802 (1963).

—, M. Federmann, and W. R. Bolle: Experimentelle Arbeiten mit Ektoparasiten der Schafe. Bekämpfung und Verhütung des Ektoparasitenbefalles bei Schafen mit Asuntol und Neguvon im Dipverfahren. Vet. Med. Nachr. 4, 179 (1959).

Berg, S., E. K. Kuchinke, and K. Fischer: Zur Kenntnis der Vergiftung mit dem Schädlingsbekämpfungsmittel Potasan. Arch. Toxicol. 16, 105 (1956).

Betker, W. R., C. J. Cohen, N. J. Beaber, and D. M. Waleski: Determination of the isomer ratio of Systox. J. Agr. Food Chem. 14, 318 (1966).

Blinn, R. C.: Metabolic fate of Abate insecticide in the rat. J. Agr. Food Chem. 17, 118 (1969).

Bolle, W. R.: Neguvon, ein äußerlich und innerlich anwendbares Insektizid, Larvizid und Acarizid. Vet. Med. Nachr. 3, 155 (1956).

—, and B. Otte: Erfahrungen bei der oralen Anwendung von Neguvon gegen die Wanderlarven der Dasselfliege. Vet. Med. Nachr. 5, 211 (1958).

Bombinski, T. J., and K. P. Dubois: Toxicity and mechanism of action of Di-Syston. Arch. Ind. Health 17, 192 (1958).

Bourke, J. B., E. J. Broderik, L. R. Hackler, and P. C. Lippold: Comparative metabolism of malathion-C^{14} in plants and animals. J. Agr. Food Chem. 16, 585 (1968).

Bowman, J. S., and J. E. Casida: Further studies on the metabolism of Thimet by plants, insects and mammals. J. Econ. Entomol. 51, 838 (1958).

Bowman, M. C., M. Beroza, C. H. Gordon, R. W. Miller, and N. O. Morgan: A method of analyzing the milk and feces of cows for Coumaphos for control of house fly larvae. J. Econ. Entomol. 61, 358 (1968).

BOYD, N. R., and B. W. ARTHUR: Biological degradation of O,O-diethyl-O-naphthalimido phosphorothioate. J. Econ. Entomol. **53**, 848 (1960).

BRADY, U. E., and B. W. ARTHUR: Metabolism of O,O-dimethyl-O-[4-(methyl-thio)-*m*-tolyl] phosphorothioate by white rats. J. Econ. Entomol. **54**, 1232 (1961).

— — Biological and chemical properties of dimethoate and related derivates. J. Econ. Entomol. **56**, 477 (1963).

—, H. W. DOROUGH, and B. W. ARTHUR: Selective toxicity and animal systemic effectiveness of several organophosphates. J. Econ. Entomol. **53**, 6 (1960).

BRAUN, H., and D. R. KLIMMER: 1. Die Entwicklung des chemischen Pflanzenschutzes und ihre Auswirkungen. 2. Toxikologische Probleme im Pflanzenschutz. Arbeitsgemeinschaft für Forschung des Landes Nordrhein-Westfalen. Köln/Opladen: Westdeutscher Verlag (1966).

BRODERICK, E. J., E. F. TASCHENBERG, L. J. HICKS, A. W. AVENS, and J. B. BOURKE: Rapid method for surface residues of organosphosphorus pesticides by total phosphorus. J. Agr. Food Chem. **15**, 454 (1967).

BRODEUR, J., and K. P. DU BOIS: Studies on factors influencing the acute toxicity of malathion and malaoxon in rats. Canad. J. Phys. Pharm. **45**, 621 (1967).

BROGDON, J. L., and E. H. DAWSON: Flavor evaluations of meat from Ruelene-treated animals. J. Econ. Entomol. **58**, 169 (1965).

—, M. E. KIRKPATRICK, and E. H. DAWSON: Flavor of meat from animals treated with malathion, Ronnel, or Co-Ral. J. Agr. Food Chem. **10**, 34 (1962).

BRUCE, W. N.: Detector cell for measuring picogram quantities of organophosphorus insectizides, pyrethrin synergists and other compounds by gas chromatography. J. Agr. Food Chem. **15**, 178 (1967).

BULL, D. L.: Metabolism of Di-Syston by insects, isolated cotton leaves and rats. J. Econ. Entomol. **58**, 249 (1965).

— Metabolism of O,O-dimethyl phosphorodithioate *S*-ester with 4-(mercaptomethyl)-2-methoxy-Δ^2-1,3,4 thiadiazolin-5-one. J. Agr. Food Chem. **16**, 610 (1968).

—, and D. A. LINDQUIST: Metabolism of 3-hydroxy-*N,N*-dimethylcrotonamide dimethylphosphate by cotton plants, insects and rats. J. Agr. Food Chem. **12**, 310 (1964).

— — Metabolism of 3-hydroxy-*N*-methyl-cis-crotonamide dimethylphosphate (Azodrin) by insects and rats. J. Agr. Food Chem. **14**, 103 (1966).

— —, and R. R. GRABBE: Comparative fate of the geometric isomers of phosphamidon in plants and animals. J. Econ. Entomol. **60**, 332 (1967).

—, and R. L. RIDGWAY: Metabolism of trichlorfon in animals and plants. J. Agr. Food Chem. **17**, 837 (1969).

BUNYAN, B. J., D. M. JENNINGS, and A. TAYLOR: Organophosphorus poisoning. J. Agr. Food Chem. **16**, 322 (1968).

— — — Organophosphorus poisoning: Chronic feeding of some common pesticides to pheasants and pigeons. J. Agr. Food Chem. **17**, 1027 (1967).

— — — Esterase inhibition in pheasants poisoned by O,O-diethyl *S*-(ethylthiomethyl)-phosphorodithioate (Thimet). J. Agr. Food Chem. **14**, 132 (1966).

BURGER, E.: Beitrag zum Nachweis von E 605. Arch. Toxicol. **16**, 401 (1957).

—, and W. JANSSEN: Akute tödliche Phosdrinvergiftung. Arch. Kriminol. **135**, 34 (1965).

BURNS, E. C., S. E. MCCRAINE, and D. W. MOODY: Ronnel and Co-Ral for horn fly control on cable-type back rubbers. J. Econ. Entomol. **52**, 648 (1959).

BUTTRAM, J. R., and B. W. ARTHUR: Absorption and metabolism of Bayer 22408 by dairy cows and residues in the milk. J. Econ. Entomol. **54**, 446 (1961 a).

— — Magnitude and nature of residues in tissues and eggs of poultry receiving Ruelene in the feed. J. Econ. Entomol. **54**, 456 (1961 b).

CAMP, H. B., T. R. FUKUTO, and R. L. METCALF: Selective toxicity of isopropyl parathion. J. Agr. Food Chem. **17**, 249 (1969).

CASIDA, J. M.: Metabolism of organophosphorus insecticides in relation to their antiesteraseactivity, stability and residual properties. J. Agr. Food Chem. **4**, 772 (1956).

—, T. C. ALLEN, and M. A. STAHMANN: Mammalian conversion of octamethylpyrophosphoramide to a toxic phosphoramide *N*-oxide. J. Biol. Chem. **210**, 607 (1954).

CASIDA, J. M., P. E. GATTERDAM, L. W. GETZIN, jr., and R. K. CHAPMAN: Residual properties of the systemic insecticide O,O-dimethyl 1-carbomethoxy-1-propen-2-yl phosphate. J. Agr. Food Chem. **4,** 236 (1956).
— —, J. B. KNAAK, R. D. LANCE, and R. P. NIEDERMEIER: Bovine metabolism of organophosphate insecticides. Subacute feeding studies with O,O-dimethyl 1-carbomethoxy-1-propen-2-yl phosphate. J. Agr. Food Chem. **6,** 658 (1958).
—, and D. M. SANDERSON: Reaction of certain phosphorothionate insecticides with alcohol and potentiation by breakdown products. J. Agr. Food Chem. **11,** 91 (1963).
CASSIDY, J. E., R. T. MURPHY, A. M. MATTSON, and R. A. KAHRS: Fate of *S*-[(2-methoxy-5-oxo-Δ^2-1,3,4-thiadiazolin-4-yl)methyl] O,O-dimethyl phosphorodithioate (Supracide) in a lactating cow. J. Agr. Food Chem. **17,** 571 (1969).
CESARO, A. N., A. GRANATA, and D. GERMANO: Altération des oxydases par les substances phytopharmaceutiques parasiticides. Application pratique pour une évaluation toxicologique. Arch. Mal. Prof. **25,** 481 (1964).
CHAMBERLAIN, W. F.: Excretory pattern and chromatography of urine, urine extracts, and residues from milk of cow treated with C^{14}-labeled phosphamidon. Ciba Druckschrift CCL No. 1440 D (1960).
— The metabolism of P^{32}-labelled Shell SD-4294 in a lactating ewe. J. Econ Entomol. **57,** 119 (1964 a).
— The metabolism of P^{32}-labeled Ciodrin in a lactating goat. J. Econ. Entomol. **57,** 329 (1964 b).
— A study of the dermal treatment of a steer with C^{14}-labeled Imidan. J. Econ. Entomol. **58,** 51 (1965).
—, P. E. GATTERDAM, and D. E. HOPKINS: Metabolism of P^{32}-Delnav in cattle. J. Econ. Entomol. **53,** 672 (1960).
— — — The metabolism of P^{32}-labeled dimethoate in sheep. J. Econ. Entomol. **54,** 733 (1961).
—, and D. E. HOPKINS: Absorption and elimination of General Chemical 4072 applied dermally to cattle. J. Econ. Entomol. **55,** 86 (1962).
CHENG, K. K.: A technique for total hepatectomy in the rat and its effect on toxicity of octamethyl pyrophosphoramide. Brit. J. Expt. Pathol. **31,** 44 (1951).
CHENG, T. H., D. E. H. FREAR, and H. F. ENOS, Jr.: Fly control in dairy barns sprayed with dimethoate and the determination of dimethoate residues in milk. J. Econ. Entomol. **54,** 740 (1961).
CHRISTEN, P. J., and E. M. COHEN: Stereospecificity of the enzymatic hydrolysis of Sarin in rat plasma. Acta Physiol. Pharmacol. Neerl. **12,** 286 (1963).
—, and J. A. C. M. VAN DEN MUYSENBERG: The enzymatic isolation and fluoride catalysed racemisation of optically active Sarin. Biochim. Biophys. Acta **110,** 217 (1965).
CLABORN, H. V., R. C. BUSHLAND, H. D. MANN, M. C. IVEY, and R. D. RADELEFF: Meat and milk residues from livestock sprays. J. Agr. Food Chem. **8,** 439 (1960 a).
—, R. A. HOFFMAN, W. D. MANN, and D. D. OEHLER: Residues of Dursban and its oxygen analog in the body tissues of treated cattle. J. Econ. Entomol. **61,** 983 (1968).
—, and M. C. IVEY: Colorimetric determination of Nemacide and Ronnel in animal tissues. J. Assoc. Official Agr. Chemists **47,** 871 (1964).
— — Determination of O,O-dimethyl O-2,4,5-trichlorphenyl phosphorothioate in animal tissues and milk. J. Agr. Food Chem. **13,** 353 (1965 a).
— — Determination of 2-chloro-1-(2,4-dichlorphenyl)vinyl diethyl phosphate and 2,2′,4′-trichloroacetophenone in animal tissues and milk. J. Agr. Food Chem. **13,** 354 (1965 b).
— —, and H. D. MANN: A colorimetric method for the determination of Co-Ral in animal tissues. J. Econ. Entomol. **53,** 263 (1960 b).
—, H. D. MANN, I. L. BERRY, and R. A. HOFFMAN: Comparisons of residues in milk resulting from two types of spray applications of DDT, Shell Compound 4072, and Ronnel. J. Econ. Entomol. **58,** 922 (1965 c).
— —, and R. D. RADELEFF: Pesticide residues in meat and milk: A research report. Agr. Research Service, *United States Department of Agriculture* (1960).

CLABORN, H. V., H. D. MANN, R. L. YOUNGER, and R. D. RADELEFF: Diazinon residues in the fat of sprayed cattle. J. Econ. Entomol. **56**, 858 (1963).
—, R. D. RADELEFF, H. F. BECKMAN, and G. T. WOODARD: Malathion in milk and fat from sprayed cattle. J. Agr. Food Chem. **4**, 941 (1956).
CLARK, D. E., R. L. YOUNGER, and C. H. AYALA: Toxicosis and residues in Bromophos-dipped sheep. J. Agr. Food Chem. **14**, 608 (1966).
v. CLARMANN, M., and M. GELDMACHER-V. MALLINCKRODT: Über eine erfolgreich behandelte akute orale Vergiftung durch Fenthion und dessen Nachweis in Mageninhalt und Harn. Arch. Toxicol. **22**, 2 (1966).
CLEMONS, G. P., and R. E. MENZER: Oxidative metabolism of phosphamidon in rats and a goat. J. Agr. Food Chem. **16**, 2 (1968).
CLEVELAND, F. P., and J. F. TREON. Response of experimental animals to Phosdrin insecticide in their daily diets. J. Agr. Food Chem. **9**, 484 (1961).
COCHRANE, D. G.: A new insecticide based on DDVP. J. Agr. Vet. Chemicals **4**, 72 (1963).
COHEN, J. A., P. J. CRISTEN, and E. MOBACH: The mode of action of diacetylmonoxime (DAM) as an antidote against Sarin poisoning. Biochem. Pharmacol. **8**, 120 (1961).
—, and M. G. P. J. WARRINGA: The fate of P^{32}-labelled diisopropylfluorophosphonate in the human body and its use as a labelling agent in the study of the turnover of blood plasma and red cells. J. Clin. Invest. **33**, 459 (1954).
CONROY, H. W.: Report on malathion. J. Assoc. Official Agr. Chemists **40**, 230 (1957).
COOK, J. W.: Report on the determination of insecticides by enzymatic methods. J. Assoc. Official Agr. Chemists **37**, 561 (1954).
— *In vitro* destruction of some organophosphate pesticides by bovine rumen fluid. J. Agr. Food Chem. **5**, 859 (1957).
— Persistence of residues in food. In C. O. CHICHESTER (ed.): Research in pesticides, p. 211. New York-London: Academic Press (1965).
—, and S. W. WILLIAMS: Pesticide residues. Anal. Chem. **37**, 130R (1965).
COREY, R. A., S. C. DORMAN, W. E. HALL, L. C. GLOVER, and R. R. WHETSTONE: Diethyl 2-chloroviny phosphate and dimethyl 1-carbomethoxy-1-propen-2-yl phosphate — Two new systemic phosphorus pesticides. Science **118**, 28 (1953 a).
— — — — Translocation studies with two new phosphate insecticides. J. Econ. Entomol. **46**, 386 (1953 b).
CORLEY, C., and M. BEROZA: Gas chromatographic determination of malathion and its oxygen analog, malaoxon. J. Agr. Food Chem. **16**, 2 (1968).
COX, D. D., A. D. ALLAN, and M. T. MULLEE: Ein Überblick über die pharmakologischen Eigenschaften des Tiguvon für die Anwendung beim Rind. II. Vet. Med. Nachr. **4**, 293 (1967).
CUMMINGS, J. G.: Pesticide residues in total diet samples. Assoc. Official Anal. Chemists **48**, 1177 (1965).
DAHM, P. H., F. C. FONTAINE, and J. E. PANKASKIE: The experimental feeding of parathion to dairy cows. Science **112**, 254 (1950 a).
— — —, R. C. SMITH, and F. W. ATKESON: The effects of feeding parathion to dairy cows. J. Dairy Sci. **33**, 747 (1950 b).
—, and N. L. JACOBSON: Effects of feeding Systox-treated alfalfa hay to dairy cows. J. Agr. Food Chem. **4**, 150 (1956).
DALE, W. E., and J. W. MILES: Gas chromatographic determination of Abate using flame photometric and electron-capture detectors. J. Agr. Food Chem. **17**, 60 (1969).
DANGSCHAT, H.: Zur Frage der Rückstände von Alkylphosphaten in der Muskulatur. Vet. Diss., München (1965).
DAUTERMAN, W. C., J. G. CASIDA, J. B. KNAAK, and T. KOWALCZYK: Bovine metabolism of organophosphorus inseticides. Metabolism and residues associated with oral administration of dimethoate to rats and three lactating cows. J. Agr. Food Chem. **7**, 188 (1959).
DAVISON, A. N.: The conversion of schradan (OMPA) and parathion into inhibitors of cholinesterase by mammalian liver. Biochem. J. **61**, 203 (1955).

DECKER, G. C.: Significance of pesticide residues in milk and meat. J. Agr. Food Chem. **7**, 681 (1959).

DEDEK, W.: Beiträge zur Analytik systemischer insektizider Phosphorsäureester in biologischen Medien mit Hilfe P^{32}-markierter Verbindungen. Vet. Habil., Leipzig (1966).

—, and M. KÜHNERT: Radioaktiv markierte Phosphorsäureester. III. Mttlg. Isotopentechnik **2**, 307 (1962).

—, and H. SCHWARZ: Studien zum Metabolismus und zur Applikation von Trichlorphon in der Veterinärmedizin. Atompraxis **12**, 603 (1966 a).

— — Untersuchungen zur Ausscheidung von P^{32}-markiertem Trichlorphon und seinen Abbauprodukten in der Milch nach unterschiedlicher Applikation am Rind. Arch. Expt. Vet. Med. **20**, 849 (1966 b).

— — Studien zur Applikation des mindertoxischen P^{32}-markierten Phosphorsäureesters Butonate beim Rind. Arch. Expt. Vet. Med. **21**, 1023 (1967).

DE FOLIART, G. R., M. W. GLENN, and T. R. ROTT: Field studies with systemic insecticides against cattle grubs and lice. J. Econ. Entomol. **51**, 876 (1958).

DEICHMANN, W. B., and S. WITHERUP: The immediate toxicity of hexaethyltetraphosphate, tetraethylpyrophosphate, and hexaoctyltetraphosphate to rabbits and rats. Federation Proc. **6**, 322 (1947).

DIGGLE, W. M., and J. C. GAGE: Cholinesterase inhibition by parathion *in vivo*. Nature **168**, 998 (1951).

DIRKSEN, G., and F. RADEMACHER: Erste Ergebnisse der Allgemeinbehandlung der Stephanofilariose des Rindes mit Antimosan und Neguvon. Dtsch. tierärztl. Wschr. **67**, 70 (1960).

DISHBURGER, H. J., J. R. RICE, W. S. MCGREGOR, and J. PENNINGTON: Residues of Dursban insecticide in tissues from turkeys confined on soil treated for chigger control. J. Econ. Entomol. **62**, 181 (1969).

DORMAL, S.: Nutritional aspects of pesticides and the use of agricultural chemicals. Effects of Processing and Additives on Foods **2**, 23 (1960).

DOROUGH, H. W., and B. W. ARTHUR: Distribution and solubility properties of phosphoric and O,O-diethyl phosphorodithioic acids fed to laying hens. J. Econ. Entomol. **54**, 1140 (1961).

—, U. E. BRADY, Jr., J. A. TIMMERMAN, Jr., and B. W. ARTHUR: Residues in tissues and eggs of poultry dusted with Co-Ral (Bayer 21/199). J. Econ. Entomol. **54**, 25 (1961 a).

— — — — Residues in tissues and eggs of poultry receiving Co-Ral (Bayer 21/199) in the feed. J. Econ. Entomol. **54**, 97 (1961 b).

DOUGLAS, J. J., and N. F. BAKER: Ruelene, an organic phosphate, as an anthelmintic in sheep. J. Amer. Vet. Med. Assoc. **135**, 567 (1959).

— —, and P. H. ALLEN: Trial with a new organic phosphate as an anthelmintic in sheep. Amer. J. Vet. Research **20**, 442 (1959).

DRUDGE, J. H., and J. SCANTO: Controlled test of the anthelmintic activity of Thiabendazole and an organic phosphate (38,023) in lambs. Amer. J. Vet. Research **24**, 337 (1963).

DRUMMOND, R. O.: Tests with dimethoate for systemic control of cattle grubs. J. Econ. Entomol. **52**, 1004 (1959).

— Preliminary evaluation of animal systemic insecticides. J. Econ. Entomol. **53**, 1125 (1960).

— Tests with sprays of General Chemical 4072 for systemic control of cattle grubs. J. Econ. Entomol. **54**, 1047 (1961 a).

— Tests with General Chemical 3582 and 4072 for the control of ticks affecting livestock. J. Econ. Entomol. **54**, 1051 (1961 b).

— Further evaluation of animal systemic insecticides, 1966. J. Econ. Entomol. **60**, 733 (1967).

—, and O. H. GRAHAM: Dowco 109 as an animal systemic insecticide. J. Econ. Entomol. **52**, 749 (1959).

— — Low-volume dermal applications and injections of Co-Ral for systemic control of cattle grubs. J. Econ. Entomol. **55**, 255 (1962).

Drummond, R. O., and B. Moore: Ronnel sprays for systemic control of cattle grubs. J. 52, 1029 (1959).
— — Systemic insecticides as feed additives for cattle grub control. J. Econ. Entomol. 53, 682 (1960).
Du Bois, K. P.: Potentiation of the toxicity of insecticidal organic phosphates. Amer. Med. Assoc. Arch. Ind. Health 18, 488 (1958).
— Lowel-level organophosphate residues in the diet. Their potential hazards. Arch. Environ. Health 10, 837 (1965).
—, and G. J. Cotter: Studies on the toxicity and mechanism of action of Dipterex. Amer. Med. Assoc. Arch. Ind. Health 11, 53 (1955).
—, J. Doull, and J. M. Coon: Studies on the toxicity and pharmacological action of octamethyl pyrophosphoramide (OMPA; Pestox III). J. Pharm. Expt. Therap. 99, 376 (1950).
—, J. Doull, P. R. Salerno, and J. M. Coon: Studies on the toxicity and mechanism of action of *p*-nitrophenyl diethyl thionophosphate (parathion). J. Pharm. Expt. Therap. 95, 79 (1949).
—, and F. Kinoshita: Acute toxicity and anticholinesterase action of O,O-dimethyl-O-(4-methylthio)-*m*-tolyl phosphorothioate (DMTP; Baytex) and related compounds. Toxicol. Applied Pharmacol. 6, 86 (1964).
—, S. D. Murphy, and D. R. Thursh: Toxicity and mechanism of action of some metabolites of Systox. Amer. Med. Assoc. Arch. Ind. Health 13, 606 (1956).
—, and G. J. Plzak: The acute toxicity and anticholinesterase action of O,O-dimethyl *S*-ethyl-2-sulfinylethyl phosphorothioate (Meta-Systox R) and related compounds. Toxicol. Applied Pharmacol. 4, 621 (1962).
—, D. R. Thursh, and S. D. Murphy: Studies on the toxicity and pharmacologic actions of the dimethoxy ester of benzotriazine dithiophosphoric acid (DBD, Guthion). J. Pharm. Expt. Therap. 119, 208 (1957).
Duggan, R. E., H. C. Barry, and L. Y. Johnson: Pesticide residues in total-diet samples. Science 151, 101 (1966).
— — —, and S. Williams: Pesticide analytical manual, Vol. II. *U. S. Department of Health, Education, and Welfare*, Food and Drug Administration (1967).
—, and J. R. Weatherwax: Dietary intake of pesticide chemicals. Science 157, 1006 (1967).
Durbin, C. G.: The veterinarian and food additive problems. Ber. XVII, Welttierärztekongreß 2, 315 (1963).
Durham, W. F.: Pesticide residues in foods in relation to human health. Residue Reviews 4, 32 (1963).
— The interaction of pesticides with other factors. Residue Reviews 18, 21 (1967).
—, T. B. Gaines, R. H. McCauley, Jr., V. A. Sedlak, A. M. Mattson, and W. J. Hayes, Jr.: Studies on the toxicity of O,O-dimethyl-2,2-dichlorvinyl phosphate (DDVP). Amer. Med. Assoc. Arch. Ind. Health 15, 340 (1957).
Eberle, D. O., R. G. Delley, G. G. Szekely, and K. H. Stammbach: Residue determination of GS 13005, a new insecticide. J. Agr. Food Chem. 15, 213 (1967).
Eddy, G. W.: Laboratory tests of residues of organophosphorus compounds against house flies. J. Econ. Entomol. 54, 386 (1961).
Egan, H.: Pesticide residues. J. Assoc. Official Anal. Chemists 50, 1067 (1967).
—, E. W. Hammond, and J. Thomson: The analysis of organophosphorus pesticide residues by gas chromatography. Analyst 89, 75 (1964).
Eichler, W.: Handbuch der Insektizidkunde. Berlin: Volk und Gesundheit (1965).
v. Eicken, S.: Zur Ausscheidung von p-Nitrophenol im Urin nach Einwirkung von Pflanzenschutzmittel „E 605". Angew. Chem. 66, 551 (1954).
Enders, A.: Beitrag zum Nachweis des E 605 im Leichenmaterial. Arch. Toxicol. 15, 313 (1954/55).
Endrejat, E.: Ein Überblick über die wirtschaftliche Bedeutung der wichtigsten Ektoparasiten des Schafes und über die Möglichkeiten ihrer Bekämpfung. Vet. Med. Nachr. 2/3, 99 (1967).

ERDÖS, E. G., and L. E. BOGGS: Hydrolysis of paraoxon in mammalian blood. Nature **190**, 716 (1961).

ESSER, H. O., and P. W. MÜLLER: Metabolism of GS 13005., a new insecticide. Experientia **22**, 36 (1966).

EVERETT, L. J., C. A. ANDERSON, and D. MCDOUGALL: Nature and extent of Guthion residues in milk and tissues resulting from treated forage. J. Agr. Food Chem. **14**, 47 (1966).

FALLSCHEER, H. O., and J. W. COOK: Report on enzymatic methods for insecticides. J. Assoc. Official Agr. Chemists **39**, 691 (1956).

FARAGÓ, A.: Tödliche, suicidale Phosdrinvergiftung. Arch. Toxicol. **23**, 233 (1968).

FAZEKAS, I. G., and B. RENGEI: Tödliche Vergiftung mit Methyl-Parathion („Wofatox"). Arch. Toxicol. **20**, 323 (1965).

— — Methylparathiongehalt menschlicher Organe nach tödlichen „Wolfatox"-Vergiftungen. Arch. Toxicol. **22**, 381 (1967).

FENWICK, M. L., J. R. BARRON, and W. A. WATSON: The conversion of Dimefox into an anticholinesterase by rat liver *in vitro*. Biochem. J. **65**, 58 (1957).

FISKEN, A. G.: A slow release formulation of Dichlorvos. Proc. 3d Brit. Insecticide Fungicide Conf. p. 445 (1965).

FIEDLER, O. G. H.: Die Bekämpfung der Rinderzecken in Südafrika. Vet. Med. Nachr. **3**, 133 (1958).

— The development of new protecting agents against blowfly strike of sheep. J. S. African. Vet. Med. Assoc. **36**, 233 (1965).

FISCHER, K., and W. SPECHT: Kritische Bemerkungen zum Metasystoxnachweis. Arch. Toxicol. **16**, 278 (1957).

FISCHER, R.: Nachweis und quantitative Bestimmung von Phosphor-Insecticiden in biologischem Material. III. Mittlg. Arch. Toxicol. **23**, 129 (1968).

—, and PLAZER-ALTENBURG: Nachweis von Phosphor-Insecticiden in biologischem Material. IV. Mittlg. Arch. Toxicol. **25**, 216 (1969).

—, and C. PLUNGER: Nachweis und quantitative Bestimmung von Phosphor-Insecticiden im biologischen Material. II. Mittlg. Arch. Toxicol. **21**, 101 (1965).

FITZHUGH, O. G.: Response of mammalian species to pesticides. In C. O. CHICHESTER: Research in pesticides, p. 59. New York-London: Academic Press (1965).

FLEISHER, J. H., and B. J. JANDORF: Metabolism of octamethyl pyrophosphoramide (OMPA) by liver slices and homogenates. Fed. Proc. **11**, 212 (1952).

FLUCKE, W.: Über prophylaktische Maßnahmen zur Bekämpfung der Hautmyiasen von Wollschafen. Pflanzenschutz-Nachrichten **21**, 92 (1968).

FORD, I. M., J. J. MENN, and G. D. MEYDING: Metabolism of *n*-(mercapto-methyl)-phthalimide-carbonyl-C^{14}-*S*-(O,O-dimethyl-phosphorodithioate) (Imidan-C^{14}): Balance study in the rat. J. Agr. Food Chem. **14**, 83 (1966).

FRAWLEY, J. P.: Synergism and antagonism. In C. O. CHICHESTER: Research in pesticides, p. 69. New York-London: Academic Press (1965).

—, and H. N. FUYAT: Effect of low dietary levels of parathion and Systox on blood cholinesterase of dogs. J. Agr. Food Chem. **5**, 346 (1957).

—, E. C. HAGAN, and O. G. FITZHUGH: A comparitive pharmacological and toxicological study of organic phosphate-anticholinesterase compounds. J. Pharm. Expt. Therap. **105**, 156 (1952).

— — —, H. N. FUYAT, and W. J. JONES: Marked potentation in mammalian toxicity from simultaneous administration of two anticholinesterase compounds. J. Pharm. Expt. Therap. **121**, 96 (1957 a).

— — — — — Marked potentation in mammalian toxicity from simultaneous administration of two anticholinesterase compounds. J. Pharm. Expt. Therap. **119**, 147 (1957 b).

—, R. WEIR, T. TUSING, K. DU BOIS, and J. C. CALANDRA: Toxicological investigations on Delnav. Toxicol. Applied Pharmacol. **5**, 605 (1963).

FREAR, D. E. H.: Pesticide index, 3rd ed. State College, Pa.: College Science Publishers (1965).

Frear, D. E. H., and S. Friedmann: Pesticide handbook-Entoma, 20th ed. State College, Pa.: College Science Publishers (1968).

— —, and T. De Martino: Pesticide handbook-Entoma, 21st ed. State College, Pa.: College Publishers (1969).

Fredriksson, T.: Studies on the percutaneous absorption of parathion and paraoxon. V. Rate of absorption of paraoxon. J. Invest. Dermatol. **38**, 233 (1962).

—, and J. K. Bigelow: Tissue distribution of P^{32}-labeled parathion. Arch. Environm. Health **2**, 663 (1961).

French, F. E., E. S. Raun, and J. B. Herrick: Trolene and Dowco 109 as feed additive for grub control. Iowa State Col. J. Sci. **33**, 119 (1958).

Fretwurst, F., and W. Naeve: Beitrag zum Nachweis des E 605 im Leichenmaterial. Arch. Toxicol. **15**, 185 (1954/55).

Friedberg, K. D., and F. Sakai: Spezifischer Nachweis von Vergiftungen mit Alkylphosphaten (E 600, E 605, Systox) in Blut und Hirngewebe mit Hilfe eines fermentaktivierenden Antidots. Dtsch. Z. für gerichtl. Medizin **47**, 580 (1958).

Führer, G., G. Fechner, and H. Ackermann: Eine einfache Methode zur Bestimmung von Trichlorphon in der Milch. Monh. Vet. Med. **22**, 908 (1967).

Furmann, D. P., and C. J. Weinmann: Toxicity of malathion to poultry and their ectoparasites. J. Econ. Entomol. **49**, 447 (1956).

Gage, J. C.: A cholinesterase inhibitor derived from O,O-diethyl O-*p*-nitrophenyl thiophosphate *in vivo*. Biochem. J. **54**, 426 (1953).

Gaines, T. B.: The acute toxicity of pesticides to rats. Toxicol. Applied Pharmacol. **2**, 88 (1960).

— Poisoning by organic phosphorus pesticides potentiated by phenothiazine derivates. Science **138**, 1260 (1962).

—, R. Kimbrough, and E. R. Laws, Jr.: Toxicology of Abate in laboratory animals. Arch. Environm. Health **14**, 283 (1967).

Galley, R. A. E.: Dichlorvos residue analysis. J. Assoc. Official Agr. Chemists **50**, 1067 (1967).

Galvin, T. J., R. R. Bell, and R. D. Turk: The efficacy and toxicity of certain organic phosphates and a carbamide as anthelmintics in ruminants. Amer. J. Vet. Research **20**, 784 (1959).

Gardiner, J. E., and B. A. Kilby: Biochemistry of organic phosphorus insecticides. 1. The mammalian metabolism of bis-(dimethylamino)-phosphonous anhydride (schradan). Biochem. J. **51**, 78 (1952).

Gardocki, J. F., and L. W. Hazleton: Urinary excretion of the metabolic products of parathion following its intravenous injection. J. Amer. Pharm. Assoc. **40**, 491 (1951).

Garner, J. R.: Veterinär-Toxikologie. Jena: VEB Fischer (1968).

Gatterdam, P. E., W. F. Chamberlain, and D. E. Hopkins: Studies with P^{32}-labeled Bayer 22408 in steers and guinea pigs. J. Econ. Entomol. **55**, 326 (1962).

—, L. A. Wozniak, M. W. Bullock, G. L. Parks, and J. E. Boyd: Absorption, metabolism, and excretion of tritium-labeled Famphur in the sheep and calf. J. Agr. Food Chem. **15**, 845 (1967).

Geldmacher-Mallinckrodt, M., and U. Weigel: Nachweis von Systox und Metasystox durch Schwermetallkomplexverbindungen. Arch. Toxicol. **20**, 114 (1963).

Giachetti, A., C. Grasso, and G. Bernardi: Verbleiben von O,O-Diäthyl-O-*p*-nitrophenylphosphat (Paraoxon) im Hirn der mit einer subtoxischen Einzeldosis Parathion behandelten Albinoratte. Boll. Soc. ital. Biol. sperim. **42**, 1625 (1966); through Chem. Zentralbl. **139**, 190 (1968).

Giang, B. Y., and H. Beckmann: Thin-layer chromatographic determination of Bidrin, Azodrin, and their metabolites. J. Agr. Food Chem. **17**, 63 (1969).

Giang, P. A.: Fluorometric method for estimation of residues of Bayer 22408. J. Agr. Food Chem. **9**, 42 (1961).

Good, F. D. T., and P. Cantor: Organo-phosphorus warble-fly dressings. Vet. Record **77**, 402 (1965).

GORDON, H. M. L.: Studies on anthelmintics for sheep. Some organicphosphorus compounds. Australian Vet. J. **34**, 104 (1958).

GRAHAM O. H.: The primary evaluation of three organophosphorus compounds for possible use in the control of livestock insects. J. Econ. Entomol. **54**, 1046 (1961).

—, B. MOORE, M. J. WRICH, S. KUNZ, J. W. WARREN, and R. O. DRUMMOND: Comparison of Ronnel and Co-Ral sprays for screw-worm control. J. Econ. Entomol. **52**, 1217 (1959).

GREGOIRE C., H. KOCH, A. DEBERDT, C. COTTELFER, and R. L. POUPLARD: Syntheses de pathologie parasitaire. VI. Aspects nouveaux de la lutte contre l'hypodermose bovine. Annales de Med. Vet. **103**, 452 (1959).

GROB, H., R. GASSER, and M. A. RUZETTE: Further investigations with "Supracide" for use in orchards and vineyards (activity, metabolism, residues toxicology). Proc. 3rd Brit. Insecticide Fungicide Conf. (1965).

GUARDA F.: Beitrag zur experimentellen Vergiftung mit E 605 forte bei Hühnern. (Toxikologie, Klinik, pathologische Anatomie und Histologie). Wien tierärztl. Mschr. **47**, 842 (1960).

GUNTHER, F. A.: Status of analytical methods for residues. J. Agr. Food Chem. **5**, 498 (1957).

—, and R. C. BLINN: Analysis of insecticides and acaricides. New York-London: Interscience (1955).

—, and D. E. OTT: Automated pesticide residue analysis and screening. Residue Reviews **14**, 14 (1966).

— —, and F. E. HEARTH: The oxidation of parathion to paraoxon in aqueous media by silver oxide (AgO). Bull. Environ. Contam. Toxicol. **3**, 49 (1968).

GUTENMANN, W. H., L. E. ST JOHN, Jr., and D. J. LISK: Metabolic studies with O,O-diethyl O-(3,5,6-trichloro-2-pyridyl) phosphorothioate (Dursban) insecticide in a lactating cow. J. Agr. Food Chem. **16**, 45 (1968).

HANSEN, D., E. SCHAUM and O. WASSERMANN: Organverteilung und Stoffwechsel von Diisopropyl-fluoro-phosphat (DFP) beim Meerschweinchen. Arch. Toxicol. **23**, 73 (1968 a).

— — — Serum level and excretion of diisopropylfluorophosphate (DFP) in cats. Biochem. Pharmacol. **17**, 1159 (1968 b).

HASSAN, A., and S. M. A. D. ZAYED: Metabolism of organophosphorus inseticides. III. Canad. J. Biochem. **43**, 1271 (1965).

— —, and F. M. ABDEL,HAMID: Metabolism of organophosphorus insecticides. II. Canad. J. Biochem. **43**, 1263 (1965 a).

— —, and S. HASHISH: Metabolism of organophosphorus insecticides. VI. Mechanism of detoxification of Dipterex in the rat. Biochem. Pharmacol. **14**, 1692 (1965 b).

HARBOUR, E. H.: Experience with organophosphorus compounds as anthelmintics. Ber. **XVII**, Welttierärztekongreß, Hannover **1**, 751 (1963).

HARDEE, D. D., G. KEENAN, G. G. GYRISCO, D. J. LISK, F. H. FOX, R. F. HOLLAND, and G. W. TRIMBERGER: Effects of feeding low levels of dimethoate on milk and whole blood cholinesterase activity of dairy cattle. J. Dairy Sci. **46**, 510 (1963).

HARRIS, T. H.: The opinion on residues. J. Agr. Food Chem. **4**, 413 (1956).

HARVEY, T. L., and J. R. BRETHOUR: Effectiviness of Ruelene and Ronnel for ear tick compared with cattle grub control. J. Econ. Entomol. **54**, 814 (1961).

HAUSCHILD, F.: Toxikologische Prüfung der Insektizide. In: Handbuch der Insektizidkunde. Berlin: Volk und Gesundheit (1965).

HAZLETON, L. W.: Review of current knowledge of toxicity of cholinesterase inhibitor insecticides. J. Agr. Food Chem. **3**, 312 (1955).

—, and E. G. HOLLAND: Pharmacology and toxicology of parathion. Adv. Chem. Series **1**, 31 (1950).

— — Toxicity of malathon. Arch. Ind. Hyg. Occupat. Med. **8**, 399 (1953).

HEBDEN, S. P., and C. A. HALL: Rametin as an anthelmintic for sheep. Vet. Record **77**, 207 (1965).

HECHT, G., and W. WIRTH: Zur Pharmakologie der Phosphorsäureester. Arch. Pathol. Pharmacol. **211**, 264 (1950).

HEILBRONN, E., I.-E. APPELGREN, and A. SUNDWALL: The fate of Tabun in atropine and atropine-oxime treated rats and mice. Biochem. Pharmacol. **13**, 1189 (1964).

HEINEMANN, H. E. O., H. O. JAYNES, and J. L. HEFLIN: Pesticides — A dairy industry problem. J. Dairy Sci. **49**, 509 (1965).

HERLICH, H., and D. A. PORTER: An anthelmintic for cattle and sheep. Vet. Med. **53**, 343 (1958).

— —, and R. S. ISENSTEIN: Anthelmintic activity of Ruelene administered to cattle orally and topically. Vet. Med. **56**, 219 (1961).

HEWITT, R., A. BREBBIA, and E. WALETZKY: Carbamoyl alkyl phosphorodithoates as chemotherapeutic agents: Screening by aedicidal properties in laboratory mammals, lambs and calves. J. Econ. Entomol. **51**, 126 (1958).

HIRANO, Y., and T. TAMURA: Spectrophotometric microdetermination of Lebaycid, O,O-dimethyl-O-[4-(methylthio)-*m*-tolyl]-phosphorothioate. Anal. Chem. **86**, 800 (1964).

HJELT, E., and A. B. MUKULOS: The spectrophotometric determination of parathion and *p*-nitrophenol. Analyst **83**, 283 (1958).

HODGE, H. C., E. A. MAYNARD, L. HURWITZ, V. DI STEFANO, W. L. DOWNS, C. K. JONES, and H. J. BLANCHET, Jr.: Studies of the toxicity and of the enzyme kinetics of ethyl *p*-nitrophenyl thionobenzenephosphonate (EPN) J. Pharm. Expt. Therapeut. **112**, 29 (1954).

HODGSON, E, and J. E. CASIDA: Mammalian enzymes involved in the degradation of 2,2-dichlorovinyl dimethyl phosphate. J. Agr. Food Chem. **10**, 208 (1962).

HOFFMANN, R. A., and R. O. DRUMMOND: Control of lice on livestock and parasites on poultry with General Chemical 4072. J. Econ. Entomol. **54**, 1052 (1961).

HOFMANN-CREDNER, D., and H. SIEDEK: Distribution and fate of schradan (bis-dimethyl-aminophosphonous anhydride) in mammals, using a radioactive compound. Arch. Internat. Pharmacodyn. **89**, 74 (1952).

HOLLINGWORTH, R. M.: Dealkylation of organophosphorus esters by mouse liver enzymes *in vitro* and *in vivo*. J. Agr. Food Chem. **17**, 987 (1969).

—, T. R. FUKUTO, and R. L. METCALF: Selectivity of Sumithion compared with methyl parathion. Influence of structure on anticholinesterase activity. J. Agr. Food Chem. **15**, 235 (1967 a).

—, R. L. METCALF, and T. R. FUKUTO: The selectivity of Sumithion compared with methyl parathion. Metabolism in the white mouse. J. Agr. Food Chem. **15**, 242 (1967 b).

HOLMES, J. H.: Clinical studies of exposures to the organophosphorus insecticides. In C. O. CHICHESTER: Research in pesticides, p. 315. New York-London: Academic Press (1965).

HOLMSTEDT, B.: Pharmacology of organophosphorus cholinesterase inhibitors. Pharm. Reviews **11**, 567 (1959).

HÖTZEL, D.: Ermittlung von Toleranzwerten für Rückstände von Pflanzenschutzmitteln in Nahrungsmitteln. Arzneimittelforschg. **15**, 573 (1965).

HUNT, L. M., B. N. GILBERT, and J. C. SCHLINKE: Rapid gas chromatographic method for analysis of O,O-diethyl O-3,5-6-trichloro-2-pyridyl phosphorothioate (Dursban) in turkey and chicken tissues. J. Agr. Food Chem. **17**, 1166 (1969).

HUTSON, D. H., D. A. A. AKINTONWA, and D. E. HATHWAY: The metabolism of 2-chloro-1-(2′,4′-dichlorophenyl) vinyl diethyl phosphate (Chlorfenvinphos) in the dog and rat. Biochem. J. **102**, 133 (1967).

IRUDAYASAMY, A., and A. R. NATARAJAN: Determination of Baytex in biological materials. Current Sci. **33**, 82 (1964).

IVERSON, L. G. K.: Pesticides, their use and misuse. J. Amer. Vet. Med. Assoc. **151**, 1806 (1967).

IVEY, M. C., H. V. CLABORN, R. A. HOFFMANN, O. H. GRAHAM, J. S. PALMER, and R. D. RADELEFF: Residues of Shell Compound 4072 in the body tissues of sprayed cattle. J. Econ. Etomol. **59**, 379 (1966).

— —, and R. L. YOUNGER: Residues of V–C 13 Nemacide in animal tissues. J. Econ. Entomol. **57**, 8 (1964).

IREY, M. C., J. L. ESCHLE, H. V. CLABORN, and O. H. GRAHAM: Ronnel residues in the meat and milk of cattle exposed to Ronnel-impregnated back rubbers used for horn fly control. J. Econ. Entomol. **60**, 712 (1967).
—, R. A. HOFFMANN, and H. V. CLABORN: Residues of Gardona in the body tissues of cattle sprayed to control Hypoderma spp. J. Econ. Entomol. **61**, 1647 (1968).
— — —, and B. F. HOGAN: Residues of Gardona in the body tissues and eggs of laying hens exposed to treated litter and dust boxes for control of external arthropod parasites. J. Econ. Entomol. **62**, 1003 (1969).
JACKSON, J. B., R. D. RADELEFF, R. H. ROBERTS, L. M. HUNT and W. B. BUCK: Acute toxicity of Delnav and its residues in tissues of livestock. J. Econ. Entomol. **55**, 699 (1962).
JACOBS, D. E.: Experiences with a broad-spectrum anthelmintic, Dichlorvos, in the adult pig. Vet. Record **83**, 160 (1968).
JAGLAN, P. S., and F. A. GUNTHER: Comparison of several liquid phases in gas liquid chromatography of methyl parathion and metabolites. Bull Environ. Contam. Toxicol. **5**, 98 (1970).
JANDORF, B. J., and P. D. MCNAMARA: Distribution of radiophosphorus in rabbit tissues after injection of phosphorus-labeled diisopropyl fluorophosphate. J. Pharm. Exp. Therapeut. **98**, 77 (1950).
JAQUES, R., and H. J. BEIN: Toxikologie und Pharmakologie eines neuen systemisch wirksamen Insektizids der Phosphorsäureester-Reihe, Phosphamidon (2-Chlor-2-diäthyl-carbamoyl-1-methylvinyl-dimethylphosphat). Arch. Toxicol. **18**, 316 (1960).
JENSEN, J. A., W. F. DURHAM, and G. W. PEARCE: Studies on fate of parathion in rabbits, using radioactive isotope techniques. Arch. Ind. Hyg. Occup. Med. **6**, 326 (1952).
—, and G. W. PEARCE: Synthesis of radioactive parathion using S^{35}. J. Amer. Chem. Soc. **74**, 3184 (1952).
JOLLY, D. W.: The toxicity of organic phosphorus insecticides. Vet. Record **69**, 796 (1957).
JONES, C. M.: Cattle grub control with Ronnel. J. Econ. Entomol. **52**, 524 (1959).
—, and J. MATSUSHIMA: Effects of Ronnel on control of cattle grubs and weight gains of beef cattle. J. Econ. Entomol. **52**, 488 (1959).
JUNG, H. F., H. KÜKENTHAL, and G. TECHNAU: Baytex (S 1752, Bayer 29493) ein neues Hygiene-Insektizid aus der Gruppe der mindertoxischen Phosphorsäureester. Höfchen-Brief **13**, 13 (1960).
KADOUM, A. M.: Application of the rapid micromethod of sample cleanup for gas chromatographic analysis of common organic pesticides in ground water, soil, plant and animal extracts. Bull. Environ. Contam. Toxicol. **3**, 65 (1968 a).
— Cleanup procedure for water, soil, animal and plant extracts for the use of electron-capture detector in the gas chromatographic analysis of organophosphorus insecticide residues. Bull. Environ. Contam. Toxicol. **3**, 247 (1968 b).
— Partitioning method for sample cleanup for gas chromatographic analysis of common organic pesticide residues in biological materials. Bull. Environ. Contam. Toxicol. **4**, 184 (1969).
KAEMMERER, K.: Zyklusbeeinflussung durch Phosphorsäureester. Unveröffentlicht, hinterlegt bei der landw. Fakultät Bonn (1961).
— Toxikologische Fragen beim Einsatz von Phosphorsäureestern als Anthelmintica. Proc. Symp. Evaluation of Anthelmintics. Hannover (1963).
— Die Bedeutung von unbekannten Metaboliten von Feed Additives für die Gesundheit des Nutztieres und des Lebensmittelverbrauchers. Ber. Internat. Ern. Kongress Hamburg, 1966 (publ. 1967).
KAISER, H., and W. LANG: Beitrag zur qualitativen und annähernd quantitativen Bestimmung von E 605 im Blut. Dtsch. Apoth. Ztg. **93**, 394 (1953).
KAPLANIS, J. N., D. E. HOPKINS, and G. H. TREIBER: Dermal and oral treatments of cattle with phosphorus-32-labeled Ro-Ral. J. Agr. Food Chem. **7**, 483 (1959 a).
—, W. E. ROBBINS, D. I. DARROW, D. E. HOPKINS, R. E. MONROE, and G. TREIBER: The metabolism of dimethoate in cattle. J. Econ. Entomol. **52**, 1190 (1959 b).

KARLOG, O., and E. POULSEN: Spontaneous and pyridinaldoxime-induced re-activation of brain cholinesterase in the chicken after fatal nitrostigmine (parathion) poisoning. Acta Pharmacol. et Toxicol. **20**, 174 (1963).

KEDENBURG, C. P.: Untersuchungen zur Frage der ernährungshygienischen Unbedenklichkeit des Einsatzes von Ruelene und Neguvon bei der Dasselbekämpfung. Diss. München (1965).

KEITH, R. V.: Subcutaneous injection of an organic phosphorus compound as an anthelmintic procedure for cattle. Australian Vet. J. **40**, 402 (1964).

KENAGA, E. E., W. K. WHITNEY, J. L. HARDY, and A. E. DOTY: Laboratory tests with Dursban insecticide. J. Econ. Entomol. **58**, 1043 (1965).

KIMMERLE, G., and D. LORKE: Die Toxikologie der insektiziden Phosphorsäureester. Pflanzenschutz-Nachrichten **21**, 111 (1968).

KINGMA, F. J.: Residue problems compounded by big feedlots. J. Amer. Vet. Med. Assoc. **151**, 741 (1967).

KINKEL, J., G. MUAČEVIĆ, R. SEHRING, and G. BODENSTEIN: Zur Toxikologie von Bromophos. Arch. Toxicol. **22**, 36 (1966).

KIRKLAND, J. J., and H. L. PEASE: Determination of ethyl-*p*-nitrophenylthionobenzene phosphonate (EPN) residues by electron-capture gas chromatography. J. Agr. Food Chem. **15**, 187 (1967).

KLIMMER, O. R.: Rückstände von Pflanzenschutzmitteln, Insektiziden und dergleichen in der Nahrung und ihre Bedeutung für die Gesundheit. Therapiewochen **13**, 600 (1963).

— Pflanzenschutz- und Schädlingsbekämpfungsmittel. Hattingen (1964).

KLOTZSCHE, C.: Zur Toxikologie neuerer insektizider Phosphorsäureester. Arzneim.-Forsch. **5**, 436 (1955).

— Zur Toxikologie des O,O-Dimethyl-2,2-dichlorvinyl-phosphat. Z. angew. Zool. **43**, 87 (1956).

— Formothion, ein neuer systemischer Phosphorsäureester geringerer Giftigkeit. Mittlg. a. d. Gebiete der Lebensmittelhyg. **52**, 340 (1961).

— Zur toxikologischen Prüfung neuer insecticider Phosphorsäureester. Int. Arch. Gewerbepath. Gewerbehyg. **21**, 92 (1964).

— Toxikologische Untersuchungen mit dem systemischen Phosphorsäureester Formothion. Int. Arch. Gewerbepath. Gewerbehyg. **22**, 246 (1966).

KNAAK, J. B., and R. D. O'BRIEN: Effect of EPN on *in vivo* metabolism of malathion by the rat and dog. J. Agr. Food Chem. **8**, 198 (1960).

KNAPP, F. W.: Poultry tolerance to excessive amounts of Co-Ral dust. J. Econ. Entomol. **55**, 560 (1962).

— Free choice feeding of Ronnel mineral block and granules for face fly, horn fly, and cattle grub control. J. Econ. Entomol. **58**, 836 (1965).

—, N. W. BRADLEY, and W. C. TEMPLETON: Effect of Ronnel mineral block (Rid-Ezy) on control of cattle grubs and weight gain of beef cattle. J. Econ. Entomol. **60**, 1455 (1967).

—, C. J. TERHAAR, and C. C. ROAN: Systemic insecticides for cattle grub control. J. Econ. Entomol. **53**, 541 (1960).

KNIPLING, E. F., and W. E. WESTLAKE: Insecticide use in livestock production. Residue Reviews **13**, 1 (1966).

KNOWLES, C. O., and B. W. ARTHUR: Residues associated with backrubber application of Ronnel to dairy cows. J. Econ. Entomol. **59**, 752 (1966 a).

— — Metabolism of and residues associated with dermal and intramuscular application of radiolabeled Fenthion to dairy cows. J. Econ. Entomol. **59**, 1346 (1966 b).

KODAMA, J. K., H. H. ANDERSON, M. K. DUNLAP, and C. H. HINE: Toxicity of organophosphorus compounds Arch. Ind. Health **11**, 487 (1955).

—, M. S. MORSE, H. H. ANDERSON, M. K. DUNLAP, and C. H. HINE: Comparative toxicity of two vinyl-substituted phosphates. Arch. Ind. Hyg. Occup. Med. **9**, 45 (1954).

— —, and C. H. HINE: Comparative toxicity of two vinyl-substituted alkyl phosphates. Fed. Proc. **12**, 337 (1953).

KOHLER, P. H., and W. M. ROGOFF: Ruelene administered free-choice in a mineral mixture for cattle grub control. J. Econ. Entomol. **54**, 278 (1961).
— — Control for cattle grubs by pour-on, injection, and spray. J. Econ. Entomol. **55**, 539 (1962).
KOJIMA, K., and R. D. O'BRIEN: Paraoxon hydrolyzing enzymes in rat liver. J. Agr. Food Chem. **16**, 574 (1968).
KOLJAKOVA, V. Ja.: Bestimmung von Chlorophos in Milch, Fleisch und Eiern mit der Methode der Dünnschichtchromatographie. cit. nach: Landwirtschaftl. Zentralblatt **13** (III), 2394 (1968).
KÖNIG, J., I. HYNIE, and K. KÁCL: Tödliche suicidale Malathion-Vergiftung. Arch. Toxicol. **22**, 129 (1966).
KONST, H., and P. J. G. PLUMMER: Acute and chronic toxicity of parathion to warm-blooded animals. Can. T. Comp. Med. **14**, 90 (1950).
KRAEMER, P.: Relative efficacy of several materials for control of poultry ectoparasites. J. Econ. Entomol. **52**, 1195 (1959).
KRUEGER, H. R., and R. D. O'BRIEN: Relationship between metabolism and differential toxicity of malathion in insects and mice. J. Econ. Entomol. **52**, 1063 (1959 b).
—, and J. E. CASIDA: Toxicity of fifteen organophosphorus insecticides to several insect species and to rats. J. Econ. Entomol. **50**, 356 (1957).
— —, and R. P. NIEDERMEIER: Bovine metabolism of organophosphorus insecticides. Metabolism and residues associated with dermal application of Co-Ral to rats, a goat, and a cow. J. Agr. Food Chem. **7**, 182 (1959 a).
KRZEMINSKI, L. F., and W. A. LANDMANN: Methods for pesticide analysis in meat products. In G. ZWEIG (ed.): Analytical methods for pesticides, plant growth regulators, and food additives, Vol. I, p. 571. New York-London: Academic Press (1963).
KUBISTOVÁ, J.: Parathion metabolism in rat liver and kidney slices. Experientia **12**, 233 (1956).
— Parathion metabolism in female rat. Arch. Internat. Pharmacodyn. **118**, 308 (1959).
KÜHNERT, M., W. DEDEK, and H. SCHWARZ: Untersuchungen über die Stoffwechselbeeinflussung und den Ausscheidungsmechanismus des Phosphonsäureesters Trichlorphon im Handelspräparat „Bubulin" mit Hilfe P^{32}-markierten Phosphors bei der intravenösen und intramuskulären Injektion an Rindern. Arch. expt. Veterinärmed. **17**, 403 (1963).
KUTZER, E.: Versuche zur Dassellarvenbekämpfung mit dem injizierbaren Phosphorsäureester Warbex an hochträchtigen Tieren. Wien. tierärztl. Mschr. **53**, 675 (1966).
LAUE, W.: Toxikologische Fragen der Anwendung moderner Pflanzenschutzmittel. Mh. Vet. Med. **23**, 521 (1968).
LAWS, E. R.: Route of absorption of DDVP after oral administration to rats. Toxicol. Applied Pharmacol. **8**, 193 (1966).
—, F. R. MORALES, W. J. HAYES, Jr., and C. R. JOSEPH: Toxicology of Abate in volunteers. Arch. Environ. Health **14**, 289 (1967).
LEAHY, J. S.: Die Bestimmung von Rückständen des Neguvon in der Milch nach dermaler Anwendung beim Rind. Vet. Med. Nachr. **1**, 37 (1964).
LEBRUN, A., and C. CERF: Note preliminaire sur la toxicité pour l'home d'un insecticide organophosphoré (Dipterex). WHO Bull. No. 22, p. 579 (1960).
LEE, R. M., and W. R. PICKERING: The toxicity of Haloxon to geese, ducks and hens, and its relationship to the stability of the di-(2-chlorethyl)phosphoryl cholinesterase derivates. Biochem. Pharmacol. **16**, 941 (1967).
LENDLE, L.: Zu den E 605-Vergiftungen. Dtsch. med. Wschr. **79**, 725 (1954).
LEONHARDT, J.: Tödliche Vergiftung mit Insecticid E 605 (forte). Arch. Toxicol. **14**, 395 (1952).
LEVINE, N. D., V. IVENS, M. D. KLECKNER, and J. K. SONDER: Nematocidal screening tests of organic phosphorus, nitrofuran, cadmium and other compounds against horse strongyle larvae *in vitro*. Amer. J. Vet. Research **17**, 117 (1956).
LIEBEN, J., R. K. WALDMANN, and L. KRAUSE: Urinary excretion of paranitrophenol following exposure to parathion. Arch. Ind. Hyg. Occup. Med. **7**, 93 (1953).

LINDQUIST, A. W.: Uses of insecticides in the production of milk. J. Dairy Sci. **1**, 192 (1959).
— Livestock insect control. Agr. Chemicals **15**, 33 (1960).
LINDQUIST, D. A., and D. L. BULL: Fate of 3-hydroxy-*N*-methyl-cis-crotonamide dimethyl phosphate in cotton plants. J. Agr. Food Chem. **15**, 267 (1967).
—, E. C. BURNS, C. P. PANT, and P. A. DAHM: Fate of P^{32}-labeled Bayer 21/199 in the white rat. J. Econ. Entomol. **51**, 204 (1958).
LITSCHAUER, G.: Der Einfluß von Warbex auf die Cholinesterase des Rinderserums nach intramuskulärer Applikation sowie der Nachweis von Warbex im Blut nach parenteraler und peroraler Verabreichung. Vet. Diss. Wien (1964).
LORENZ, W., A. HENGLEIN, and G. SCHRADER: The new insecticide O,O-dimethyl-2,2,2-trichloro-1-hydroxy ethylphosphonate. J. Amer. Chem. Soc. **77**, 2554 (1955).
LOVINS, R. E.: Identification of pesticides in mixtures by high-resolution mass spectrometry. J. Agr. Food Chem. **17**, 663 (1969).
LUSCHIN, B.: Über die Bekämpfung der Dasselfliege mit Ruelene 25 E. Wien. tierärztl. Mschr. **53**, 194 (1966).
LYONS, E. T., J. H. DRUDGE, and F. W. KNAPP: Controlled test of anthelmintic activity of Trichlorfon and Thiabendazole in lambs, with observations on *Oestrus ovis*. Amer. J. Vet. Research **28**, 1111 (1967).
MACHATA, G.: Über den Nachweis von E 605 und Systox in der gerichtsmedizinischen Praxis. Arch. Toxicol. **16**, 119 (1956).
MAGAT, A.: Commentaires sur les applications des composés organophosphorés en médecine vétérinaire. Bull. Soc. Sci. vétérin. Med. comparée Lyon **66**, 427 (1964).
MAIER-BODE, H.: Pflanzenschutzmittel-Rückstände. Stuttgart: Ulmer (1965).
— Zur Verbreitung von Schädlingsbekämpfungsmitteln. Naturwissensch. **55**, 470 (1968).
MALONE, J. C.: The toxicity of Coroxon/Phenothiazine and Coumaphos/Phenothiazine. Research Vet. Sci. **3**, 18 (1962).
— Toxicity of Haloxon. Research Vet. Sci. **5**, 17 (1964).
MARCH, R. B., T. R. FUKUTO, R. L. METCALF, and M. G. MAXON: Fate of P^{32}-labeled malathion in the laying hen, white mouse, and American cockroach. J. Econ. Entomol. **49**, 185 (1956 a).
—, R. L. METCALF, T. R. FUKUTO, and F. A. GUNTHER: Fate of P^{32}-labeled malathion sprayed on jersey heifer calves. J. Econ. Entomol. **49**, 679 (1956 b).
MARCO, G. J., and E. G. JAWORSKI: Metabolism of O-phenyl-O′-(4-nitrophenyl) methylphosphonothionate (Colep) in plants and animals. J. Agr. Food Chem. **12**, 305 (1964).
MARESCH, W.: Die Vergiftung durch Phosphorsäureester (E 605, Parathion, Thiophos). Arch. Toxicol. **16**, 285 (1957).
MARGOT, A., and K. STAMMBACH: Diazinon. In G. ZWEIG (ed.): Analytical methods for pesticides, plant growth regulators, and food additives, Vol. II, p. 109 New York-London: Academic Press (1964).
MARQUARDT, R. P.: Ronnel. In G. ZWEIG (ed.): Analytical methods for pesticides, plant growth regulators, and food additives, Vol. II, p. 427 New York-London: Academic Press (1964).
MARQUARDT, W., C., and W. W. HAWKINS: Experimental therapy of fly strike in sheep, using a systemic insecticide. J. Amer. Vet. Med. Assoc. **132**, 429 (1958).
—, and ST. A. LOVELACE: A comparison of dimethoate administered as an injection and in supplemental feed for control of cattle grubs. J. Econ. Entomol. **54**, 252 (1961).
MARTIN, H.: Guide to the chemicals used in crop protection, 4th ed. Ottawa: Roger Duhamel (1961).
MATOUSEK, J., and J. TOMECEK: Analyse synthetischer Gifte, p. 187. Berlin: Dtsch. Militär-Verlag (1965).
MATSUMURA, F., and G. M. BOUSH: Malathion degradation by *Trichoderma viride* and a *Pseudomonas* species. Science **153**, 1278 (1966).
MATTHYSSE, J. G., W. H. GUTENMANN, and R. GIGGER: Sheep ectoparasite control. II. Toxicity to sheep, and residues of diazinon and lindane. J. Econ. Entomol. **61**, 207 (1968).

MATTHYSSE, J. G., and D. LISK: Residues of diazinon, Coumaphos, Ciodrin, methoxychlor, and rotenone in cow's milk from treatments similar to those used for ectoparasite and fly control on dairy cattle with notes on safety of diazinon and Ciodrin to calves. J. Econ. Entomol. **61**, 1394 (1968).

MATTSON, A. M., R. A. KAHRS, and R. T. MURPHY: Routine quantitative residue determinations of *S*-[(2-methoxy-5-oxo-Δ^2-1,3,4-thiadiazolin-4-yl) methyl] O,O-dimethyl phosphorodithioate (Supracide) and its oxygen analog in forage crops. J. Agr. Food Chem. **17**, 565 (1969).

—, and V. A. SEDLAK: The detection and measurement of malathion-derived materials in the urine of man and rats. Communication from the producer (1959).

—, J. T. SPILLANE, and G. W. PEARCE: Dimethyl 2,2-dichlorovinyl phosphate (DDVP), an organic phosphorus compound highly toxic to insects. J. Agr. Food Chem. **3**, 319 (1955).

MAZUR, A.: An enzyme in animal tissues capable of hydrolyzing the phosphorus-fluorine bond of alkyl fluorophosphates. J. Biol. Chem. **164**, 271 (1946).

McBAIN, J. B., J. J. MENN, and J. E. CASIDA: Metabolism of carbonyl-C^{14}-labeled Imidan, *N*-(mercaptomethyl) phthalimide-*S*-(O,O-dimethyl phosphorodithioate), in rats and cockroaches. J. Agr. Food Chem. **16**, 813 (1968).

McCARTY, R. T., M. HAUFLER, and C. A. McBETH: Acute toxicity of carbophenothion and demeton in sheep. Amer. J. Vet. Research **28**, 507 (1967).

McCOLLISTER, D. D., F. OYEN, and V. K. ROWE: Toxicological studies of O,O-dimethyl O-(2,4,5-trichlorophenyl) phosphorothioate (Ronnel) in laboratory animals. J. Agr. Food Chem. **7**, 689 (1959).

McDOUGALL, D.: Baytex, p. 43; Co-Ral, p. 83; Dylox, p. 199; Guthion, p. 231; and Meta-Systox, p. 295. In G. ZWEIG (ed.): Analytical methods for pesticides, plant growth regulators and food additives Vol. II. New York-London: Academic Press (1964).

—, and T. E. ARCHER: Di-Syston. In G. ZWEIG (ed.): Analytical methods for pesticides, plant growth regulators, and food additives, Vol. II, p. 187 New York-London: Academic Press (1964).

— —, and W. L. WINTERLIN: Systox. In G. ZWEIG (ed.): Analytical methods for pesticides, plant growth regulators, and food additives, Vol. II, p. 451 New York-London: Academic Press (1964).

McGIRR, J. L.: Present day toxicity problems — A review. Vet. Record **68**, 902 (1956).

—, and D. S. PAPWORTH: Toxic hazards of the newer insecticides and herbicides. Vet. Record **65**, 857 (1953).

McGREGOR, W. S., and R. C. BUSHLAND: Tests with Dow ET-57 against two species of cattle grubs. J. Econ. Entomol. **50**, 246 (1957).

—, P. D. LUDWIG, and L. L. WADE: Progress report on Ruelene for cattle grub control. Down to Earth **15**, 2 (1959).

—, R. D. RADELEFF, and R. C. BUSHLAND: Some phosphorus compounds as systemic insecticides against cattle grubs. J. Econ. Entomol. **47**, 465 (1954).

—, L. L. WADE, and R. W. COLBY: Systemic control of *Dermatobia hominis* in Central and South American cattle with Narlene insecticide. J. Econ. Entomol. **51**, 725 (1958).

McKINLEY, W. P., and S. I. READ: Esterase inhibition technique for the detection of organophosphorus pesticides. J. Assoc. Official Agr. Chemists **45**, 467 (1962).

McLAUGHLIN, J. E.: Studies in pesticide residues. 3. Ronnel residues in the perirenal and omental fat of cattle following dermal application. Landwirtschftl. Zentralblatt **14**, (III), 3 (1969).

McLEOD, H. A., G. MULKINS, and S. L. N. RAO: Gas chromatographic analysis of Phorate and five metabolites in monkey liver homogenates. Bull. Environ. Contam. Toxicol. **4**, 224 (1969).

MEDLEY, J. G., and R. O. DRUMMOND: Polymerization as a mean of prolonging effectiveness of orally administered systemic insecticides. J. Econ. Entomol. **55**, 118 (1962).

— —, and O. H. GRAHAM: Field tests with low-level feeding of Ronnel for control of cattle grubs and hornflies. J. Econ. Entomol. **56**, 500 (1963).

Menn, J. J., G. G. Patchett, and G. H. Batchelder: Trithion. In G. Zweig (ed.): Analytical methods for pesticides, plant growth regulators, and food additives, Vol. II, p. 545. New York-London: Academic Press (1964).

Menzer, R. E., and J. E. Casida: Nature of toxic metabolites formed in mammals, insects, and plants from 3-(dimethoxyphosphinyloxy)-*N*,*N*-dimethyl-*cis*-crotonamide and its *N*-methyl analog. J. Agr. Food Chem. **13**, 102 (1965).

Metcalf, R. L., and R. B. March: Further studies on the mode of action of organic thionophosphate insecticides. Ann. Entomol. Soc. Amer. **46**, 63 (1953).

— —, T. R. Fukuto, and M. G. Maxon: Metabolism of Systox-isomers in bean and citrus plants. J. Econ. Entomol. **47**, 1045 (1955).

— — — — The nature and significance of Systox residues in plant materials. J. Econ. Entomol. **48**, 355 (1956).

Metelica, V. K.: Studium der Toxizität des Ruelen für Tiere. Landwirtschftl. Zentralblatt **14**, (IV), 79 (1969).

Michel, H. O., and S. Krop: The reaction of cholinesterase with diisopropyl fluorophosphate. J. Biol. Chem. **190**, 119 (1951).

Millar, K. R.: Detection and distribution of P^{32}-labelled diazinon in dry tissue, after oral administration. New. Zeal. Vet. J. **11**, 141 (1963).

— Residues in tissues of sheep following oral dosing and tip spraying with P^{32}-labelled Ronnel. N. Z. J. Agr. Research **8**, 302 (1964).

—, and W. M. Aitken: Residues in meat following exposure to P^{32}-labelled dichlorvos vapour in an enclosed space. N. Z. J. Agr. Research **8**, 350 (1965).

Mills, P. A.: Pesticide residue contents. J. Assoc. Offical Anal. Chemists **46**, 762 (1963).

Miyamoto, J., Y. Sato, T. Kadota, A. Fujinami, and M. Endo: Studies on the mode of action of organophosphorus compounds. Part I. Agr. Biol. Chem. **27**, 381 (1963).

Moeller, H. C., and J. A. Rider: Plasma and red blood cell cholinesterase activity as indications of the threshold of incipient toxicity of ethyl-*p*-nitrophenyl thionobenzenephosphonate (EPN) and malathion in human beings. Toxicol. Applied Pharmacol. **4**, 123 (1962).

Moffit, R. A.: Residue analysis in the dairy industry. In G. Zweig (ed.): Analytical methods for pesticides, plant growth regulators, and food additives, Vol. I, p. 545. New York-London: Academic Press (1963).

Möllhoff, E.: Die Rückstandsfrage bei der Dasselbekämpfung mit systemischen Insektiziden. Vet. Med. Nachr. **2/3**, 240 (1967).

— Metaboliten insektizider Phosphorsäureester und ihre analytische Erfassung in Lebensmitteln. Pflanzenschutz Nachr. **21**, 401 (1968).

Morse, M. S., J. K. Kodama, and C. H. Hine: Cholinesterase-inhibiting properties of two vinyl-substituted phosphates. Proc. Soc. Expt. Biol. Med. **83**, 765 (1953).

Mounter, L. A.: Metabolism of organophosphorus anticholinesterase agents. Handbuch exp. Pharmakologie (Berlin) **15**, 486 (1963).

—, R. F. Baxter, and A. Chanutin: Dialkylfluorophosphatases of microorganisms. J. Biol. Chem. **215**, 699 (1955 a).

—, L. T. H. Dien, and A. Chanutin: The distribution of dialkylfluorophosphatase in the tissues of various species. J. Biol. Chem. **215**, 691 (1955 b).

—, and V. P. Whittaker: The hydrolysis of esters of phenol by cholinesterases and other esterases. Biochem. J. **54**, 551 (1953).

Mücke, W., K. O. Alt, and H. O. Esser: Degradation of C^{14}-labeled diazinon in the rat. J. Agr. Food Chem. **18**, 208 (1970).

Mühlmann, R., and G. Schrader: Hydrolyse der insektiziden Phosphorsäureester. Z. Naturforschg. **12 b**, 196 (1957).

Murphy, S. D.: Liver metabolism and toxicity of thiophosphate insecticides in mammalian, avian and piscine species. Proc. Soc. Expt. Biol. Med. **123**, 392 (1966).

Nabb, D. P., W. J. Stein, and W. J. Hayes: Rate of skin absorption of Parathion and Paraoxon. Arch. Envir. Health **12**, 501 (1966).

Naeve, W.: Tödliche akute Vergiftung mit dem Pflanzenschutzmittel Systox. Arch. Toxicol. **15**, 167 (1954/55).

NAEVE, W.: Zur Dsis letalis des E 605. Arch. Toxicol. **15**, 359 (1954/55).
NAGATSUGAWA, T., N. M. TOLMAN, and P. A. DAHM: Degradation and activation of parathion analogs by microsomal enzymes. Biochem. Pharmacol. **17**, 1517 (1968).
NEAL, R. A., and K. P. DU BOIS: Studies on the mechanism of detoxification of cholinergic phosphorothioates. J. Pharmacol. Expt. Therapeut. **148**, 185 (1965).
NEEL, W. W.: Field tests with systemic inseticides for the control of cattle grubs. J. Econ. Entomol. **51**, 793 (1958).
NELSON, D. L., A. D. ALLEN, J. O. MOZIER, and R. G. WHITE: Toxikologie des Tiguvon beim Rind. Teil I. Vet. Med. Nachr. **2/3**, 280 (1967).
—, R. G. WHITE, J. O. MOZIER, and A. D. ALLEN: Toxicity of larger-than-recommended doses of Naphthalophos to cattle, sheep and goats. Amer. J. Vet. Research **31**, 199 (1970).
NESHEIM, E. D., and J. W. COOK: Cholinesterase inhibition method of analysis for organic phosphate pesticides: Effect of enzyme-inhibitor reaction time upon inhibition. J. Assoc. Official Agr. Chemists **42**, 187 (1959).
NETHERY, A., G. B. WILSON, and R. HOOPINGARNER: Cytological and genetic studies on the effects of Ruelene. J. Econ. Entomol. **58**, 511 (1965).
NIESSEN, H., H. TIETZ, and H. FREHSE: Papierchromatographische Trennung aromatischer Phosphorsäureester-Insektizide. J. Chromatog. **9**, 111 (1962).
— —, G. HECHT, and G. KIMMERLE: Über Vorkommen von Sulfoniumverbindungen in Metasystox (i) und Metasystox R und ihre physiologische Wirkung. Arch. Toxicol. **20**, 44 (1963).
NORRIS, M. V., E. W. EASTER, L. T. FULLER, and E. J. KUCHAR: Colorimetric estimation of malathion residues in animals products. J. Agr. Food Chem. **6**, 111 (1958).
—, W. A. VAIL, and P. R. AVERELL: Colorimetric estimation of malathion residues. J. Agr. Food Chem. **2**, 570 (1954).
NUNNS, V. J., D. A. RAWES, and G. C. SHEARER: Field trials of Haloxon in sheep. Vet. Record **76**, 489 (1964).
O'BRIEN, R. D.: Properties and metabolism in the cockroach and mouse of malathion and malaoxon. J. Econ. Entomol. **50**, 159 (1957).
— Toxic phosphorus esters. New York-London: Academic Press (1960).
—, W. C. DAUTERMAN, and R. P. NIEDERMEIER: The metabolism of orally administered malathion by a lactating cow. J. Agr. Food Chem. **9**, 39 (1961).
—, E. C. KIMMEL, and P. R. SFERRA: Toxicity and metabolism of Famphur in insects and mice. J. Agr. Food Chem. **13**, 366 (1965).
—, and E. V. SPENCER: Metabolism of octamethylpyrophosphoramide by insects. J. Agr. Food Chem. **1**, 946 (1953).
—, and L. S. WOLFE: The metabolism of Co-Ral (Bayer 21/199) by tissues of the house fly, cattle grub, ox, rat, and mouse. J. Econ. Entomol. **52**, 692 (1959).
OETTEL, H.: Toxische Stoffe in der Luft, im Wasser und in Nahrungsmitteln? Med. Mschr. **21**, 340 (1967).
OKINAKA, A. J., J. DOULL, J. M. COON, and K. P. DU BOIS: Studies on the toxicity and pharmacological actions of bis (dimethylamido) fluorophosphate (BSP). J. Pharm. Expt. Therapeut. **112**, 231 (1954).
OSER, B. L.: The no-residue problem and the proposed solution. Proc. 7th World Nutrition Congress Hamburg, p. 740 (1966).
PACK, D. E., J. N. OSPENSON, and G. K. KOHN: Phosphamidon. In G. ZWEIG (ed.): Analytical methods for pesticides, plant growth regulators, and food additives, Vol. II, p. 375. New York-London: Academic Press (1964).
— — — Dibrom. In G. ZWEIG (ed.): Analytical methods for pesticides, plant growth regulators, and food additives, Vol. II, p. 125. New York-London: Academic Press (1964).
PALMER, J. S., and R. D. RADELEFF: The toxicological effects of dual applications of Bayer 21/199 and arsenical solution on cattle and calves. J. Amer. Vet. Med. Assoc. **143**, 1208 (1963).

PANKASKIE, J. E., F. C. FOUNTAINE, and P. A. DAHM: The degradation and detoxication of parathion in dairy cows. J. Econ. Entomol. **45**, 51 (1952).
PASARELA, N. R., R. G. BROWN, and C. B. SHAFFER: Feeding of malathion to cattle: Residue analyses of milk and tissue. J. Agr. Food Chem. **10**, 7 (1962).
—, R. E. TONDREAU, W. R. BOHN, and G. O. GALE: Gas chromatographic determination of Famphur and its oxygen analog residue in bovine milk, blood, and edible tissues. J. Agr. Food Chem. **15**, 920 (1967).
PERKOW, W.: Die Insektizide. Heidelberg: Hüthig (1956).
PLAPP, F. W., and J. E. CASIDA: Bovine metabolism of organophosphorus insecticides. J. Agr. Food Chem. **6**, 622 (1958 a).
— — Hydrolysis of the alkyl-phosphate bond in certain dialkyl aryl phosphorothioate insecticides by rats, cockroaches, and alkali. J. Econ. Entomol. **51**, 800 (1958 b).
— — Ion-exchange chromatography for hydrolysis products of organophosphate insecticides. Anal. Chem. **30**, 1622 (1958 c).
— —, W. S. BIGLEY, and D. J. DARROW: Studies on the metabolism and residue of P^{32}-labeled Delnav in a hereford steer. J. Econ. Entomol. **53**, 60 (1960 a).
— —, W. F. CHAMBERLAIN, and R. D. RADELEFF: Systemic insecticides in animals. Symp. Nature and Fate of Chemicals Applied to Soils, Plants, and Animals, Apr. 27–29 (1960 b).
POLAN, C. E., J. T. HUBER, R. W. YOUNG, and J. C. OSBORNE: Chronic feeding of *S*-[(2-methoxy-5-oxo-Δ^2-1,3,4-thiadiazolin-4-yl) methyl] O,O-dimethyl phosphorodithioate (Supracide) to rumating bull calves. J. Agr. Food Chem. **17**, 857 (1969).
PONSOLD, A., and G. BOHN: Tödliche Vergiftung mit Mevinphos. Arch. Toxicol. **21**, 163 (1965).
PORTER, P. E.: Vapona insecticide (DDVP). In G. ZWEIG (ed.): Pesticides, plant growth regulators, and food additives, Vol. II, p. 561. New York-London: Academic Press (1964).
—, YUN-PEI SUN, and T. E. ARCHER: Phosdrin. In G. ZWEIG (ed.): Pesticides, plant growth regulators, and food additives, Vol. II, p. 351. New York-London: Academic Press (1964).
PRIBILLA, O.: Vergiftungen mit E 605. Arch. Toxicol. **15**, 210 (1954).
PURDUE, L. J., J. BRYANT, and B. ORTIZ DE MONTELLANO: Analysis of pesticide residues by a dual-column, dual-electron-capture detector method. J. Agr. Food Chem. **17**, 264 (1969).
RADELEFF, R. D.: Newer insecticides. J. Amer. Vet. Med. Assoc. **136**, 529 (1960).
— Veterinary toxicology. Philadelphia: Lea & Febiger (1964).
— Toxicity of organophosphorus compounds. Ber. v. XVIII. Welttierärztekongreß, Paris, p. 89 (1967).
—, and R. C. BUSHLAND: The toxicity of pesticides for livestock. Symp. Nature and Fate of Chemicals applied to Soils, Plants, and Animals, Apr. 27–29 (1960).
—, L. W. M. HUNT, and C. P. WEIDENBACH: Toxicity studies of General Chemical 4072 and two related compounds to cattle. J. Econ. Entomol. **54**, 1051 (1961).
—, J. B. JACKSON, L. W. M. HUNT, W. B. BUCK, and M. WRICH: The acute toxicity of Ronnel applied dermally to cattle and sheep. J. Econ. Entomol. **56**, 272 (1963).
—, and G. T. WOODARD: Toxicological studies of Dow ET-57 in cattle and sheep. J. Econ. Entomol. **50**, 249 (1957 a).
— — The toxicity of organic phosphorus insecticides to livestock. J. Amer. Vet. Med. Assoc. **130**, 215 (1957 b).
RAGAB, M. T. H.: Direct fluorescent detection of organothiophosphorus pesticides and some of their sulfur-containing breakdown products after thin-layer chromatography. J. Assoc. Official Anal. Chemists **50**, 1088 (1967).
— Gas chromatographic analysis of malathion in water and in fish. Bull. Environ. Contam. Toxicol. **3**, 3 (1968).
RAHN, H. W.: Über den papierchromatographischen Nachweis von Potasan-G-flüssig. Arch. Toxicol. **19**, 359 (1962).

RAHN, H. W.: Vergleichende Untersuchungen von Phosphorsäureester-Präparaten. Arch. expt. Veterinärmed. **17,** 281 (1963).
RAMACHANDRAN, B. V.: Distribution of $DF^{32}P$ in mouse organs. I. Biochem. Pharmacol. **15,** 169 (1966 a).
— Distribution of $DF^{32}P$ in mouse organs. II. Biochem. Pharmacol. **15,** 1577 (1966 b).
— Distribution of $DF^{32}P$ in mouse organs. III. Biochem. Pharmacol. **16,** 1381 (1967).
—, and G. AGREN: Determination of DFPase in rabbit and rat tissues using $DF^{32}P$. Bio chem. Pharmacol. **13,** 849 (1964).
RAUN, E. S., and F. E. FRENCH: Practical application methods for systemic cattle grub control. J. Econ. Entomol. **54,** 428 (1961).
—, and J. B. HERRICK: Organophosphate systemics as sprays and feed additives for cattle grub control. J. Econ. Entomol. **53,** 125 (1960).
REID, B. L.: Californians told about leg weakness in poultry and agricultural toxicants. Feedstuffs **38,** 7 (1966).
RENG, G., and J. S. LIEM: Untersuchungen über den Einfluß bestimmter Insektizide auf die Verdauungsfermente der weißen Maus. Z. Pflkrankh. Pflpath. Pflschutz **73,** 180 (1966).
RICH, G. B.: Free-choice feeding of Trolene for reduction of cattle warble infestations. Canad. J. Animal Sci. **40,** 30 (1960).
—, and H. R. IRELAND: Studies of bolus and feed formulations of two systemic insecticides for reduction of cattle warble infestations. Canad. J. Animal Sci. **39,** 170 (1959).
RIEK, R. F., and R. K. KEITH: Studies on anthelmintics for cattle. IV. Australian Vet. J. **34,** 93 (1958).
ROAN, C. C., D. P. MORGAN, N. COOK, and E. H. PASCHAL: Blood cholinesterases, serum parathion concentrations and urine *p*-nitrophenol concentrations in exposed individuals. Bull. Environ. Contam. Toxicol. **4,** 362 (1969).
ROBBINS, W. E., T. L. HOPKINS, D. I. DARROW, and G. W. EDDY: Studies with P^{32}-Bayer 21/199 sprayed on cattle. J. Econ. Entomol. **52,** 214 (1959 a).
— — — Synergistic action of piperonyl butoxide with Bayer 21/199 and its corresponding phosphate in mice. J. Econ. Entomol. **52,** 660 (1959 b).
— —, and G. W. EDDY: The metabolism of P^{32}-labeled Bayer L 13/59 in a cow. J. Econ. Entomol. **49,** 801 (1956).
— — — Metabolism and excretion of phosphorus-32-labeled diazinon in a cow. J. Agr. Food Chem. **5,** 509 (1957).
ROBERTS, R. H., R. D. RADELEFF, and H. V. CLABORN: Residues in the milk of dairy cows sprayed with P^{32}-labeled General Chemical 4072. J. Econ. Entomol. **54,** 1053 (1961).
— —, and J. N. KAPLANIS: Bioassay of the blood from cattle treated with American Cyanamid 12, 880. J. Econ. Entomol. **51,** 861 (1958).
— —, and H. G. WHEELER: Malathion residues in the tissues of sheep, goats, and hogs. J. Econ. Entomol. **53,** 972 (1960).
—, M. J. WRICH, R. A. HOFFMAN, and C. M. JONES: Control of horn flies and stable flies with three General Chemical compounds. J. Econ. Entomol. **54,** 1047 (1961).
ROBINSON, J., J. C. MALONE, and B. BUSH: Residues of Supona in sheep. J. Sci. Food Agr. **17,** 309 (1966).
ROGOFF, W. M.: Control of cattle grubs by pour-on, injection and spray. J. Econ. Entomol. **55,** 539 (1962).
—, G. BRODY, A. R. ROTH, G. H. BATCHELDER, G. D. MEYDING, W. S. BIGLEY, G. H. GRETZ, and R. ORCHARD: Efficacy, cholinesterase inhibition, and residue persistence of Imidan for the control of cattle grubs. J. Econ. Entomol. **60,** 640 (1967).
—, and P. H. KOHLER: Free-choice administration of Ronnel in a mineral mixture for the control of cattle grubs. J. Econ. Entomol. **52,** 958 (1959).
— — Effectiveness of Ruelene applied as localized "pour-on" and as spray for cattle grub control. J. Econ. Entomol. **53,** 814 (1960).
— — Horn fly control by the pour-on technique using Ruelene or toxaphene. J. Econ. Entomol. **54,** 1101 (1961).
— —, and R. N. DUXBURY: The *in vivo* activity of several systemic insecticides against cattle grubs in South Dakota. J. Econ. Entomol. **53,** 183 (1960).

ROOS, C. V., and M. R. KARR: Palatability studies of rations for suckling lambs. J. Animal Sci. **19**, 1313 (1960).
ROSENBERGER, G.: Beitrag zur Frage der Verträglichkeit von systematisch wirkenden Präparaten zur Dasselbekämpfung. Schweiz. Arch. Thkd. **109**, 21 (1967).
—, R. SCHADE, and E. HEMPEL: Versuche zur Dasselbekämpfung mit den organischen Phosphorpräparaten Etrolene und Ruelene. Dtsch. tierärztl. Wschr. **68**, 547 (1961).
ROTH, A. R., and G. W. EDDY: Tests with Dow ET 57 against cattle grubs in Oregon. J. Econ. Entomol. **50**, 244 (1957).
RUZICKA, J., J. THOMSON, and B. B. WHEALS: The gas chromatographic examination of organophosphorus pesticides and their oxidation products. J. Chromatog. **30**, 92 (1967).
SALZER, W.: Vorwort. Pflanzenschutz-Nachr. **21** (1), 3 (1968).
SANDERSON, D. M., and E. F. EDSON: Toxicological properties of the organo-phosphorus insecticide dimethoate. Brit. J. Ind. Med. **21**, 52 (1964).
SANDI, E: Neue Wege zum Nachweis und zur Bestimmung der Rückstände insektizider Phosphorsäureester in Lebensmitteln. Nahrung **6**, 57 (1962).
SAUNDERS, B. C., and G. J. STACEY: Esters containing phosphorus. IV. J. Chem. Soc., p. 695 (1948).
SCHAD, G. A., R. W. ALLEN, and K. S. SAMSON: The effect of Dow ET 57 on some sheep parasites. Vet. Med. **53**, 533 (1958).
SCHARFF, D. K.: Cattle grub control with Ruelene as a dip and a pour-on treatment. J. Econ. Entomol. **55**, 191 (1962).
SCHECHTER, M. S., and M. E. GETZ: Comments on screening and analysis of multiple pesticide residues. J. Assoc. Official Anal. Chemists **50**, 1056 (1967).
SCHENK, L.: Untersuchungen zum Rückstandsverhalten von Trichlorphon im tierischen Organismus. Vet. Diss. München (1967).
—, and G. SCHREIBER: Das Rückstandsverhalten von Trichlorphon im tierischen Organismus. Vet. Med. Nachr. **3**, 194 (1969).
SCHMIDT, G.: Toxikologische Erfahrungen bei E 605-Vergiftungen. Arch. Toxicol. **15**, 361 (1954/55).
SCHNORBUS, R. R., and W. F. PHILLIPS: New extraction system for residue analyses. J. Agr. Food Chem. **15**, 661 (1967).
SCHRADER, G.: Die Entwicklung des Bayer-Präparates „S 1752". Höfchen-Briefe **13**, 1 (1960).
— Die Entwicklung neuer insektizider Phosphorsäure-Ester, 3rd ed. Weinheim/Bergstr.: Verlag Chemie GmbH (1963).
SCHREIBER, H.: Notizen zum Nachweis von E 605 nach Schwerd und Schmidt. Arch. Toxicol. **16**, 129 (1956).
— Bemerkungen zum Nachweis von E 605. Arch. Toxicol. **19**, 141 (1961).
SCHULZ, J. A., and G. WUJANZ: Verträglichkeitsuntersuchungen an Jungrindern mit dem Phosphonsäureester-Kombinationspräparat „Bubulin" unter Praxisverhältnissen. Mh. Vet. Med. **16**, 492 (1961).
SCHWARZ, H., and W. DEDEK: Untersuchungen über den Abbau und die Ausscheidungen von P^{32}-markiertem Trichlorphon beim Schwein. Zbl. Vet. Med. **B 12**, 653 (1965 a).
— — Das Verhalten von radioaktiv markiertem Trichlorphon nach Pour-on-Applikation (Aufgießverfahren) zur Dassellarvenbekämpfung beim Rind. Mh. Vet. Med. **20**, 958 (1965 b).
— — Untersuchungen zum Nachweis von P^{32}-markiertem Trichlorphon im Fleisch beim Schwein. Zbl. Vet. Med. **B 13**, 489 (1966 a).
— — Das Verhalten von radioaktiv markiertem Trichlorphon nach Rückenwäsche zur Dassellarvenbekämpfung beim Rind. Mh. Vet. Med. **21**, 945 (1966 b).
SCHWEITZER, H.: Außergewöhnlicher Verlauf einer Vergiftung mit E 605-Spritzpulver. Arch. Toxicol. **17**, 12 (1958).
SCHWERD, W., and G. SCHMIDT: Einfache Schnellreaktion im Blut zum Nachweis von Vergiftungen mit dem Schädlingsbekämpfungsmittel E 605. Dtsch. med. Wschr. **77**, 372 (1952).
SCOTT, W. N.: Pesticides toxic to vertebrates. Vet. Record **80**, 168 (1967).

Seidel, E.: Untersuchungen auf Kontaktinsektizidspuren im Tiermaterial im Jahr 1955. Mh. Vet. Med. **11**, 636 (1956).

Shafik, M. T., and H. F. Enos: Determination of metabolic and hydrolytic products of organophosphorus pesticide chemicals in human blood and urine. J. Agr. Food Chem. **17**, 1186 (1969).

Shaver, R. J., and J. F. Landram: Progress-report on Ruelene, a new anthelminitic. Down to Earth **15**, 7 (1959).

Shaw, F. R., C. T. Smith, D. L. Anderson, W. J. Fischang, W. H. Ziener and J. Hurny: The effects of Coumaphos on poultry and its residues in tissue and eggs. J. Econ. Entomol. **57**, 516 (1964).

Sherman, M., and M. T. Y. Chang: Dimethoate residue in eggs and tissues of laying hens. J. Econ. Entomol. **60**, 1552 (1967).

—, and E. Ross: Toxicity to house fly larvae of insecticides administered as single oral dosages to chicks. J. Econ. Entomol. **52**, 719 (1959).

— — Toxicity to house fly larvae of droppings from chicks administered insecticides in feed, water, and as single oral dosages. J. Econ. Entomol. **54**, 573 (1961).

— —, F. F. Sanchez, and M. T. Y. Chang: Chronic toxicity of dimethoate to hens. J. Econ. Entomol. **56**, 10 (1963).

Sinell, H. J.: Auswirkung der Arzneianwendung auf die Lebensmittel- und Milchhygiene. Dtsch. Tierärzteblatt, Sonderteil zu Nr. 1, p. 30 (1967).

Smith, C. L., and R. Richards: New insecticides for control of the cattle grub. J. Econ. Entomol. **47**, 712 (1954).

Smith, C. T., F. Shaw, R. Lavigne, J. Archibald, H. Fenner, and D. Stern: Residues of malathion on alfalfa and in milk and meat. J. Econ. Entomol. **53**, 495 (1960).

Smith, G. N., and F. S. Fischer: Use of paper partition and thin-layer chromatography for identification of activ ingredient in Dursban insecticide and its possible metabolites. J. Agr. Food Chem. **15**, 183 (1967).

—, and B. J. Thiegs: Determination of Ronnel in sheep and cattle dip solutions. J. Agr. Food Chem. **10**, 467 (1962).

—, B. S. Watson, and F. S. Fischer: The metabolism of [C^{14}] O,O-diethyl O-(3,5,6-trichloro-2-pyridyl) phosphorothioate (Dursban) in fish. J. Econ. Entomol. **59**, 1464 (1966).

— — — Investigations on Dursban insecticide. Metabolism of [Cl^{36}] O,O-diethyl O-3,5,6-trichloro-2-pyridyl phosphorothioate in rats. J. Agr. Food Chem. **15**, 132 (1967).

Smith J. N., and R. T. Williams: Studies in detoxication. 23. The fate of aniline in the rabbit. Biochem. J. **44**, 242 (1949).

Spencer, E. Y., R. D. O'Brien, and R. W. White: Permanganate oxidation products of schradan. J. Agr. Food Chem. **5**, 123 (1957).

Stenersen, J. H. V.: 2,6-Dibromobenzoequinone-4-chloroimide as a reagent for determination of dimethoate. Bull. Environ. Contam. Toxicol. **2**, 364 (1967).

Stiasni, M., D. Rehbinder, and W. Deckers: Absorption, distribution, and metabolism of O-(4-bromo-2,5-dichlorophenyl) O,O-dimethylphosphorothioate (Bromophos) in the rat. J. Agr. Food Chem. **15**, 474 (1967).

St. John, L. E., and D. J. Lisk: Determination of hydrolytic metabolites of organophosphorus insecticides in cow urine using an improved thermionic detector. J. Agr. Food Chem. **16**, 48 (1968 a).

— — Rapid, sensitive residue determination of organophosphorus insecticides by alkali thermionic gas chromatography of their methylated alkyl phosphate hydrolytic products. J. Agr. Food Chem. **16**, 408 (1968 b).

Stöckel, H., and K. H. Meinecke: Über eine gewerbliche Vergiftung durch Mevinphos. Arch. Toxicol. **21**, 284 1966).

Street, J. C.: Ecological systems: Domestic animals. In C. O. Chichester (ed.): Research in pesticides, p. 151. New York-London: Academic Press (1965).

Supperer, R., K. Onderscheka, E. Kutzer, and J. Pack: Versuche zur Dassellarvenbekämpfung mit dem injizierbaren Phosphorsäureester Warbex. Wien. tierärztl. Mschr. **51**, 729 (1964).

Sutherland, G. L.: Malathion. In G. Zweig (ed.): Analytical methods for pesticides, plant growth regulators, and food additives, Vol. II, p. 283. New York-London: Academic Press (1964).

—, P. A. Giang, and T. E. Archer: Thimet. In G. Zweig (ed.): Analytical methods for pesticides, plant growth regulators, and food additives, Vol. II, p. 487. New York-London: Academic Press (1964).

—, and R. Miskus: Parathion. In G. Zweig (ed.): Analytical methods for pesticides, plant growth regulators, and food additives, Vol. II, p. 321. New York-London: Academic Press (1964).

Szyszko, E.: Oszillopolarographische Bestimmungen von Rückständen phosphororganischer Insektizide in Lebensmitteln. III. Mittlg. Landwirtschaftl. Zentralbl. **12** (IV), 725 (1967).

Taylor, K. E.: Control of residues in meat from animals, drugs and biologicals. Ber. v. XVII. Welttierärztekongreß Hannover **2**, 939 (1963).

— Toxic residues in meat products. Proc. 69th Ann. Meeting-U. S. Livestock Sanitary Assoc., p. 294, Oct. 25–29 (1965).

Thamm, H.: Experimentelle Prüfung der Einwirkungen von Phosphorsäureester (Wofatox) auf Rinder und Schweine. Mh. Vet. Med. **13**, 193 (1958).

— Die Bedeutung der Phosphor- und Phosphonsäureester in der Veterinärmedizin vom Standpunkt der Veterinärhygiene. Halle (1962).

Thier, H. P., and K. G. Bergner: Eine Schnellmethode zum Nachweis wichtiger Schädlingsbekämpfungsmittel in Obst und Gemüse. Dtsch. Lebensmittel Rdsch. **62**, 399 (1966).

Tiews, J.: Zur Frage von Rückstandstoleranzen in Lebensmitteln tierischer Herkunft. Tierärztl. Umschau Nr. 8, 428 (1967).

— Futtermittelzusätze sind keine Lebensmittelzusätze. Ber. v. VII. Internat. Ernährungs-Kongreß, Hamburg **4**, 768 (1966).

Tolkmith, H.: Acute mamalian toxicity and structure of heterocyclic organophosphorus compounds. Annals N. Y. Acad. Sci. **136**, 59 (1966).

Tomov, A., N. Najdenow, and N. Bucvarova: Der Synergismus bei Vergiftungen von Tieren mit organischen Chlor- und Phosphorinsektiziden. Landwirtschaftl. Zentralbl. **12** (IV), 1572 (1967).

Tracy, R. L., J. G. Woodcock, and Chodroff: Toxicological aspects of 2,2-dichlorovinyl dimethyl phosphate (DDVP) in cows, horses, and white rats. J. Econ. Entomol. **53**, 593 (1960).

Treeby, P. J.: Carbophenothion as a sheep dip for the control of blowfly, lice and keds. Vet. Record **81**, 322 (1967).

Tsuyuki, H., M. A. Stahmann, and J. E. Casida: Preparation, purification, isomerization, and biological properties of octamethyl-pyrophosphoramide *N*-oxide. J. Agr. Food Chem. **3**, 922 (1955).

Turner, E. C., D. F. Watson, and F. S. McClaugherty: Anthelmintic activity of systemic insecticides used in control of cattle grubs. J. Amer. Vet. Med. Assoc. **141**, 360 (1962).

Uchida, T., W. C. Dauterman, and R. D. O'Brien: The metabolism of dimethoate by vertebrate tissues. J. Agr. Food Chem. **12**, 48 (1964).

Unterstenhöfer, G.: Lebaycid, ein neues mindertoxisches Insektizid. Höfchen-Briefe **13**, 44 (1960).

— Die Bedeutung der organischen Phosphorverbindungen für den Pflanzenschutz, Pflanzenschutz-Nachrichten **21**, 53 (1968).

Unwin, D. D.: Field trial with an organophosphorus compound against warble fly larvae in cattle. Vet. Record **77**, 593 (1965).

van Esch, G. J.: Die Beurteilung der Toxizität der Schädlingsbekämpfungsmittel. Dtsch. Lebensmittel-Rundschau **62**, 342 (1966).

van Genderen, H.: The establishment of residue tolerances and its relationship of toxicity. Bull. Inst. Agron. Stat. Récherche Gembloux, Hors Série **3**, 1233 (1960).

van Meter, W. G., and A. G. Karczman: Prophylactic and antidotal treatment of Sarin poisoning with drugs given singly and in combination. Arch. Internat. Pharmacodyn. Therap. **172**, 62 (1968).

Vardanis, A., and L. G. Crawford: Comparative metabolism of O,O-dimethyl O-*p*-nitrophenyl phosphorothioate (methyl parathion) and O,O-dimethyl O-(3-methyl-4-nitrophenyl) phosphorothioate (Sumithion). J. Econ. Entomol. **57**, 136 (1964).

Venturoli, M., and L. Tunioli: Determinazione della colinesterasi ematica in bovini normali ed in bovini sottoposti ad avvelenamento con Parathion. Atti Soc. ital. Sci. vet. **13**, 545 (1959).

Vickery, D. S., and B. W. Arthur: Animal systemic activity, metabolism, and stability of Co-Ral (Bayer 21/199). J. Econ. Entomol. **53**, 1037 (1960).

Vigne, J. P., J. Chouteau, R. L. Tabau, P. Rancien, and A. Karamanian: Sur le métabolisme d'un insecticide organo-phosphoré, le diéthylthionophosphate de 2 isopropyl 4 méthyl 6 oxypyrimidine chez la chèvre. Bull. Acad. Vét. **30**, 85 (1957).

Villeneuve ,D. C., and W. P. McKinley: Inhibition of beef liver hydrolytic enzymes by organophosphorus pesticides. J. Agr. Food Chem. **16**, 290 (1968).

—, G. J. Mulkins, H. L. Trenholm, K. A. McCully, and W. P. McKinley: Inhibition of beef liver hydrolytic enzymes by organophosphorus pesticides. J. Agr. Food Chem. **17**, 101 (1969).

—, W. E. J. Phillips, and J. Syrotiuk: Modification of microsomal enzyme activity and parathion toxicity in rats. Bull. Environ. Contam. Toxicol. **5**, 125 (1970).

Völksen, W.: Nachweis der E-605-Vergiftung. Dtsch. Apoth. Ztg. **93**, 393 (1953).

Vorhees, F. A.: Requirements of analytical data. J. Agr. Food Chem. **4**, 415 (1956).

Wallace, J. B., and E. C. Turner: Lowel-level feeding of Ronnel in a mineral salt mixture for area control of the face fly. J. Econ. Entomol. **57**, 264 (1964).

Watts, R.: Chromogenic spray reagents for the organophosphate pesticides. Residue Reviews **18**, 105 (1967).

Weber, K., and J. Matkovic: Die Bestimmung des Tabuns mit Hilfe der Chemiluminescenz des Luzigenins. Arch. Toxicol. **21**, 38 (1965).

Webley, D. J.: The determination of Fenchlorphos residues in milk. Analyst **86**, 476 (1961).

Weinig, E., H. Schmitt, and G. Schmidt: Zum Beweiswert der Reaktion von Averell und Noris beim Nachweis von E 605. Arch. Toxicol. **15**, 423 (1954/55).

Weintraub, J., G. B. Rich, and C. O. M. Thompson: Timing the treatment of cattle with Trolene for systemic control of the cattle grubs in Alberta and British Columbia. Canad. J. Animal Sci. **39**, 50 (1959 a).

—, and C. O. M. Thompson: Comparison of Ronnel, DOWCO 109, and DOWCO 105 for systemic control of cattle grubs in Alberta. J. Econ. Entomol. **54**, 79 (1961).

— —, and M. C. Qually: Low-level feeding of Trolene for control of the cattle grubs. Canad. J. Animal Sci. **39**, 58 (1959 b).

Westlake, A., F. A. Gunther, and W. E. Westlake: Conversion of the insecticide Ciodrin to acetophenone for microdetermination. J. Agr. Food Chem. **17**, 1156 (1969 a).

—, F. E. Hearth, F. A. Gunther, and W. E. Westlake: Determination of Ciodrin from fortified animal tissues by oscillopolarography of its conversion product acetophenone. J. Agr. Food Chem. **17**, 1160 (1969 b).

Westlake, W. E.: Insecticide residues in plants, animals and soils. Symp. Nature and Fate of Chemicals applied to Soils, Plants, and Animals, Apr. 27–29, ARS 20–9, (1960).

Whetstone, R. R., D. D. Phillips, Y. P. Sun, and L. F. Ward: 2-Chloro-1-(2,4,5-trichlorophenyl)vinyl dimethylphosphate, a new insecticide with low toxicity to mammals. J. Agr. Food Chem. **14**, 352 (1966).

Wilber, C. G., and R. A. Morrison: The physiological action of parathion in goats. Amer. J. Vet. Research **16**, 308 (1955).

Williams, M. W., H. N. Fuyat, J. P. Frawley, and O. G. Fitzhugh: *In vivo* effects of paired combinations of five organic phosphate insecticides. J. Agr. Food Chem. **6**, 514 (1958).

Wilson, C. W., and W. E. Baier: Toward an equitable basis for assignment of residue tolerance values. Residue Reviews **4**, 1 (1963).

Winterlin, W., G. Walker, and H. Frank: Detection of cholinesterase-inhibiting pesticides following separation on thin-layer-chromatograms. J. Agr. Food Chem. **16**, 808 (1968).

Wirth, W.: Zur Pharmakologie der Phosphorsäureester (Mintacol). Arch. expt. Pathol. Pharmakol. **207**, 547 (1949).

— Zur Pharmakologie der insektiziden Phosphorsäureester. Dtsch. med. Wschr. **79**, 1205 (1954).

— Zur Wirkung der systeminsektiziden Phosphorsäureester an Warmblütern (Systoxgruppe). Verh. IV. Internat. Pflanzenschutz-Kongreß, Hamburg **2**, 1635 (1960).

Wood, C. H. P., and D. Tyson: Formothion, a new systemic insecticide of low mammalian toxicity. Proc. 3rd Brit. Insecticide Fungicide Conf., p. 407 (1965).

Wrich, M. J., W. F. Chamberlain, and C. L. Smith: Toxicity of General Chemical compounds 3582, 3583, and 4072 to screw worms in laboratory and field tests. J. Econ. Entomol. **54**, 1049 (1961).

Yfary, R.: Public health significance of chemical residues in foods. J. Amer. Vet. Med. Assoc. **149**, 145 (1966).

Younger, R. L., R. D. Radeleff, and J. B. Jackson: Preliminary studies of the toxicity of carbophenothion and methyl Trithion in livestock. J. Econ. Entomol. **56**, 757 (1963).

Zacherl, M. K., W. Stöckl, M. Weiser, G. Litschauer, and A. Zuchi: Chemische Untersuchungen nach Applikation von Warbex. Wien. tierärztl. Mschr. **25**, 669 (1965).

Zweig, G. (ed.): Analytical methods for pesticides, plant growth regulators, and food additives, Vol. I. New York-London: Academic Press (1963).

— Analytical methods for pesticides, plant growth regulators, and food additives, Vol. II. New York-London: Academic Press (1964).

Manuscript received August 31, 1970; accepted April 4, 1972.

SUBJECT INDEX

Subject Index

Residue Reviews

Previously Published Volumes

Volume 1	0-387-02899-4	$ 6.90
Volume 2	0-387-03047-6	$ 6.90
Volume 3	0-387-03048-4	$ 6.90
Volume 4	0-387-03049-2	$ 7.60
Volume 5	0-387-03201-0	$ 8.40
Volume 6	0-387-03202-9	$ 7.60
Volume 7	0-387-03203-7	$ 7.20
Volume 8	0-387-03390-4	$ 8.00
Volume 9	0-387-03391-2	$ 7.20
Volume 10	0-387-03392-0	$ 6.60
Volume 11	0-387-03393-9	$ 8.00
Volume 12	0-387-03647-4	$ 8.60
Volume 13	0-387-03648-2	$ 7.60
Volume 14	0-387-03649-0	$ 8.00
Volume 15	0-387-03650-4	$ 8.00
Volume 16	0-387-03651-2	$ 9.10
Volume 17	0-387-03963-5	$ 10.20
Volume 18	0-387-03964-3	$ 11.90
Volume 19	0-387-03965-1	$ 9.90
Volume 20	0-387-04310-1	$ 11.90
Volume 21	0-387-04311-X	$ 10.20
Volume 22	0-387-04312-8	$ 11.60
Volume 23	0-387-04313-6	$ 12.70
Volume 24	0-387-04314-4	$ 13.20
Volume 25	0-387-04687-9	$ 19.80
Volume 26	0-387-04688-7	$ 10.00
Volume 27	0-387-04689-5	$ 9.50
Volume 28	0-387-04690-9	$ 9.50
Volume 29	0-387-04691-7	$ 13.50
Volume 30	0-387-04692-5	$ 14.50
Volume 31	0-387-05000-0	$ 12.00
Volume 32	0-387-05235-6	$ 14.80
Volume 33	0-387-05236-4	$ 14.80
Volume 34	0-387-05237-2	$ 14.80
Volume 35	0-387-05238-0	$ 14.20
Volume 36	0-387-05373-5	$ 19.80
Volume 37	0-387-05374-3	$ 14.80
Volume 38	0-387-05375-1	$ 14.20
Volume 39	0-387-05409-X	$ 13.50
Volume 40	0-387-05410-3	$ 14.20
Volume 41	0-387-05568-1	$ 14.80
Volume 42	0-387-05627-0	$ 14.80
Volume 43	0-387-05779-X	$ 14.20
Volume 44	0-387-90058-6	$ 16.50
Volume 45	0-387-90059-4	$ 16.20
Volume 46	0-387-90060-8	$ 26.00

In Preparation

Volume 47	0-387-90057-8	$ 17.80